EVIDENCE-BASED ENDOCRINOLOGY

CONTEMPORARY ENDOCRINOLOGY

P. Michael Conn, *SERIES EDITOR*

EVIDENCE-BASED ENDOCRINOLOGY

Edited by

VICTOR M. MONTORI, MD, MSc

Mayo Clinic College of Medicine, Rochester, MN

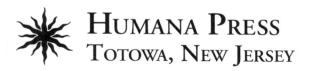

HUMANA PRESS
TOTOWA, NEW JERSEY

For additional copies, pricing for bulk purchases, and/or information about other Humana titles, contact Humana at 999 Riverview Drive, Suite 208, Totowa, NJ 07512 or at any of the following numbers: Tel: 973-256-1699; Fax: 973-256-8341; E-mail: orders@humanapr.com or visit our website at http://humanapress.com

This publication is printed on acid-free paper. ∞

ANSI Z39.48-1984 (American National Standards Institute) Permanence of Paper for Printed Library Materials.

Production Editor: Jennifer Hackworth
Cover design: Patricia F. Cleary

Printed in the United States of America. 10 9 8 7 6 5 4 3 2 1
E-ISBN 1-59745-008-1
Library of Congress Cataloging-in-Publication Data
Evidence-based endocrinology / edited by Victor M. Montori.
    p. cm. -- (Contemporary endocrinology)
  Includes bibliographical references and index.
  ISBN 1-58829-579-6 (alk. paper)
  1. Endocrinology. 2. Evidence-based medicine.   I. Montori,
 Victor M. II. Series: Contemporary endocrinology (Totowa, N.J.)
  [DNLM: 1. Endocrine System Diseases. 2. Endocrinology.
  3. Evidence-Based Medicine.   WK 140 E92 2006]
  RC649.E96 2006
  616.4--dc22

2005012487

PREFACE

This book is about evidence-based endocrinology, but it is not a "how-to-do-it" evidence-based medicine manual (indeed several other books are available that fulfill this objective optimally). It is a broad-ranging collection of essays, each with its own voice, that place evidence-based medicine in the context of endocrine practice and policy. My instruction to each one of the generous contributors to this volume was to be honest, be clear, and be bold. Some went beyond this request and submitted controversy and irritation, and I thank them for taking this risk. I expect all of these chapters to provoke thought and reflection in the curious reader who faces their content with an open but critical mind.

Evidence-Based Endocrinology is divided into four sections. An initial section outlines the past, present, and future of evidence-based medicine. A series of chapters on the practical aspects of evidence-based endocrinology follows. The third section is about the "evidence" in evidence-based medicine. The final section offers case-based discussions by practicing evidence-based clinicians. These chapters highlight both the usefulness of evidence-based medicine in endocrinology and its limitations as we currently understand these.

I selected the authors from among people I respect for their expertise, integrity, and rigor. My deepest gratitude goes to them and to their families for allowing them to produce these chapters mostly during their personal time. I hope the readers will appreciate this book as a testament of friendship, generosity, and scholarship.

I was honored to edit *Evidence-Based Endocrinology* at a particularly exciting point in my career and in my life. I ask the reader to imagine my professional life as one surrounded by the talent of those who have authored the chapters in this book. At the risk of offending those whom I am not mentioning, I want to single out three friends who have been instrumental in my personal and professional growth: Sean Dinneen introduced me to the excitement of endocrinology and systematic reviews; Steven Smith introduced me to health services research, to information technology, and to the "Jimmy Carter" way of getting things done when organizational hairballs limit progress; and Gordon Guyatt, the father of evidence-based medicine, who has shown me that genius, consequence, loyalty, friendship, citizenship, and mentorship can all be qualities of the same wonderful human being. Thank you.

My sons and my wife Claudia have been proverbially patient and extremely generous with their time, and have filled me with unconditional love. They are the best available evidence that I am the luckiest man alive. The time away from them editing this book is the greatest gift I can give to my patients who, I hope, will one day expect, demand, and benefit from the care of evidence-based endocrinologists.

Victor M. Montori, MD, MSc

CONTENTS

CONTRIBUTORS

ELIE A. AKL, MD, MPH, *Departments of Medicine and Social and Preventive Medicine, School of Medicine and Biomedical Sciences, University at Buffalo, State University of New York, Buffalo, NY*

DAVID ARON, MD, MS, *Department of Medicine, Division of Clinical and Molecular Endocrinology, Case Western Reserve University School of Medicine, and VA Health Services Research and Development Center for Quality Improvement Research, Louis Stokes Department of Veterans Affairs Medical Center, Cleveland, OH*

ELIZABETH BAYLISS, MD, MSPH, *Clinical Research Unit, Kaiser Permanente Colorado, Penrose, CO*

SUE A. BROWN, MD, *Division of Endocrinology, Department of Medicine, University of North Carolina, Chapel Hill, NC*

JASON W. BUSSE, DC, MSc, *Department of Clinical Epidemiology and Biostatistics, McMaster University, Hamilton, Ontario, Canada*

SARAH E. CAPES, MD, MS, *Department of Medicine at McMaster University, Diabetes Care and Research Center, Division of General Internal Medicine, Hamilton Health Sciences Corporation, Hamilton, Ontario, Canada*

JEANNE DALY, PhD, *Mother and Child Health Research Centre at La Trobe University, Melbourne, Australia*

SEAN F. DINNEEN, MD, MSC, FRCP(I), FACP, *National University of Ireland, and University College Hospital, Galway, Ireland*

PAUL A. ESTABROOKS, PhD, *Clinical Research Unit, Kaiser Permanente Colorado, Penrose, CO*

AMIRAM GAFNI, BSC, MSC, DSc, PhD, *Department of Clinical Epidemiology and Biostatistics, Centre for Health Economics and Policy Analysis, McMaster University, Hamilton, Ontario, Canada*

GEOFFREY S. GATES, MD, *Department of Internal Medicine, Division of Endocrinology, Mayo Clinic College of Medicine, Jacksonville, FL*

RUSSELL E. GLASGOW, PhD, *Clinical Research Unit, Kaiser Permanente Colorado, Penrose, CO*

MICHAEL L. GREEN, MD, MSc, *Department of Medicine, Yale University School of Medicine, New Haven, CT*

JANELLE GUIRGUIS-BLAKE, MD, *Department of Family and Community Medicine, Georgetown University School of Medicine, Washington, DC*

GORDON H. GUYATT, MD, MSc, *Departments of Medicine and Clinical Epidemiology and Biostatistics, McMaster University, Hamilton, Ontario, Canada*

R. BRIAN HAYNES, MD, PhD, *Department of Clinical Epidemiology and Biostatistics, Health Information Research Unit, McMaster University, Hamilton, Ontario, Canada*

WILLIAM L. ISLEY, MD, *Division of Endocrinology, Diabetes, Metabolism, and Nutrition, Mayo Clinic College of Medicine, Rochester, MN*

KURT A. KENNEL, MD, *Division of Endocrinology, Diabetes, Metabolism, and Nutrition, Mayo Clinic College of Medicine, Rochester, MN*

TECK-KIM KHOO, MD, *Department of Internal Medicine, Mayo Clinic College of Medicine, Rochester, MN*

YOGISH C. KUDVA, MD, MBBS, *Division of Endocrinology, Mayo Clinic College of Medicine, Rochester, MN*

FRANCE LÉGARÉ, MD, PhD, CCFP, FCFP, *Département de Médecine Familiale, Université Laval, Québec City, Québec, Canada*

L. JOSEPH MELTON III, MD, MPH, *Division of Epidemiology, Department of Health Sciences Research, Division of Endocrinology, Department of Medicine, Mayo Clinic College of Medicine, Rochester, MN*

EVELYN MENTARI, MD, *Division of Nephrology, Department of Medicine, Case Western Reserve University School of Medicine, Cleveland, OH*

EDWARD J. MILLS, MSc, *Department of Clinical Epidemiology, Canadian College of Naturopathic Medicine, Toronto, Ontario, Canada, and Department of Clinical Epidemiology and Biostatistics, McMaster University, Hamilton, Ontario, Canada*

VICTOR M. MONTORI, MD, MSc, *Knowledge and Encounter Research Unit, Divisions of Endocrinology, Diabetes, and Internal Medicine, Mayo Clinic College of Medicine, Rochester, MN*

ANNETTE M. O'CONNOR, RN, MScN, PhD, *Ottawa Health Research Institute, The Ottawa Hospital, University of Ottawa, Ottawa, Ontario, Canada*

EDUARDO ORTIZ, MD, MPH, *Department of Veterans Affairs, Washington DC VA Medical Center, Washington, DC, and Division of Health Sciences Informatics, Johns Hopkins University School of Medicine, Baltimore, MD*

BETH RACHLIS, BSc, *Department of Clinical Epidemiology, The Canadian College of Naturopathic Medicine, Toronto, Ontario, Canada*

W. SCOTT RICHARDSON, MD, *Department of Internal Medicine, Wright State University School of Medicine, Dayton, OH*

BERND RICHTER, MD, PhD, *Department of Endocrinology, Diabetology, and Rheumatology, Coordinating Editor Metabolic and Endocrine Disorders Cochrane Review Group, Heinrich-Heine University, Duesseldorf, Germany*

CLIFFORD J. ROSEN, MD, *Maine Center for Osteoporosis Research and Education, St. Joseph Hospital, Bangor, ME, and The Jackson Laboratory, Bar Harbor, ME*

HOLGER J. SCHÜNEMANN, MD, PhD, *McMaster University, Hamilton, Ontario, Canada, Departments of Medicine and Social and Preventive Medicine, School of Medicine and Biomedical Sciences, University at Buffalo, State University of New York; Buffalo, NY, and National Cancer Institute, Rome, Italy*

DUGALD SEELY, ND, *Department of Clinical Epidemiology, The Canadian College of Naturopathic Medicine, Toronto, Ontario, Canada*

ROBERT K. SEMPLE, MA, MB, BCHIR, *Department of Clinical Biochemistry, Addenbrooke's Hospital, Cambridge, UK*

STEVEN A. SMITH, MD, *Division of Endocrinology, Diabetes, Nutrition, and Metabolism, Division of Health Care Policy and Research, Department of Internal Medicine, Medical Director, Section of Patient Education, Mayo Clinic College of Medicine, Rochester, MN*

DAWN STACEY, MScN, RN, PhD, *Ottawa Health Research Institute, The Ottawa Hospital, Ottawa, University of Ottawa, Ontario, Canada*

PETER J. TEBBEN, MD, *Division of Pediatric Endocrinology, Department of Adolescent and Pediatric Medicine, Mayo Clinic College of Medicine, Rochester, MN*

CYNTHIA J. WALKER-DILKS, MLS, *Department of Clinical Epidemiology and Biostatistics, Health Information Research Unit, McMaster University, Hamilton, Ontario, Canada*

1

The New Endocrinologist
Evidence-Based Medicine Meets Endocrine Practice

Victor M. Montori, MD, MSc

CONTENTS

INTRODUCTION

Why evidence-based endocrinology? The practice of evidence-based medicine (EBM) requires the conscientious and judicious application of the best available evidence from clinical care research toward making clinical decisions. It requires expertise in order to understand the context of the patient and to incorporate the patient's values and preferences into evidence-based decisions. This approach to clinical practice is new to medicine *(1)* and to endocrinology *(2–4)* (*see* Chapter 2 for a brilliant account of the history of EBM). This chapter will place the contents of this volume in context while identifying five key contributions that EBM can make to the practice of endocrinology.

EVIDENCE-BASED ENDOCRINOLOGY HELPS PRACTICING ENDOCRINOLOGISTS KEEP UP TO DATE

There are at least 88 journals that focus on endocrinology; 10 of these publish more than 5000 articles every year. Of course, there are also endocrine-related articles

From: *Contemporary Endocrinology: Evidence-Based Endocrinology*
Edited by: V. M. Montori © Mayo Foundation for Medical Education and Research

published in clinical (surgical, radiological, pathological, and general medical) journals, clinical investigation journals, and basic science journals. There is simply no hope that dedicated endocrinologists who want to stay up to date will ever know the totality of research published every day.

Most abnegated specialists read a few journals that share a specific focus with the specialist, a few additional generic journals in their area of clinical practice (usually the table of contents plus selected original articles chosen in some haphazard way, editorials, and reviews), and a few other more general publications. Despite this approach, endocrinologists often see an accumulation of journals in their offices, electronically delivered table of contents in their e-mail inboxes, photocopies, PDFs, and torn-apart articles in their files. Clearly, this approach does not work. Furthermore, if the clinician gets to these articles, he or she clearly has accessed a section of the literature that may not include critical evidence pertinent to his or her practice.

Many prioritization systems are available. One could read journals that are widely recognized as publishing great papers or practical reviews; journals that come to us because of subscription, gift, or entitlement of our membership in a specialty society; or journals that offer their full content on the Internet. None of these approaches, however, select material for review on the basis of how valid and relevant the results are to the practicing endocrinologist.

How does one scan the literature in search of the valid and relevant evidence that could and should impact one's practice? Haynes and his Health Information Research Unit at McMaster University have made several critical contributions toward this goal. Haynes was among the pioneers of the structured abstract that allows the reader to have access to the methods and results of a study rather than the narratives that obscure what matters in these reports *(5)*. Also, Haynes and his team have developed "hedges" that allow the search in MEDLINE and other electronic databases containing high-quality reports in diagnosis, prognosis, etiology, therapy, systematic reviews, health services research, qualitative research, economic studies, and other areas *(6–12)*.

Secondary journals that scan the literature and identify and highlight the most valid and relevant evidence (e.g., *American College of Physicians [ACP] Journal Club, Evidence-Based Medicine*) are another contribution of his team. The reader is enthusiastically referred to their chapter in this volume. Thus, having a set of skills enabling one to quickly scan literature to which we have access, or having access to services that scan the literature—using a transparent method with a goal consistent with the physician's goal of keeping up to date—appear to be better solutions. However, a secondary journal with a focus solely on endocrinology does not exist. Is there enough high-quality and relevant evidence out there to justify one?

EVIDENCE-BASED ENDOCRINOLOGY CALLS FOR MOVING THE RESEARCH AGENDA UP THE HIERARCHY OF EVIDENCE

In Chapter 3, Guyatt—the creator of the term "evidence-based medicine"—and Busse outline the current understanding of the philosophy of EBM. The synthesis of this paradigm shift into two principles facilitates our understanding of what EBM means. The first of these principles recognizes a hierarchy of evidence. One such hierarchy places large and rigorous randomized trials that render accurate and precise estimates of the efficacy of therapies on outcomes that matter to patients at the top. Given that evidence-based practitioners, who want to make recommendations on stronger grounds, need evidence from the top of the hierarchy, evidence-based endocrinology invites clinical researchers and responsive funding agencies to recast the research agenda. In the case of therapy questions, for instance, the path of discovery from basic research, to physiological investigations, to clinical trials needs to move faster—in order to fully understand how treatments work. This is imperative because it is clinical trials that measure the extent to which the treatment, as used by its target patients in usual practice, affects outcomes that matter to patients. Two chapters in this volume are pertinent to this discussion. In a lucid and critical chapter, Isley identifies some of the contemporary issues in the distal part of this process, the space between clinical investigation and large clinical trials that are particular to endocrinology. Glasgow and colleagues offer their expert view of the research that is more proximal to clinical practice and community interventions: translational research in Chapter 16.

Evidence not only informs clinical practice; evidence ought to inform health policy. Integrative or synthetic forms of evidence are particularly useful. In Chapter 12, Richter offers us the opportunity to consider the role of systematic reviews of the literature, as those prepared by the Cochrane Collaboration. Building on these, consideration of how important the outcomes are either in terms of impact on health or on health care costs lead to decision analyses and cost-effectiveness analyses. Aron and collaborators discuss these forms of evidence, and we learn from Gafni, in Chapter 15, that clouded thinking may threaten policy decisions when based on cost-effectiveness analyses.

EVIDENCE-BASED ENDOCRINOLOGY RECASTS THE DEFINITION OF NORMAL

Practicing endocrinologists may find that, for common conditions, they are deriving comfort in the wisdom of the collective and unsystematic experience of colleagues that their interventions lead, on average, to more good than harm (consider the management of Addison or Graves disease). I think that one of the reasons for this belief is that we have measurable hormones with levels that change in predictable ways in response to our interventions. So, if we know what is normal and a patient has an abnormal hormone level that we can normalize with our intervention then we are likely doing more good than harm. However, when we consider how "normal" gets defined we should be concerned. If one takes 500 healthy volunteers, measures hormone levels, and takes the 95% of the distribution around the mean and defines this as normal, 5% of completely normal volunteers will immediately enter the abnormal category. Also, this assumes that the hormone levels take a Gaussian distribution, able to take negative values and have limits at infinity on the positive and negative ends. Most problematic though is the issue of spectrum; we are not interested in differentiating people with disease from healthy volunteers. We are interested in identifying folks with an endocrine condition among those who present to us. The need to diagnose endocrine disease in acutely ill patients illustrates this issue. The need for terms such as euthryoid sick syndrome or relative adrenal insufficiency reflects the uselessness of the normal range in such patients. The diagnosis of pheochromocytoma illustrates another problem with the use of the referential normal range; clinicians recommend a value of total urinary metanephrines that is twofold higher than the upper limit of normal *(13)*.

Thus, for evidence-based diagnosis, other definitions of normal are potentially more useful; a prognostic definition of normal will alert clinicians and patients of the relation between a given hormone level and their risk of disease manifestations or complications that are important to patients. A fasting glucose level in excess of 120 mg/dL clearly indicates an increase in the risk of developing retinopathy among patients with diabetes (14). The folkloric 1000 mg/dL triglycerides threshold, above which the risk of pancreatitis increases substantially, is another example.

A therapeutic definition of normal is even more attractive. This refers to the level of abnormality beyond which taking the treatment will yield more good than harm. The ongoing debate between treating to goal of low-density lipoprotein (LDL) vs just taking a meaningful dose of statins is an example. Some clinicians would not consider starting a statin in a patient at high cardiovascular risk with LDL cholesterol below 100 mg/dL; thus, they operate as if this was the upper limit of the therapeutic definition of normal for the LDL-cholesterol level. The MRC/BHF Heart Protection Study suggested that people benefit to the same extent from statin therapy regardless of their level of LDL (15), suggesting that a therapeutic definition of normal may not exist, and that there is, indeed, no need for a normal range for clinical decision making limited to the use of statins to reduce cardiovascular risk.

Unless the objective of the test is to monitor the degree of derangement—for example, how we use tests in the intensive care setting, as dashboard indicators of the patient's physiology—the diagnostic test result ought to help clinicians and patients determine the likelihood that the patient they are evaluating has the target condition. The performance measure of the test that indicates the extent to which the likelihood of the target condition before we obtained the test changes with the given test result is the likelihood ratio.

Imagine a laboratory report that, instead of offering the normal range for a given test, offered the likelihood ratio that corresponds to the test result obtained. This would be very helpful in situations where patients with extremely low likelihood of having an endocrine problem receive test results that are abnormal (remember that, because of our usual definition of normal, each time a patient is tested they run at least a 5% chance of having an abnormal test result); one could decide about further testing if the post-test probability (derived from the joint consideration of the pretest probability and the likelihood ratio) exceed a threshold above which we are no longer comfortable forgoing testing. Indeed, I believe that explicit and quantitative evidence-based diagnosis will not take place until such information (i.e., likelihood ratios for the test results) is routinely presented in laboratory reports (16). However, other forms of evidence enter the diagnostic process and offer hope for evidence-based diagnostic processes slightly different from the one just outlined. In this volume, Richardson has successfully presented a holistic consideration of evidence-based diagnosis.

An even more radical concern with the issue of normal values is that they are sometimes used to define disease. For example, what is subclinical hypothyroidism? What is diabetes? What is hypogonadism? Whereas it would be easy to identify individuals who are markedly myxedematous, who have uncontrolled diabetes, and have marked hypogonadism, more subtle presentations are often defined exclusively by abnormal laboratory values. And if these laboratory parameters are weakly linked to patient important outcomes, what is the value of these laboratory-based diagnoses? No surprise that we are yet to know if hormone replacement improves patient-important outcomes in patients with subclinical hypothyroidism, hypogonadism, or newly diagnosed diabetes.

EVIDENCE-BASED ENDOCRINOLOGY CAN RECAST THE OBJECTIVES OF TREATMENT—FROM NORMALIZATION OF PHYSIOLOGY TO PATIENT-IMPORTANT OUTCOMES

When asked why patients with microalbuminuria should take angiotensin-converting enzyme (ACE) inhibitors, diabetologists used to say that these agents caused a vasodilation of the efferent arteriole in the glomeruli, which in turn decreased the filtration pressure and delayed progression to proteinuria. Most diabetologists today will answer that same question, I hope, pointing out that ACE inhibitors in patients with diabetes and microalbuminuria can reduce the risk of death, stroke, and heart attacks (17). Furthermore, I suspect that patients will be more likely to decide to take this agent if they are given the latter rather than the former reason. We say outcomes are patient important when patients are willing to consider interventions when the only effect they have is on these outcomes. In general, patient-important outcomes refer to mortality and morbidity that affect patients' present or future quality of life. Although the pain and visual disability of Graves ophthalmopathy are patient-important outcomes, a reduction in the level of antithyroid antibodies is not.

Schünemann and Akl discuss the features of quality of life measures in patients with endocrine conditions in Chapter 13. Instead of focusing on surrogate outcomes (such as LDL cholesterols, HbA1c, thyroid stimulating hormone [TSH], cortisol levels, or bone mineral density) that patients cannot perceive, clinicians and patients may prefer to focus on patient-important outcomes (cardiovascular events, microvascular events, bone fractures, and quality of life) when making choices. Thus, evidence that does not allow us to assess the extent to which our interventions affect patient-important outcomes is not very useful in clinical decision making. In other words, one is not on strong ground when making a recommendation based on evidence that links the intervention with a surrogate outcome. This surrogate outcome may not completely capture the impact of the intervention through the multiple causal paths that lead to impact on the outcome of interest (bone mineral density is a reliable surrogate for bone fracture prevention with biphosphonates, but not for 75 mg/d of sodium fluoride [18]). Indeed, this form of evidence leads to variation in practice (19) (e.g., does it matter if we normalize thyroid tests using antithyroid medication, radioactive iodine, or surgery in patients with Graves disease?), and to catastrophic errors (20,21) (e.g., do reductions of Lp(a) associated with use of hormone replacement therapy for postmenopausal women predict that this intervention will reduce the risk of cardiovascular events?).

One is also on weak ground when making recommendations based on randomized trials that measure the effect of therapy on a composite endpoint—a design often used to allow investigators the opportunity to identify treatment effects with fewer events—than on a single endpoint. The critical issue is that the composite may combine individual outcomes that are quite important to some patients and relatively less important to others. For example, is the need for dialysis as important as duplication in creatinine levels, both components of the composite outcome of a trial of angiotensin receptor blockers for patients with diabetic nephropathy (21)?

When there is no gradient in treatment effect across the component endpoints then gradients in patient importance across the component endpoints become irrelevant; this, however, is uncommon.

I expect that, in refocusing on patient important outcomes and away from the normalization of a physiologic parameter, endocrine research will find the n-of-1 randomized trial design attractive (22). This design can determine the unbiased effect of a treatment (compared to a control intervention) on reversible outcomes in an otherwise stable and symptomatic patient. Consider the difficult decision of determining the ideal dose of steroid replacement in a patient with adrenal insufficiency, thyroid replacement in patients with hypothyroidism, and testosterone replacement in patients with hypogonadism. The opportunity to carefully test different regimens, with random crossover to the control intervention and with blinded patient ascertainment of symptom control and quality of life, could provide the definitive evidence on the efficacy of the regimen for short-term relief of the clinical syndrome. It should follow that the long-term outcomes associated with endocrine therapies will only be determined through careful conduct of large randomized trials with many subjects. Perhaps, a series of n-of-1 trials can determine the range of treatment that usually results in response across a range of random patients. Large clinical trials will require collaboration of endocrinologists and pharmacists, multi-center collaboration, and adequate nonprofit funding.

Once these findings become available, how do we bring the evidence to bear at the point of care? Smith and Gates discuss some strategies to make this happen in their contribution to this volume. Also, O'Connor and her colleagues discuss strategies to support patient decisions in their essay on patient decision aids.

EVIDENCE-BASED MEDICINE CAN LAUNCH THE NEW ENDOCRINOLOGIST

Endocrinologists are considered cognitive specialists, physicians who use their intellect to diagnose, prognosticate, treat, and rehabilitate patients with endocrine abnormalities. For the most part, the use of genomics, molecular biology, physiology, pathophysiology, and pharmacology distinguish these clinicians from their colleagues. With the advent of EBM, clinical reasoning on the basis of this evidence is considered flawed to the extent that it ignores how open these forms of evidence are to bias and error. Thus, as medicine moves towards evidence-based practice, endocrinologists face a tough choice—to become a relic or to lose identity.

I believe endocrinologists have a third path: to embrace evidence-based endocrinology as the new basis for self-identity. Consider the advent of genomics and the possibility of early testing for endocrine diseases, highly personalized treatments that consider genetic predictors of treatment response and toxicity, and of precise prognostic information. Endocrinologists will have to understand how to appraise the medical literature that makes use of genetic, proteonomic, and metabolomic markers as diagnostic or prognostic tests and as guides for therapy. Understanding of the mechanism will be less important than understanding how a given genetic profile increases or decreases the likelihood of disease, how a proteonomic signature increases the likelihood of developing a complication after adjusting for other predictors, and to what extent treatment dosing that takes into account the patient's drug metabolism is more effective and safer than single-dose interventions (23,24). I predict that endocrinologists will be at the forefront of rigorous clinical care research in diagnosis, prognosis, and therapy, and that clinical investigations with a few patients in the Clinical Research Center will cease to be the gold standard of endocrine research. I predict that the transition from research findings to clinical action will be swift and safe as research design mimics clinical practice (for instance, by conducting pragmatic clinical trials *[25]*, or by evaluating the efficacy of diagnostic algorithms in test-and-treat trials) and clinical practice mimics research settings. These new skills will require endocrinologists to be trained differently. Michael Green offers some insights into how we should do that in his contribution to this volume.

I think the evidence-based endocrinologists will expand their role as clinicians that care for those who, in turn, care for patients with common endocrine conditions *(26)*. I am thinking of the large number of patients with obesity, diabetes, osteoporosis, and thyroid abnormalities for who endocrine care will be delivered in the primary care setting by professionals closely supported by an endocrinologist. Thus, a small number of endocrinologists working in a smarter way will be able to ensure that these patients receive evidence-based care every time. This practice model will also free up endocrinologists to see the rare cases that require their expertise (e.g., Cushing disease, acromegaly, pheochromocytoma) *(27)*. The evidence-based endocrinologist will need to have a different model of reimbursement than that which devalues the contributions of safe and effective clinicians who need no knife or catheter to enhance the health of their patients.

Finally, the evidence-based endocrinologist should seriously consider their relationship with interests that are not those of the patient. In their brilliant contribution to this volume, Ortiz and colleagues (Chapter 9) outline the intersection between evidence and policy with attention to the interplay between stakeholders and guidelines. Many individuals, and several organizations of endocrinologists, have made the terrible mistake of closely aligning with the commercial interests of for-profit organizations involved in the commercialization of endocrine testing procedures (assays, imaging) and hormone replacement formulations and related treatments. As a result, their expert opinion appears, to an ever increasingly cynical society, to be severely conflicted. We need to remember why we went into health care. It was, and I hope it will continue to be, because of our calling to heal patients. It is imperative that we practice with only the interest of the patient at heart, that we remain mindful of the influences of the very powerful interests that would like to impact our behavior, and that we remain true to the original calling to apply our ability, our passion, and our intellect to heal the sick and advance the science.

REFERENCES

1. Guyatt G. Evidence-based medicine. ACP J Club 1991;114:A16.
2. Montori V, Guyatt G. What is Evidence-based Medicine? Endocrinol Metabol Clin N Am 2002; 31:521–526.
3. Montori V. Evidence-based endocrinology. How far have we gone? Treat Endocrinol 2004;3:1–10.
4. Montori VM. Evidence-based endocrine practice. Endocr Pract 2003;9:321–323.
5. Haynes RB, Mulrow CD, Huth EJ, Altman DG, Gardner MJ. More informative abstracts revisited. Ann Intern Med 1990;113:69–76.
6. Haynes RB, Wilczynski NL. Optimal search strategies for retrieving scientifically strong studies of diagnosis from Medline: analytical survey. BMJ 2004;328:1040.
7. Montori VM, Wilczynski NL, Morgan D, Haynes RB. Optimal search strategies for retrieving systematic reviews from Medline: analytical survey. BMJ 2005;330:68.

8. Wilczynski NL, Haynes RB. Developing optimal search strategies for detecting clinically sound causation studies in MEDLINE. AMIA Annu Symp Proc 2003:719–723.

9. Wilczynski NL, Haynes RB. Developing optimal search strategies for detecting clinically sound prognostic studies in MEDLINE: an analytic survey. BMC Med 2004;2:23.

10. Wilczynski NL, Haynes RB, Lavis JN, Ramkissoonsingh R, Arnold-Oatley AE. Optimal search strategies for detecting health services research studies in MEDLINE. CMAJ 2004;171:1179–1185.

11. Wong SS, Wilczynski NL, Haynes RB. Developing Optimal Search Strategies for Detecting Clinically Relevant Qualitative Studies in MEDLINE. Medinfo 2004;2004:311–316.

12. Wong SS, Wilczynski NL, Haynes RB, Ramkissoonsingh R. Developing optimal search strategies for detecting sound clinical prediction studies in MEDLINE. AMIA Annu Symp Proc 2003:728–732.

13. Kudva YC, Sawka AM, Young WF, Jr. Clinical review 164: the laboratory diagnosis of adrenal pheochromocytoma: the Mayo Clinic experience. J Clin Endocrinol Metab 2003;88:4533–4539.

14. American Diabetes Association. Diagnosis and classification of diabetes mellitus. Diabetes Care 2005; 28:S37–S42.

15. Heart Protection Study Collaborative Group. MRC/BHF Heart Protection Study of cholesterol lowering with simvastatin in 20,536 high-risk individuals: a randomised placebo-controlled trial. Lancet 2002;360:7–22.

16. Montori VM, Guyatt GH. Summarizing studies of diagnostic test performance. Clin Chem 2003;49: 1783–1784.

17. Gerstein HC. Reduction of cardiovascular events and microvascular complications in diabetes with ACE inhibitor treatment: HOPE and MICRO-HOPE. Diabetes Metab Res Rev 2002;18:S82–S85.

18. Riggs BL, O'Fallon WM, Lane A, et al. Clinical trial of fluoride therapy in postmenopausal osteoporotic women: extended observations and additional analysis. J Bone Miner Res 1994;9:265–275.

19. Tominaga T, Yokoyama N, Nagataki S, et al. International differences in approaches to 131I therapy for Graves' disease: case selection and restrictions recommended to patients in Japan, Korea, and China. Thyroid 1997;7:217–220.

20. Shlipak MG, Chaput LA, Vittinghoff E, et al. Lipid changes on hormone therapy and coronary heart disease events in the Heart and Estrogen/progestin Replacement Study (HERS). Am Heart J 2003; 146:870–875.

21. Lewis E, Hunsicker L, Clarke W, et al. Renoprotective effect of the angiotensin-receptor antagonist irbesartan in patients with nephropathy due to type 2 diabetes. N Engl J Med 2001;345:851–860.

22. Guyatt G, Keller J, Jaeschke R, Rosenbloom D, Adachi J, Newhouse M. The n-of-1 randomized controlled trial: clinical usefulness. Our three-year experience. Ann Intern Med 1990;112:293–299.

23. Ransohoff DF. Evaluating discovery-based research: when biologic reasoning cannot work. Gastroenterology 2004;127:1028.

24. Ransohoff DF. Rules of evidence for cancer molecular-marker discovery and validation. Nat Rev Cancer 2004;4:309–314.

25. Schwartz D, Lellouch J. Explanatory and pragmatic attitudes in therapeutical trials. J Chronic Dis 1967;20:637–648.

26. Montori VM, Smith SA. From artisan to architect: the specialist and systems of provision of diabetes care in 2001. Endocr Pract 2001;7:287–292.

27. Rizza RA, Vigersky RA, Rodbard HW, et al. A model to determine workforce needs for endocrinologists in the United States until 2020. J Clin Endocrinol Metab 2003;88:1979–1987.

I PAST, PRESENT, AND FUTURE

2

A Short History
of Evidence-Based Medicine
Issues for the Clinician

Jeanne Daly, PhD

CONTENTS

INTRODUCTION

Evidence-based medicine (EBM) has made a clear contribution to medicine in a short 10 yr or so. Why then should we stop and consider where it came from and who the people were who generated this new direction? We do not expect any intervention in medicine, whether theoretical or therapeutic, to be perfect. The enthusiasm that greets a new approach gradually gives way to critique with the aim of improving it, of setting limits to its use, or of discarding it. There has sometimes been vehement criticism of EBM, countered with a, sometimes, evangelistic defense. The furor seems to have died down and now is a good time to take stock. What does EBM offer to the clinician in a field like endocrinology, and where might improvements be sought?

If we think of the progression of EBM, then there are traditions that fed into its genesis. There were certainly people who made decisions about the direction in which it should develop; but these decisions were constrained, if not determined, by circumstances: social, professional, and economic. Re-examining this history now gives access to some of the directions that could have been explored yet were not. Are there productive activities that can be introduced in the present time more easily than in the past?

My account draws on research that I conducted over the past 15 yr, interviewing the pioneers of EBM if they were still alive or using archival material to flesh out the

From: *Contemporary Endocrinology: Evidence-Based Endocrinology*
Edited by: V. M. Montori © Mayo Foundation for Medical Education and Research

activities of those who had died. The methods and more detailed discussion are to be found in my book, *Evidence-Based Medicine and the Search for a Science of Clinical Care (1)*. Here I provide a discussion of those aspects of the history that seem relevant to the clinician in the field of endocrinology.

My argument is that EBM was formed from the interweaving of two distinct strands, one arising in the United Kingdom and one in North America. Each of those strands drew on a different intellectual tradition in medicine and when they came together it created a powerful new approach. The examples I use are those of the Cochrane Collaboration and the McMaster University School of Clinical Epidemiology and Biostatistics. Before discussing these two approaches, I outline the intellectual heritage that existed in the 1960s, those researchers whose intellectual contribution underpins EBM.

THE INTELLECTUAL PIONEERS

The two major figures whose work inspired EBM are Archie Cochrane in the United Kingdom and Alvan Feinstein in the United States. These two men both cast long shadows. Both of them were attracted to laboratory medicine, which was dominant in medical schools at the time, but instead they turned to the research that underpins much of EMB. Their careers initially took them in diametrically opposed directions.

Archie Cochrane

Archie Cochrane believed that he could not be a laboratory scientist because of his social conscience. This is the view of Cochrane held by his contemporary, Sir Richard Doll:

> "*Archie Cochrane was a man of the 1930s. His character and lifelong convictions were formed by the cataclysmic events that brought Hitler to power and plunged the greater part of the world into a devastating six-year war. In this he was not alone. What distinguished him from so many others of his generation was the depth of his emotional and intellectual reaction to these events and his fiery independence of mind, which prevented him from accepting any of the easy political solutions and kept him a rationalist to the day of his death.*" (2)

In the 1930s, Cochrane interrupted his clinical studies to volunteer in the Spanish Civil War for the republican Spanish Medical Aid Field Ambulance Unit, supporting the International Brigade. He was a prisoner of war for 4 yr during World War II, within which time he had to care for fellow prisoners suffering the effects of malnutrition and infectious diseases. All he had to treat them with was aspirin, antacid, and skin antiseptic. The German command was of the opinion that doctors were superfluous so Cochrane meticulously observed the prisoners' health needs and used a primitive trial of yeast supplementation *(3)* to argue for improved rations. In another camp he had to care for prisoners with tuberculosis. Later he concluded that he had enjoyed being a caring doctor, he found it intellectually satisfying, but he felt desperately worried that he was making decisions about interventions without knowing whether he was doing more harm than good. "I had never heard of 'randomized controlled trials' but I knew there was no real evidence that anything we had to offer had any effect on tuberculosis, and I was afraid that I shortened the lives of some of my friends by unnecessary intervention." *(4)*

After leaving the army, Cochrane was awarded a Rockefeller fellowship in preventive medicine. He first studied at the London School of Hygiene and Tropical Medicine where he was taught medical statistics by Austin Bradford Hill. In the 1930s, Bradford Hill had designed a randomized controlled trial for application to medical care *(5)* and this was put to use after the war in a trial of streptomycin in the treatment of tuberculosis *(6)*. The drug was in short supply, there was only enough to treat 50 patients, and a randomized controlled trial was seen as the best way of allocating this scarce resource and of getting a definitive answer about effect.

The second stage of Cochrane's fellowship was spent in the United States where Birkelo et al. *(7)* had published a study of differences between radiologists in the interpretation of the same chest films. At the Henry Phipps Clinic, Cochrane studied tuberculosis, including the problem of medical error in the interpretation of X-rays, related to prognosis *(8)*. He returned to the United Kingdom with a fierce interest in medical error and accepted a position in the Pneumoconiosis Research Unit of the Medical Research Council, in Cardiff, South Wales, one of the poorest areas in the country. Cochrane's role was to improve classification of the chest X-rays of coal miners and to conduct surveys of mining populations.

Near Cardiff, there were two mining valleys with a population of about 30,000 people and here Cochrane started his Rhondda Fach studies of factors affecting the progression of lung disease *(9,10)*. Cochrane immersed himself and his researchers in the area. They lived there, based themselves in the small hospital in Llandough (where the Cochrane archives are now located) and set about X-raying the entire adult population and testing all schoolchildren for exposure. Their field workers were from the area and there were regular meetings reporting back to the community. Cochrane's strategies for maintaining response rates of never less than 90% became legendary—including fetching recalcitrant research participants from their homes in his Daimler.

The 20 yr of effort required to maintain the studies deepened Cochrane's commitment to the eradication of error and bias in research. Cochrane had become an epidemiologist. He showed that a team such as his could achieve measurements with a precision matching that of laboratory studies and his main concern became that population studies representative of a community should be rigorous and fully exploited. The Rhondda Fach studies failed to achieve their main aim because the introduction of streptomycin changed the pattern of lung disease, but by then a number of other studies had been nested around this original purpose.

He also became impatient. Lord Cohen of Birkenhead was later to recall, "Bias, indeed, in all its forms, scientific or otherwise, became almost a personal enemy, and once it was detected, he was ruthless in exposing it." Cohen added, "He cannot always have been the easiest of colleagues." *(11)*

Cochrane had been deeply influenced by his participation in the Spanish Civil War. He had concluded that pacifism was impossible in the face of fascism, but he also developed an aversion to communists who, he believed, did not know how to run either a country or a revolution *(12)*. On the other hand, he was committed to social medicine and a passionate supporter of the National Health Service introduced in the United Kingdom after World War II. He was moved by the "gloomy picture" of inconsistent and inadequate health care in South Wales and realized the importance of the randomized controlled trial in measuring the effectiveness of therapies. It "offered clinical medicine an experimental approach to the validation of its practices and treatments. It was high time that medicine and the National Health Service monitored and accounted for how they were serving the public. Too much that was being done in the name of health care lacked scientific validation." *(12)*

While Cochrane extolled the randomized controlled trial as a "very beautiful technique" *(4)* for resolving issues of bias, he proceeded to target his colleagues for substandard care, on local and national committees. In the process, he became notorious as a gadfly but caught the attention of the health bureaucracies. In 1972, he was invited to deliver the Rock Carling lecture, simultaneously published as *Effectiveness and Efficiency: Random Reflections on Health Services (4)*. The book enjoyed immediate popular acclaim for what seemed to many to be a sensible message: that medical care is expensive, that any procedures that could not be shown to be effective should be eradicated and the savings should be committed to proper care for underserved communities. Ten years later, *The Times Health Supplement* (January 22, 1982) reported that Cochrane's medical colleagues were still reeling under the onslaught.

In the United States, Kerr White, who considered Cochrane to be "an icon and an iconoclast," introduced the Cochrane book to the newly established Institute of Medicine *(13)*. There was the perception that Cochrane's book was seen as useful "to halt a lot of costly pie-in-the-sky nonsense from the hi-tech aristocrats aching to get into the health scene, who were very much in the ascendancy in the United States, after the moon landing." *(14)*

The randomized controlled trial was at the heart of Cochrane's radical proposals. Cochrane then went further, calling on each medical specialty to maintain a list of all trials that related to its own practice and to ensure that this list was regularly updated. At this stage, in the 1970s, Cochrane met Iain Chalmers who was to carry this program through to form the international Cochrane Collaboration in the 1990s.

Alvan Feinstein

Like Cochrane, Alvan Feinstein was respected but feared. The targets of his criticisms had to suffer his capacity to coin eloquent new terms to denigrate opponents. An over-commitment to the randomized controlled trial was described as "randophilia;" his critique of clinical biostatistics decried "the haze of Bayes, the aerial palaces of decision analysis, and the computerized Ouija board;" *(15)* meta-analysis was described as "statistical alchemy for the 21st century." *(16)*

Unlike Cochrane, Feinstein was not interested in the health system and he did not want to destabilize the medical establishment: "I am willing to utter heretical remarks, in the inner councils but I don't break up the service in the church." On the other hand, he was in favour of dissidents: "Harold McMillan when he was prime minister of England, made a remark that is one of my guiding lights, he said that whenever the establishment is unanimous in a particular position, he noted that carefully because they were almost invariably wrong. So you always want to have some dissidents." Feinstein certainly was a dissident.

Feinstein first trained in mathematics. When he found that he was unable to make the leaps in understanding of a great mathematician, he switched to medicine. To his surprise, he found that he enjoyed being a doctor and he was good at it. Medicine also gave access to "some wonderful goldmines" both financial and intellectual. In search of this gold, he said, he moved to New York, to the Rockefeller Institute where all good academicians trained. Feinstein was something of a raconteur and could sing self-composed ditties about having to run endless tests on urine and feces while being treated as "somebody's lab boy." Instead he decided to aim for private practice in New York and so he became Clinical Director at Irvington House, a rheumatic fever hospital and convalescent home. Here researchers were conducting a trial of prophylactic treatment for prevention of a recurrence of rheumatic fever. Feinstein's task was to collect the clinical data for the study. He was hooked.

Like Cochrane, Feinstein was immediately concerned about the disagreement in the interpretation of heart sounds and uncertainty in the diagnosis of rheumatic fever. Laboratory tests could establish the presence of a streptococcal infection but the diagnosis of rheumatic fever rested on clinical interpretation of the difference in heart sound between a normal heart (sometimes with a normal murmur) and the heart sound of an affected child. The textbooks were little help and when he tried to get clinicians to state the criteria for a diagnosis, he was told, "Just stay with me and you will learn it." After much "sticking around" he concluded that diagnosis was all too often based on the idiosyncratic views of authoritative clinical teachers. His first aim was reduce inter-observer error.

> *"The first step was to recognize what we heard. I'd say, 'Look, do you agree that what you hear sounds like lubsshh, lubsshh, lubsshh, lubsshh?' 'Yeah, that's what it sounds like.' 'Okay, then what do you think is the lub and what do you think is the sshh? Or do you agree that it sounds like lp dp, lp dp, lp dp?' 'Yeah, yeah.' 'Okay what do you think is the lur, up, the dd and the pp.' This type of cardiophonetics led my colleagues and me to agree on what we heard. We could then go on from there."* (1, p 28)

In time, the researchers on the team developed explicit criteria for classification for each of the manifestations of rheumatic fever. Feinstein then classified patients into subgroups, based on various combinations of symptoms, signs, and test results. He found that overlapping circles were a convenient way of illustrating these subgroups. "I used a circle to represent patients who all had a single common property (such as arthritis) and another, overlapping circle to represent patients with another property (such as carditis). The overlap of the circle would denote patients with both properties; the non-overlapping sectors would denote patients who had one property or the other but not both *(17)*."

When a prognosis was obtained for each of these classificatory groups, it was clear that there was a spectrum of the disease. Antibiotics were found to be effective in preventing recurrence of rheumatic fever in children with abnormal heart sounds but children with the first attack of rheumatic fever who did not have abnormal heart sounds were not at increased risk *(18)*. These were important findings. Prolonged bed-rest was prescribed for any child with rheumatic fever, seriously disrupting their lives. Feinstein celebrated his victory over the "cardiopathic doctors." "Quit keeping them in bed, quit keeping them from athletics, quit keeping them from having children!" As a result of this research, he claims, Irvington House was closed. "They couldn't keep the beds full!"

In the process of conducting this study, Feinstein realized that there was a fundamental problem in clinical research. The study, a trial, was funded to test effectiveness of antibiotic prophylaxis. Feinstein's clinical research addressed practical clinical problems but was regarded as intellectually inferior. Whereas the statisticians on the team categorized data according to demographic variables, they rejected clinical data as unreliable and only considered these data when Feinstein devised ways of making them reliable. But he also realized that the familiar demographic variables were mutually exclusive whereas clinical variables were overlapping. Then Feinstein, the mathematician, saw the solution. "I did not have to remove the overlap; I could preserve and classify it. Boolean algebra and Venn diagrams were a perfect intellectual mechanism for classifying overlap; they were an ideal way to distinguish multiple properties that could be present or absent, alone or in combination." *(17)*

From 1964 onwards, Feinstein was publishing articles on the scientific methods to be used in conducting research specific to clinical care *(19–22)*. Clinicians, Feinstein argued, understand the heterogeneity of clinical practice. It was this heterogeneity that should be accurately observed, classified, and used to determine prognosis and treatment. Clinicians think in terms of overlapping categories and in terms of a systematic taxonomic classification of disease; his 1967 book describing this approach was called *Clinical Judgment (17)*. He described the book as a labor of love, providing a way for clinicians to analyze their own practice. This was the real goldmine. The benefits to clinical practice were clear: there would there be research directly relevant to clinicians' concerns and, in the process, they would gain an additional basic science specific to clinical care *(23)*, additional to the medicine of the laboratory.

By now located at Yale University, Feinstein had defined his life's work. It was not a minor undertaking. He was passionately opposed to the idea that clinician-researchers would borrow research methods from other disciplines. "Clinicians should make use of all the effective, consultative help they can get, but should not abandon fundamental challenges that require direct clinical solutions from wise intellects." *(24)*

He saw the benefits of the randomized controlled trial but he did not define himself as an epidemiologist; since he had entered epidemiology by the "clinical backdoor," he described what he was doing as "clinical epidemiology." *(25–27)*

Feinstein set out a challenging program but, as he himself recognized, his initiative was overtaken by developments at McMaster University. With characteristic vigor he opposed what he saw as their preoccupation with the randomized controlled trial, which, he argued, answered regulatory rather than clinical questions. Although he "dearly loved the gang at McMaster," he felt that the fascination with trials had displaced the program he outlined in *Clinical Judgment*:

> "Clinical Judgment *is dead. This generation has never heard of it. Everything that I recommended in* Clinical Judgment *has been utterly ignored in most of the clinical epidemiology today. What I talked about in that book was a need for clinicians to develop a scientific taxonomy for what they do, and that taxonomy has been utterly ignored during the infatuation with mathematical models, which is why the randomised trial is so powerful because if you don't want to think the randomised trial is a perfect way to avoid thinking. I am not attacking randomised trials, mind you, they have made some wonderful contributions and I am all for them, but it is just absolute folly to think that you are going to answer the questions in clinical practice with randomised trials."*

Despite these views, he had a close relationship with academics at the Department of Clinical Epidemiology and Biostatistics at McMaster University and spent 2 yr there, urging them on to greater scientific rigor.

DAVID SACKETT AND THE DEPARTMENT
OF CLINICAL EPIDEMIOLOGY AND BIOSTATISTICS

It is with the founding of the new medical school at McMaster University that clinical epidemiology became a separate medical discipline and it is here that EBM emerged.

When the new medical school was established in the 1970s, there was concern about the rising cost of health care and, in the next 20 yr, this grew into a sense of crisis especially in the United States *(28)*. There was evidence of regional variations in practice that cast doubt on clinical decision making *(29)*. Medical students joined into the student revolt by questioning the medical curriculum, and began to consider careers outside the traditional academic pathways. Feinstein foresaw that the effectiveness of clinical care was going to be evaluated and he wanted clinicians to do this work. Cochrane saw the randomized controlled trial as well suited for the task of administering a health system. McMaster University combined the two approaches.

In North America there was a tension between clinical care and public health, sometimes so intense as to be described as a schism *(30)*. Although public health addressed issues in the population at large, clinicians saw their own role differently. David Sackett, who was appointed as the first chair of the new department, had the experience of working in a "terrible outfit," the Heart Disease Control Program, when he was drafted into the US Public Health Service during the Cuban missile crisis in 1962. He had to be trained in epidemiology and biostatistics in order to conduct surveys of disease outbreaks and found the work soul-destroying. Then, in 1963, he read Feinsteins's paper *Boolean Algebra and Clinical Taxonomy (31)* and was converted to try to work at the interface between clinical medicine and epidemiology and biostatistics.

In 1967 Sackett was at the State University of New York, Buffalo, establishing himself in the Department of Medicine, when he was invited to come for an interview to McMaster University. He was asked what sort of Department of Social, Community, and Preventive Medicine he thought they should have, and he proposed instead that they should have a department that would do research but serve as a resource for people doing research of all kinds in the medical school and to induct family physicians into critical clinical reasoning about measurement issues and prediction. He was appointed to the new Department of Clinical Epidemiology and Biostatistics.

In the present time, what Sackett proposed may not seem very revolutionary but, at the time, these ideas encountered stiff opposition. Biomedical colleagues thought that what the new department proposed was "not really science"; they saw science as firmly located in the laboratory. What the department needed was somebody to persuasively sell their message. David Sackett filled the role to perfection.

The first people whom Sackett appointed to the department were two statisticians. They joined this risky new venture, persuaded by Sackett. Repeatedly in interview the early recruits to the department recount how they were converted and joined the new Department because of Sackett's vision. Repeatedly these early recruits talk about meeting a charismatic man who was proposing a challenging new program. Here is the account of Mike Gent, statistician and later second chair of the department: "The single thing that moved me here was Sackett. I couldn't believe Sackett! He actually interviewed me, lying on one elbow on the floor. He had outrageous ideas, half of which would never work, but if only 10% worked it would be fantastic. All the concepts about clinical epidemiology were there including getting together a group that was really going to shape the thinking of medical colleagues." *(1*, p 58)

The material generated is now familiar to us under the term "clinical epidemiology." They promoted their approach in journals, in textbooks and in a seemingly endless series of international presentations. They persuaded the Rockefeller Foundation to fund the International Clinical Epidemiology Network (INCLEN) to train international fellows in the new approach. Their approach is set out in the textbook that they published (32) and later updated (33). The books give a common sense approach to the scientific principles underlying diagnosis and management in clinical care. They taught clinicians to be critical in their decision making, for example, factoring into diagnosis the effects of the sensitivity and specificity of a diagnostic test and the prevalence of disease in the community. The methods they described could be used to conduct critical appraisal of the medical literature, and this evidence could then be applied to their own clinical practices. What they proposed was a scientific approach to replace clinical intuition promulgated by clinical authorities:

> *"Our underlying assumption, once again, is that medicine is rational and so are you. That is, your clinical acts of diagnosis and management reflect your assessment of the evidence that this or that diagnostic test is valid and will do more good than harm. If this view of clinical practice is correct, then you should constantly be seeking evidence, not just conclusions or, worse still, authoritarian opinions. Just as your ability to achieve accurate diagnosis and efficacious therapy determines your clinical effectiveness today, it is your skills in self-assessment and in tracking down and assessing biomedical knowledge (most of which resides in the journals) that will more and more determine your clinical effectiveness tomorrow." (32, p 246)*

Sackett gives a humorous summary of why they succeeded. "A group of us came here in the late sixties, rebels with a cause. We set this thing up. We said, 'We know a lot of stuff about medical education (we think it's crap) and we ain't going to do any of that.' We had an idea about how it might work. We got it all done'" (1, p 57). But he also points out that clinical epidemiology provided a scientific discipline for general internal medicine, that it was a source of interesting new research and, finally, that it allowed Departments of Medicine "to justify themselves to the public, to their universities and to funding agencies as doing things with direct payoff to patients."

THE EMERGENCE OF EVIDENCE-BASED MEDICINE

It was in this department that the idea of EBM arose. In common with Cochrane and Feinstein, there was distrust of traditional clinical authority and the search for a more scientific and systematic approach to clinical decision making. From the Cochrane agenda came the emphasis on the randomized controlled trial and its capacity to demonstrate what works. From the Feinstein agenda came the focus not on the health service or public health epidemiology but on the decision making of clinicians, studied by clinicians.

The randomized controlled trial gave a solid foundation for the new discipline. To Feinstein it was an unfortunate choice because it was an epidemiological tool and delivered an outcome based on a population average. In the process the heterogeneity of patient care was obliterated. This problem was to dog the new discipline; clinicians found it difficult to decide how the results of a trial were to be applied to one particular patient. The N of one trial was a response to this problem (34). But the randomized controlled trial design had other advantages. It was difficult to establish the scientific credibility of the new initiative and only in a new medical school would the substantial challenge to traditional medicine even be possible. The trial used an experimental design, allied to the experimental approach of the dominant paradigm of laboratory medicine. It provided a common sense basis for the educational efforts of the department, here described by Gordon Guyatt:

"What we talk about is applying certain rules and concepts of science to clinical experience and systematizing it. 'How do you know that treatment x works?' 'Well I gave it out and the person did well.' OK. And then you say, 'But to what extent can you be confident?' You find out very quickly that you can't be confident at all. And then you say, 'OK, well how can I be more systematic in my accumulation of clinical information to strengthen my inference?' And if you push it, you end up with a double blind randomized trial as a systematic way of accumulating clinical experience. The problem isn't clinical experience, the problem is that we were so unsystematic, intuitive and with no notion of scientific principles in our accumulation of clinical experience. And now is clinical experience worthless? No, but with the appropriate level of skepticism and knowing how things go wrong." (1, p 88).

In 1990, Guyatt was Director of the Internal Medicine Residency program. He saw their approach as a "new brand of medicine," "scientific medicine," an approach so important that it could be seen as a paradigm shift in clinical thinking:

"What were the assumptions of the old paradigm? First, that clinical experience was a valid way of obtaining knowledge about prognosis, the value of diagnostic tests and therapy. Second, that one could work out the appropriate way of treating people just on the basis of physiology and physiological principles. If you knew the physiology and you knew how the drug affected the physiology, you could predict its clinical effects. The third assumption is the high value on authority, and the fourth is that good medical training and commonsense allows you to be appropriately critical about the medical literature. Those are the four assumptions of the old paradigm.

The assumptions within the new paradigm are different in all four. The new paradigm suggests that clinical experience has severe limitations as a guide to understanding the properties of diagnostic tests, whether treatment works, or prognosis. Second, medical training and commonsense are very inadequate guides to deciding whether something is scientifically valid. One needs rules of evidence that are, essentially, clinical epidemiology. Third, reasoning on the basis of physiology often proves misleading without empirical testing and, fourth, following from all this, a much lower value in authority and, in fact, a sort of iconoclasm.

At the point where you say I'm going to be tremendously rigorous and systematic in my accumulation of clinical evidence, you're into the new paradigm and you're into doing science." (1, pp 88–89)

Guyatt was criticized when he called the new approach "scientific medicine." He then called it "evidence-based medicine," evidence being, after all, what they had doing been emphasizing in their approach all along. "Evidence" is what clinical epidemiology produced, and EBM is the practical application of clinical epidemiology to patient care. Guyatt first used the term in 1990 in an information document for residents. In 1991, he defined it as "the application of scientific method in determining the optimal management of the individual patient *(35)*."

In the 20 yr after the department was established, the number of published randomized controlled trials rapidly increased. Brian Haynes, also in the department, was alert to the problem that this burgeoning literature was posing a substantial challenge to clinicians in terms of keeping up to date with the latest developments in a field. He initiated the *American College of Physicians (ACP) Journal Club*. This publication gave clinicians access to the abstracts of selected studies from medical journals, articles that were relevant to internal medicine and that met explicit criteria for validity. A team of researchers worked to extract the articles and a clinical commentator placed the article in the context of other relevant work. Clinicians could breathe a sigh of relief, he believed, especially when this resource and a growing number of others, were produced in readily accessible electronic format.

In the 1970s, Archie Cochrane had called for every medical specialty to collect, and prepare critical summaries of all trials relevant to their field of practice. A parallel initiative in which this was also being done was the Cochrane Collaboration.

THE COCHRANE COLLABORATION

Central to the activities of the Cochrane Collaboration was the work of another North American, Tom Chalmers who had developed meta-analysis as a way of statistically combining the results of multiple different trials of the same intervention. Many published trials were too small to show a statistically significant result. Combining these trials, argued Chalmers, was better than trying to conduct a bigger trial. If meta-analyses were done as soon as trials were completed, the cumulative effect could be assessed so that there was no delay in implementing the evidence (36). A famous example shows that intravenous streptokinase as thrombolytic therapy for acute myocardial infarction could have been demonstrated to be effective in 1973, before a single trial demonstrated this effect and long before clinical opinion changed (37).

The work done by Tom Chalmers provided one of the methodological skills needed to fulfill Archie Cochrane's plea that each clinical specialty should keep an up-to-date summary of work in their field. Iain Chalmers was an obstetrician who had encountered the problem of bias in his own practice, and his research. Three carefully designed consecutive studies had failed to find any effect but he was not sure that he had managed to exclude bias and this bothered him (38–40). Then he read Archie Cochrane's book, met him, and committed himself to the Cochrane agenda in the field of obstetrics.

Iain Chalmers was persuaded that randomized controlled trials would have an important role in changing practice but the cumulative effect would be even more powerful. "Once you start to get trials which show, for example, that 50 yr of radical mastectomies have not been justified, then you can start to see what a powerful weapon such evidence is for those who wish to challenge authority" (1, p 161). From 1978, a team comprising Chalmers, Murray Enkin (an obstetrician from Hamilton and McMaster University), and Eleanor Enkin (a librarian) collected and classified over 3000 reports of trials from 250 journals. They surveyed 42,000 obstetricians and pediatricians in 18 countries, obtaining data on 395 unpublished trials. To deal with the problem of publication bias they set up registers for published, unpublished trials and planned trials. They collected overviews or meta-analyses, conducted according to explicit procedures and regularly updated.

They published their work in an edited collection, *Effective Care in Pregnancy and Childbirth (41)* with the database itself published as the *Oxford Database of Perinatal Trials (42)*. Contributors to the book had access to the Database, which was expanded to include any further trials that authors wanted to use. The emphasis was on combining the results of trials, where possible. A standard format for displaying results included the graph that represents point estimates and confidence intervals for each of the trials of an intervention; it became the logo for the Cochrane Collaboration. The book includes a telling chapter by Peter Goldstein, Henry Sacks and Thomas Chalmers that demonstrates that the prescription of diethylstilbestrol for the maintenance of pregnancy would have been stopped by 1955 by a large well-designed randomized controlled trial or by a systematic review of properly controlled trials.

In 1992, the National Health Service Research and Development Programme decided to support this effort by funding the Cochrane Centre, a small group based in Oxford, independent of the university and part of the National Health Service, to conduct similar work in other areas of clinical care. Chalmers knew that the task could not be done by one center. It needed an international collaboration of researchers and reviewers to voluntarily commit their time to generating reviews according to specific criteria (43), regularly updated. There are now about 50 international review groups, each with a coordinating editor supported by an editorial team, focusing their research on an issue of interest to the group. There are 14 Cochrane Centers with national or regional responsibilities for supporting and coordinating Cochrane initiatives. Brian Haynes established the Canadian Cochrane Centre at McMaster University.

WHERE TO FROM HERE?

EBM is iconoclastic. In both the North American and British contexts it set out to generate an alternative to an unthinking acceptance of traditional clinical authority. Clinicians should assess traditional clinical claims critically, using an additional science, additional to biomedicine, a science that addresses the application of biomedical knowledge to the care of live patients. Over decades a powerful new approach was developed and justified.

The question now is what the status is of EBM as a science of clinical care. Especially at McMaster University, it is argued to represent a new paradigm. This claim is not controversial if by "new paradigm" we mean a new way of doing things, additional to the old, requiring some fine new skills with new benefits to reap from improved patient care. But a "new paradigm" can also mean that there has been a fundamental shift in the way in which we understand clinical decision making so that the old way of doing things is no longer acceptable. It may even mean that the way in which we speak about clinical care has changed so that the things that were said in the past are no longer intelligible to those practicing in the new paradigm. It is the latter meaning that raises concern.

If there has been a shift to a fundamentally new understanding of clinical care, then there are serious disadvantages for clinicians practicing in those areas of clinical care where the evidence from randomized controlled trial and systematic reviews is thin on the ground. Clearly there should be a concerted attempt to generate the evidence, but this takes time. Some areas of clinical care are beset with complexity that does not readily yield a single issue for testing by randomized controlled trial and here EBM may be particularly difficult to practice. One of the problems encountered in clinical care is the need to take account of the social contexts of patients. In a comprehensive textbook from the Evidence-based Medicine Working Group (44), these additional issues are captured under a description of the way in which clinicians and patients negotiate about patient values and preferences. Clearly evidence about the ways in which knowledge of social context enters into clinical decision making is difficult to address in a randomized controlled trial. The risk is that such knowledge will be seen as dispensable to the research agenda.

In contrast, if we mean that EBM represents a new, additional way of proceeding, one that allows for other evidences additional to the evidence produced by randomized controlled trial, then a more complex resolution is possible.

David Armstrong (45) presents a sociological analysis of the way in which general practitioners incorporate new drugs into clinical practice. He shows that it is a gradual process over time, not one that is set in place by a single decision based on new evidence of the effectiveness of a drug. Clinicians took account of their own small personal experiments with the drug to see on which patients it seemed to have the best effect, adjusting their prescribing to take account of what they knew about the psychosocial needs of specific patients.

Armstrong's conclusion is that this way of gradually testing and incorporating a new treatment is complex and changeable and "seems inimical to the logic of evidence-based medicine." (45) In other words, clinicians take account of other evidences than the evidence of effectiveness. This raises the question of the scientific status of these other evidences and also raises the issue that we may need a broader repertoire of methods if we are to judge these other evidences generated by methods other than the randomized controlled trial. We might even revisit the Feinstein project of basing analysis on the carefully defined spectrum of disease instead of a population average. We might return to Archie Cochrane's aim of diverting funds from those interventions that do not work to those geographic areas that are underserved.

If Feinstein was right and clinical practice is a goldmine for researchers, much ore has now been mined. But we can take heart, there is still a rich vein or two left to mine.

REFERENCES

1. Daly J. Evidence-Based Medicine and the Search for a Science of Clinical Care. University of California Press, Berkeley and Milbank Memorial Fund, New York, 2005.
2. Doll R. Foreword to A. L. Cochrane with M. Blythe. One Man's Medicine: An Autobiography of Professor Archie Cochrane. BMJ Publishing Group, 1989, London, pp. ix.
3. Cochrane AL. Sickness in Salonica, my first, worst and most successful clinical trial. Br Med J 1984; 289:1726–1727.
4. Cochrane AL. Effectiveness and Efficiency: Random Reflections on Health Services. The Nuffield Provincial Hospitals Trust, London, 1972.
5. Bradford Hill A. Principles of Medical Statistics. Lancet, London, 1937.
6. Medical Research Council. Streptomycin treatment of pulmonary tuberculosis. Br Med J 1948;2: 769–782.
7. Birkelo CC, Chamberlain WE, Phelps PS, Schools PE, Zacks D. Tuberculosis case findings: a comparison of the effectiveness of various Roentgenographic and photofluorographic methods. JAMA 1947;133:359–365.
8. Cochrane AL, Campbell HW, Steen SC. The value of roentgenology in the prognosis of minimal tuberculosis. AJR Am J Roentgenol 1949;61:153–165.
9. Cochrane AL, Cox JG, Jarman TF. Pulmonary tuberculosis in the Rhondda Fach: an interim report of a survey of a mining community. Br Med J 1952;18:843–853.
10. Atuhaire IK, Campbell MJ, Cochrane AL, Jones M, Moore F. Specific causes of death in miners and ex-miners in the Rhondda Fach, 1959–1980. Br J Ind Med 1986;43:497–49.
11. Cohen D. Introduction to Cochrane, AL with M. Blythe, One Man's Medicine: An Autobiography of Professor Archie Cochrane. BMJ Publishing Group, London, 1989, pp. xvi.
12. Cochrane, AL, Blythe M. One Man's Medicine: An Autobiography of Professor Archie Cochrane. BMJ Publishing Group, London, 1989.
13. White KL. Archie Cochrane's legacy: An American perspective. In: Maynard A, Chalmers I, eds. Non-random Reflections on Health Services Research: On the 25th anniversary of Archie Cochrane's Effectiveness and Efficiency. BMJ Publishing Group, London, 1997, pp. 3–6.

14. McLachlan G. Archie and the Nuffield Hospitals Trust. In: Maynard A, Chalmers I, eds. Non-random Reflections on Health Services Research: On the 25th anniversary of Archie Cochrane's Effectiveness and Efficiency. BMJ Publishing Group, London, 1997, pp. 14–16.

15. Feinstein AR. Clinical Biostatistics: XXXIX, The haze of Bayes, the aerial palaces of decision analysis, and the computerized Ouija board. Clin Pharmacol Ther 1977;21:482–496.

16. Feinstein AR. Meta-analysis: Statistical alchemy for the 21st century. J Clin Epidemio 1995;48:71–79.

17. Feinstein AR. Clinical Judgment. Robert E Krieger Publishing Company, Malabar, 1967.

18. Feinstein AR, Di Massa R. Prognostic significance of valvular involvement in acute rheumatic fever. N Engl J Med 1959;260:1001–1007.

19. Feinstein AR. Scientific methodology in clinical medicine: introduction, principles and concepts. Ann Intern Med 1964;61:564–579.

20. Feinstein AR. Scientific methodology in clinical medicine: classification of human disease by clinical behavior. Ann Intern Med 1964;61:4:757–781.

21. Feinstein AR. Scientific methodology in clinical medicine: the evaluation of therapeutic response. Ann Intern Med 1964;61:944–965.

22. Feinstein AR. Scientific methodology in clinical medicine: acquisition of clinical data. Ann Intern Med 1964;61:1162–1193.

23. Feinstein AR. An additional basic science for clinical medicine: Parts I–III. Ann Intern Med 1983;99: 393–397; 544–550; 705–712.

24. Feinstein AR. Mathematical models and clinical practice. In: Daly J, ed. Ethical Intersections: Health Research, Methods and Researcher Responsibility. Allen and Unwin, Sydney, Australia, 1996, pp. 203–210.

25. Feinstein AR. Clinical epidemiology: I. The populational experiments of nature and man in human illness. Ann Intern Med 1968;69:807–820.

26. Feinstein AR. Clinical epidemiology: II. The identification rates of disease. Ann Intern Med 1968;69: 1037–1061.

27. Feinstein AR. Clinical epidemiology: III. The clinical design of statistics in therapy. Ann Intern Med 1968;69:1287–1311.

28. Shapiro DW, Lasker RD, Bindman AB, Lee PR. Containing costs while improving quality of care: The role of profiling and practice guideline. Annu Rev Public Health 1993;14:219–241.

29. Wennberg JE, Gittelsohn AM. Small area variations in health care delivery. Science 1973;182: 1102–1108.

30. White KL. Healing the Schism: Epidemiology, Medicine and the Public's Health. Springer-Verlag, New York, 1991.

31. Feinstein AR. Boolean algebra and clinical taxonomy: I. Analytic synthesis of the general spectrum of a human disease. N Engl J Med 1963;269:929–938.

32. Sackett DL, Haynes RB, Tugwell P. Clinical Epidemiology: A Basic Science for Clinical Medicine. Little Brown, Boston, 1985.

33. Sackett DL, Haynes RB, Guyatt GH, Tugwell P. Clinical Epidemiology: A Basic Science for Clinical Medicine, 2nd ed. Little Brown, Boston, 1991.

34. Guyatt GH, Sackett D, Taylor DW, Chong J, Roberts R, Pugsley S. Determining optimal therapy— randomized trials in individual patients. N Engl J Med 1986;314:889–892.

35. Guyatt GH. Evidence-based medicine. Ann Intern Med 1991;114:A-16.

36. Lau J, Chalmers TC. The rational use of therapeutic drugs in the 21st century. Important lessons from cumulative meta-analysis of randomized control trials. Int J Technol Assess Health Care 1995;11: 509–522.

37. Antman EM, Lau J, Kupelnick B, Mosteller F, Chalmers TC. A comparison of results of meta-analyses of randomized control trials and recommendations of clinical experts. Treatments for myocardial infarction. JAMA 1992;268:240–248.

38. Chalmers I, Campbell H, Turnbull AC. Evaluation of different approaches to obstetric care, Part 1. Br J Obstet Gynaecol 1976;83:921–929.

39. Chalmers I, Campbell H, Turnbull AC. Evaluation of different approaches to obstetric care, Part II. Br J Obstet Gynaecol 1976;83:930–934.

40. Chalmers I, Zlosnik JE, Johns KA, Campbell H. Obstetric practice and outcome of pregnancy in Cardiff residents, 1965–1973. Br Med J 1976;1:735–738.

41. Chalmers I, Enkin M, Keirse MJNC, eds. Effective Care in Pregnancy and Childbirth. Oxford University Press, Oxford, UK, 1989.

42. Chalmers I, ed. The Oxford Database of Perinatal Trials. Oxford University Press, Oxford, UK, 1988.
43. Oxman A. Checklists for reviewing articles. In: Chalmers I, Altman DG, eds. Systematic Reviews. BMJ Publishing Group, London, 1995, pp. 75–85.
44. Guyatt GH, Rennie D, eds. Users' Guides to the Medical Literature: A Manual for Evidence-Based Clinical Practice. AMA Press, Chicago, IL, 2001.
45. Armstrong D. Clinical autonomy, individual and collective: the problem of changing doctors' behaviour. Soc Sci Med 2002;55:1771–1777.

3

The Philosophy
of Evidence-Based Medicine

Gordon H. Guyatt, MD, MSc
and Jason W. Busse, DC, MSc

CONTENTS

INTRODUCTION

This chapter is drawn largely from a chapter in another book, the *Users' Guide to the Medical Literature (1)*. As the first reference to evidence-based medicine (EBM) in the published literature makes evident, EBM is about solving clinical problems *(2)*. Historically, clinicians found solutions to problems in manuals, textbooks, or in counsel from senior colleagues. Time and experience were seen as sufficient to impart clinical wisdom. As it turned out, however, this paradigm of education and practice resulted in wide practice variations across institutions. At the same time, although important clinical research was available, few clinicians had the skillset required to critically evaluate that literature and decide on the best way to incorporate findings into clinical practice.

For example, in 1998 a survey asked both American and European experts in the field of thyroidology about their recommendations for management on the same case involving a solitary thyroid nodule *(3)*. The survey demonstrated several differences in both examination and treatment. For example, 43% of Europeans and 5% of North American clinicians measured calcitonin levels, and 58% of Europeans, vs 13% of North American experts, pursued ultrasound and scintigraphy. Furthermore, 23% of European thyroidologists elected to excise the nodule surgically compared with only 1% of their

From: *Contemporary Endocrinology: Evidence-Based Endocrinology*
Edited by: V. M. Montori © Mayo Foundation for Medical Education and Research

North American colleagues. As this example illustrates, the historical model of incorporating evidence led to marked variation in practice.

In 1992, in recognition of the historical barriers to incorporating evidence into clinical practice, a group of clinician scientists and clinical teachers described EBM as a shift in medical paradigms *(4)*. In contrast to the traditional paradigm of medical practice, EBM acknowledges that intuition, unsystematic clinical experience, and pathophysiological rationale are insufficient grounds for clinical decision making and it stresses the examination of evidence from clinical research. In addition, EBM suggests that a formal set of rules must complement medical training and common sense for clinicians to interpret the results of clinical research effectively. It requires the judicious application of research findings in the patient context, a sense of the availability of resources, and an understanding of the values of persons involved in the clinical decision. Finally, EBM places a lower value on authority than does the traditional medical paradigm.

This paradigm shift continues to be one useful way of conceptualizing EBM. The world, however, is often complex enough to invite more than one useful way of thinking about an idea or a phenomenon. In this chapter, we will describe an alternative conceptualization. We will explain two key principles of EBM relating to the value-laden nature of clinical decisions, along with a hierarchy of evidence. We will describe some of the additional skills necessary for optimal clinical practice, and conclude with a discussion of the challenges facing EBM in the new millennium.

TWO FUNDAMENTAL PRINCIPLES OF EVIDENCE-BASED MEDICINE

As a distinctive approach to patient care, EBM involves two fundamental principles. First, evidence alone is never sufficient to make a clinical decision *(5)*. Decision makers must always trade the benefits and risks, inconvenience, and costs associated with alternative management strategies, and in doing so consider the patient's values *(6)*. Second, EBM posits a hierarchy of evidence to guide clinical decision making.

CLINICAL DECISION MAKING: EVIDENCE IS NEVER ENOUGH

Picture a patient with chronic pain resulting from terminal cancer. She has come to terms with her condition, has resolved her affairs and said her goodbyes, and she wishes to receive only palliative therapy. The patient develops pneumococcal pneumonia. Evidence that antibiotic therapy reduces morbidity and mortality from pneumococcal pneumonia is strong *(7)*. Almost all clinicians would agree, however, even evidence this convincing does not dictate that this particular patient should receive antibiotics. Despite the fact that antibiotics might reduce symptoms and prolong the patient's life, her values are such that she would prefer a rapid and natural death.

Envision a second patient, an 85-yr-old man with severe dementia, who is incontinent, contracted, and mute, without family or friends, who spends his days in apparent discomfort. This man develops pneumococcal pneumonia. Although many clinicians would argue that those responsible for this patient's care should not administer antibiotic therapy because of his circumstances, others, by contrast, would suggest that they should do so. Again, evidence of treatment effectiveness does not automatically imply that treatment should be administered. The management decision requires a judgment about the trade-off between risks and benefits, and because values or preferences differ, the best course of action will vary from patient to patient and among clinicians.

Finally, picture a third patient, a healthy, 30-yr-old mother of two children who develops pneumococcal pneumonia. No clinician would doubt the wisdom of administering antibiotic therapy to this patient. However, this does not mean that an underlying value judgment has been unnecessary. Rather, our values are sufficiently concordant, and the benefits so overwhelm the risks, that the underlying value judgment is unapparent.

In current health care practice, judgments often reflect clinical or societal values concerning whether intervention benefits are worth the cost. Consider the decisions regarding administration of anticoagulants vs aspirin to patients with atrial fibrillation, or administration of clopidigrel vs aspirin to patients with transient ischemic attack. In both cases, evidence from large randomized trials suggests that that aspirin is less effective in reducing strokes than the alternative agents. Nevertheless, many patients with atrial fibrillation will choose aspirin over warfarin to reduce bleeding risks. Most guidelines suggest aspirin rather than clopidigrel as the first line agent for transient ischemic attacks, largely because it is less expensive and experts presumably believe society's resources would be better used in other ways. Implicitly, they are making a value or preference judgment about the tradeoff between deaths and strokes prevented, and resources allocated.

By *values* and *preferences*, we mean the underlying processes we bring to bear in weighing what our patients and our society will gain—or lose—when we make a management decision. The explicit enumeration and balancing of benefits and risks that is central to EBM brings the underlying value judgments involved in making management decisions into bold relief.

Acknowledging that values play a role in every important patient care decision highlights our limited understanding of how best to elicit and incorporate societal and individual values. Whereas health economists have played a major role in developing a science of measuring patient preferences, and their techniques are suitable for measuring societal preferences (8,9), they are not practical in the clinical setting. Decision aids that provide structured presentations of options and outcomes for conditions such as breast cancer, cardiovascular risk modification, and stroke prevention may be practical and useful for the clinical setting (10). If patients truly understand the potential risks and benefits that the decision aid aims to convey, their decisions will likely reflect their preferences.

These developments constitute a promising start. Nevertheless, many unanswered questions remain concerning how to elicit preferences and how to incorporate them in clinical encounters already subject to crushing time pressures. Addressing these issues constitutes an enormously challenging frontier for EBM (11).

A HIERARCHY OF EVIDENCE

What is the nature of the "evidence" in EBM? A broad definition is most appropriate: any empirical observation about the apparent relation between events constitutes potential evidence. Thus, the unsystematic observations of the individual clinician constitute one source of evidence; physiological experiments constitute another source. Unsystematic observations can lead to profound insight, and experienced clinicians develop a healthy respect for the reflections of their senior colleagues on issues of clinical observation, diagnosis, and relations with patients and colleagues. Some of these insights can be taught, yet rarely appear in the medical literature.

At the same time, unsystematic clinical observations are limited by small sample size and, more importantly, by deficiencies in human processes of making inferences (12). Predictions about intervention effects on patient-important outcomes (13) based on physiological experiments usually are right, but occasionally are disastrously wrong (14).

Given the limitations of unsystematic clinical observations and physiological rationale, EBM suggests a hierarchy of evidence. Table 1 presents a hierarchy of study designs for treatment issues; very different hierarchies are necessary for issues of diagnosis or prognosis. Consider the study design at the top of the hierarchy, a randomized trial that involves only one patient. Because few, if any, interventions are effective in all patients, we would ideally test a treatment in a patient to whom we would like to apply it. Thus clinicians often make use of conventional open trials of therapy, in which they ask patients to take a medication and then return to evaluate its impact. Unfortunately, numerous factors can lead clinicians astray as they try to interpret the results of such conventional open trials of therapy. These include natural history, placebo effects, patient and health worker expectations, and the patient's desire to please.

The same strategies that minimize bias in conventional therapeutic trials involving multiple patients can guard against misleading results in studies involving single patients (15). In the N-of-1 randomized control trial (RCT), patients undertake pairs of treatment periods in which they receive a target treatment in one period of each pair, and a placebo or alternative in the other. Patients and clinicians are blind to allocation, the order of the target and control are randomized, and patients make quantitative ratings of their symptoms during each period. The N-of-1 RCT continues until both the patient and clinician conclude that the patient is, or is not, obtaining benefit from the target intervention. N-of-1 randomized trials are often feasible (16,17), can provide definitive evidence of treatment effectiveness in individual patients, and may lead to long-term differences in treatment administration (18).

When considering any other source of evidence about treatment, clinicians are applying generalized results of other people to their patients, inevitably weakening inferences about treatment impact and introducing complex issues of how trial results apply to individual patients. Inferences may nevertheless be very strong if results come from a systematic review of methodologically strong RCTs with consistent results. Inferences will, in general, be weaker if only a single RCT is being considered, unless it is very large and has enrolled a diverse patient population (Table 1).

Because observational studies may under- or, more typically, over-estimate treatment effects in an unpredictable fashion (19), their results are far less trustworthy than those of randomized trials. Nonrandomized clinical trials may exaggerate the estimates for a given intervention by up to 150% or underestimate effectiveness by up to 90% (20). For example, many large observational studies suggested that hormone replacement therapy in postmenopausal women reduced their relative risk of coronary death by up to 35% (21). However, the results of the first randomized trial of hormone replacement therapy in postmenopausal women at high risk of coronary events found no benefit (22), as did the first large trial in lower risk women (23). Physiological studies and unsystematic clinical observations provide the weakest inferences about treatment effects.

Evidence from the top of the hierarchy in Table 1 should have greater impact on clinical decision making that lower level observations; however, this hierarchy is not

Table 1
A Hierarchy of Strength of Evidence for Treatment Decisions

- *N*-of-1 randomized trial.
- Systematic reviews of randomized trials.
- Single randomized trial.
- Systematic review of observational studies addressing patient-important outcomes.
- Single observational study addressing patient-important outcomes.
- Physiological studies (studies of blood pressure, cardiac output, exercise capacity, bone density).
- Unsystematic clinical observations.

absolute. If treatment effects are sufficiently large and consistent, for instance, observational studies may provide more compelling evidence than most RCTs. By way of example, observational studies have allowed extremely strong inferences about the efficacy of insulin in diabetic ketoacidosis or that of hip replacement in patients with debilitating hip osteoarthritis. At the same time, instances in which RCT results contradict consistent results from observational studies reinforce the need for caution. Defining the extent to which clinicians should temper the strength of their inferences when only observational studies are available remains one of the important challenges for EBM. The challenge is particularly important given that much of the evidence regarding the harmful effects of our therapies comes from observational studies.

The hierarchy implies a clear course of action for physicians addressing patient problems: they should look for the highest available evidence from the hierarchy. The hierarchy makes clear that any statement to the effect that there is no evidence addressing the effect of a particular treatment is a non sequitur. The evidence may be extremely weak—it may be the unsystematic observation of a single clinician, or a generalization from physiological studies that are only indirectly related—but there is always evidence.

Next we will briefly comment on additional skills that clinicians must master for optimal patient care and the relation of those skills to EBM.

CLINICAL SKILLS, HUMANISM, SOCIAL RESPONSIBILITY, AND EVIDENCE-BASED MEDICINE

The evidence-based process of resolving a clinical question will be fruitful only if the problem is formulated appropriately. A colleague of ours, a secondary care internist, developed a lesion on his lip shortly before an important presentation. He was quite concerned and, wondering if he should take acyclovir, proceeded to spend the next 2 h searching for the highest quality evidence and reviewing the available RCTs. When he began to discuss his remaining uncertainty with his partner, an experienced dentist, she quickly cut short the discussion by exclaiming, "But, my dear, that isn't herpes!"

This story illustrates the necessity of obtaining the correct diagnosis before seeking and applying research evidence in practice, the value of extensive clinical experience, and the fallibility of clinical judgment. The essential skills of obtaining a history and conducting a physical examination and the astute formulation of the clinical problem come only with thorough background training and extensive clinical experience. The clinician makes use of evidence-based reasoning—applying the likelihood ratios associated with positive or negative physical findings, for instance—to interpret the results of the history and physical examination. Clinical expertise is further required to define the relevant treatment options before examining the evidence regarding the expected benefits and risks of those options.

Finally, clinicians rely on their expertise to define features that impact on the generalizability of the results to the individual patient. We have noted that, except when clinicians have conducted N-of-1 RCTs, they are attempting to generalize (or, one might say, particularize) results obtained in other patients to the individual patient before them. The clinician must judge the extent to which differences in treatment (local surgical expertise or the possibility of patient noncompliance, for instance), the availability of monitoring, or patient characteristics (such as age, comorbidity, or concomitant treatment) may impact estimates of benefit and risk that come from the published literature.

Thus, knowing the tools of evidence-based practice is necessary, but not sufficient, for delivering the highest quality patient care. In addition to clinical expertise, the clinician requires compassion, sensitive listening skills, and broad perspectives from the humanities and social sciences. These attributes allow understanding of patients' illnesses in the context of their experience, personalities, and cultures. The sensitive understanding of the patient relates to evidence-based practice in a number of ways. For some patients, incorporation of patient values for major decisions will mean a full enumeration of the possible benefits, risks, and inconvenience associated with alternative management strategies that are relevant to the particular patient. For some of these patients and problems, this discussion should involve the patients' family. For other problems—the discussion of screening with prostate-specific antigen with older male patients, for instance—attempts to involve other family members might violate strong cultural norms.

Application of evidence also must account for the patient's particular circumstances. For instance, the mentally disabled and institutionalized patient with type I diabetes mellitus will be unlikely to benefit from insulin treatment if the institution cannot organize frequent glucose checks and insulin injections and be prepared to diagnose and treat hypoglycemic episodes.

Many patients are uncomfortable with an explicit discussion of benefits and risks, and object to having what they perceive as excessive responsibility for decision making being placed on their shoulders (13). In such patients, who would tell us they want the physician to make the decision on their behalf, the physician's responsibility is to develop insight to ensure that choices will be consistent with patients' values and preferences. Understanding and implementing the sort of decision-making process patients desire and effectively communicating the information they need requires skills in understanding the patient's narrative and the person behind that narrative (14,15). A continuing challenge for EBM—and for medicine in general—will be to better integrate the new science of clinical medicine with the time-honored craft of caring for the sick.

Ideally, evidence-based physicians' technical skills and humane perspective will lead them to become effective advocates for their patients both in the direct context of the health system in which they work and in broader health policy issues. Most physicians see their role as focusing on health care interventions for their patients. Even when they consider preventive therapy, they focus on individual patient behavior. However, we consider this focus to be too narrow.

Observational studies have documented the strong and consistent association between socioeconomic status and health. Societal health may be more strongly associated with income gradients than with the total wealth of the society. In other words, the overall health of the populace may be higher in poorer countries with a relatively equitable distribution of wealth than in richer countries with larger disparities between rich and poor. These considerations suggest that physicians concerned about the health of their patients as a group, or about the health of the community, should consider how they might contribute to reducing poverty.

Observational studies have shown a strong and consistent association between pollution levels and respiratory and cardiovascular health. Physicians seeing patients with chronic obstructive pulmonary disease will suggest that they stop smoking. But should physicians also be concerned with the polluted air that patients are breathing? We believe they should.

ADDITIONAL CHALLENGES FOR EVIDENCE-BASED MEDICINE

In 1992, we identified skills necessary for evidence-based practice. These included the ability to precisely define a patient problem and to ascertain what information is required to resolve the problem, conduct an efficient search of the literature, select the best of the relevant studies, apply rules of evidence to determine their validity, extract the clinical message, and apply it to the patient problem *(1)*. To these we would now add an understanding of how the patient's values impact the balance between advantages and disadvantages of the available management options, and the ability to appropriately involve the patient in the decision.

A further decade of experience with EBM has not changed the biggest challenge to evidence-based practice: time limitation. Fortunately, new resources to assist clinicians are available and the pace of innovation is rapid. One can consider a classification of information sources that comes with a mnemonic device, 4S: the individual *study*, the *systematic review* of all the available studies on a given problem, a *synopsis* of both individual studies and summaries, and *systems* of information. By systems we mean summaries that link a number of synopses related to the care of a particular patient problem (acute upper gastrointestinal bleeding) or type of patient (the diabetic outpatient) (Table 2). Evidence-based selection and summarization is becoming increasingly available at each level (*see* Finding the Evidence).

The acceptance of EBM presents further challenges, especially when the findings from rigorous studies conflict with current practices *(24)*, or challenge powerful special interest groups *(25)*. Recently, one of us was involved in a systematic overview to determine whether a difference in adjusted mortality rates exists between hemodialysis patients receiving care in private for-profit vs private not-for-profit dialysis centers *(26)*. The results suggested that there are annually 2500 (with a plausible range of 1200–4000) excessive premature deaths in United States for-profit dialysis centers. Approximately 75% of facilities that provide hemodialysis care in the United States are private for-profit, and those involved in these profit-making facilities strongly resisted our findings *(27–30)*.

This chapter deals primarily with decision making at the level of the individual patient. Evidence-based approaches can also inform health policymaking *(16)*, day-to-day decisions in public health, and systems-level decisions such as those facing hospital managers. In each of these arenas, EBM can support the appropriate goal of gaining the greatest health benefit from limited resources. On the other hand, *evidence*—as an

Table 2
A Hierarchy of Preprocessed Evidence

Studies	Preprocessing involves selecting only those studies that are both highly relevant and that are characterized by study designs that minimize bias and thus permit a high strength of inference.
Summaries	Systematic reviews provide clinicians with an overview of all of the evidence addressing a focused clinical question.
Synopses	Synopses of individual studies or of systematic reviews encapsulize the key methodologic details and results required to apply the evidence to individual patient care.
Systems	Practice guidelines, clinical pathways, or evidence-based textbook summaries of a clinical area provide the clinician with much of the information needed to guide the care of individual patients.

ideology, rather than a focus for reasoned debate—has been used as a justification for many agendas in health care, ranging from crude cost cutting to the promotion of extremely expensive technologies with minimal marginal returns.

In the policy arena, dealing with differing values poses even more challenges than in the arena of individual patient care. Should we restrict ourselves to alternative resource allocation within a fixed pool of health care resources, or should we be trading off health care services against, for instance, lower tax rates for individuals, or lower health care costs for corporations? How should we deal with the large body of observational studies suggesting that social and economic factors may have a larger impact on the health of populations than health care delivery? How should we deal with the tension between what may be best for a person and what may be optimal for the society of which that person is a member? The debate about such issues is at the heart of evidence-based health policymaking, but, inevitably, it has implications for decision making at the individual patient level.

REFERENCES

1. Guyatt GH, Haynes B, Jaeschke, et al. The philosophy of evidence-based medicine. In: Users' Guides to the Medical Literature. Guyatt G, Rennie D, eds. AMA Press, Chicago, IL, 2002.
2. Guyatt, G. Evidence-Based Medicine. Ann Intern Med 1991;14:A–16.
3. Bennedbaek FN, Hegedus L. Management of the solitary thyroid nodule: results of a North American survey. J Clin Endocrinol Metab 2000;85:2493–2498.
4. Evidence-Based Medicine Working Group. Evidence-based medicine. A new approach to teaching the practice of medicine. JAMA 1992;268:2420–2425.
5. Sackett DL, Rosenberg WM, Gray JA, Haynes RB, Richardson WS. Evidence-based medicine: what it is and what it isn't. BMJ 1996;312:71–72.
6. Guyatt G, Schunemann H, Cook D, Jaeschke R, Pauker S, Bucher H; American College of Chest Physicians. Grades of recommendation for antithrombotic agents. Chest 2001;119:3S–7S.
7. Bru JP, Leophonte P, Veyssier P. Levofloxacine for the treatment of pneumococcal pneumonia: results of a meta-analysis. Rev Pneumol Clin 2003;59:348–356.
8. O'Brien B, Drummond M, Richardson WS, Levine M, Heyland D, Guyatt G. Economic analysis. In: Users' Guides to the medical literature. Guyatt G, Rennie D, eds. AMA Press, Chicago, IL, 2002.
9. Feeny D, Furlong W, Barr RD. Multiattribute approach to the assessment of health-related quality of life: Health Utilities Index. Med Pediatr Oncol 1998;Suppl 1:54–59.
10. O'Connor AM, Legare F, Stacey D. Risk communication in practice: the contribution of decision aids. BMJ 2003;327:736–740.

11. Guyatt G, Straus S, McCalister F, et al. Incorporating patient values. In: Users' Guides to the Medical Literature. Guyatt G, Rennie D, eds. AMA Press, Chicago, IL, 2002.
12. Nisbett RE, Ross L. Human Inference: Strategies and Shortcomings of Social Judgment. Prentice-Hall, Englewood Cliffs, 1980.
13. Guyatt, GM, Montori V, Devereaux P, Schunemann H, Bhandari M. Patients at the centre: In our practice, and in our use of language. ACP J Club 2004;140:A–11.
14. Lacchetti C, Guyatt G. Surprising results from randomized controlled trials. In: Users' Guides to the Medical Literature. Guyatt G, Rennie D, eds. AMA Press, Chicago, IL, 2002.
15. Guyatt G, Sackett D, Taylor DW, Chong J, Roberts R, Pugsley S. Determining optimal therapy—randomized trials in individual patients. N Engl J Med 1986;314:889–892.
16. Guyatt GH, Keller JL, Jaeschke R, Rosenbloom D, Adachi JD, Newhouse MT. The n-of-1 randomized controlled trial: clinical usefulness. Our three-year experience. Ann Intern Med 1990;112:293–299.
17. Larson EB, Ellsworth AJ, Oas J. Randomized clinical trials in single patients during a 2-year period. JAMA 1993;270:2708–2712.
18. Mahon J, Laupacis A, Donner A, Wood T. Randomised study of n of 1 trials versus standard practice. BMJ 1996;312:1069–1074.
19. Guyatt GH, DiCenso A, Farewell V, Willan A, Griffith L. Randomized trials versus observational studies in adolescent pregnancy prevention. J Clin Epidemiol 2000;53:167–174.
20. Kunz R, Oxman AD. The unpredictability paradox: review of empirical comparisons of randomized and non-randomised clinical trials. BMJ 1998;317:1185–1190.
21. Stampfer MJ, Colditz GA. Estrogen replacement therapy and coronary heart disease: a quantitative assessment of the epidemiologic evidence. Prev Med 1991;20:47–63.
22. Hulley S, G.D., Bush T, Furberg C, Herrington D, Riggs B, Vittinghoff E. Randomized trial of estrogen plus progestin for secondary prevention of coronary heart disease in postmenopausal women. Heart and Estrogen/progestin Replacement Study (HERS) Research Group. JAMA 1998;280:605–613.
23. Rossouw JE, Andersen GL, Prentice RL, et al.; Writing Group for the Women's Health Initiative Investigators. Risks and benefits of estrogen plus progestin in healthy postmenopausal women: principal results From the Women's Health Initiative randomized controlled trial. JAMA 2002;288: 321–333.
24. Moseley JB, OMalley K, Petersen NJ, et al. A controlled trial of arthroscopic surgery for osteoarthritis of the knee. N Engl J Med 2002;347:81–88.
25. Deyo RA, Psaty BM, Simon G, Wagner EH, Omenn GS. The messenger under attack—intimidation of researchers by special-interest groups. N Engl J Med 1997;336:1176–1180.
26. Devereaux PJ, Schunemann HJ, Ravindran N, et al. Comparison of mortality between private for-profit and private not-for-profit hemodialysis centers: a systematic review and meta-analysis. JAMA 2004;288:2449–2457.
27. Bosch J, HakimRM, Lazarus JM, McAllister CJ. Quality of care in profit vs not-for-profit dialysis centers [letter]. JAMA 2003;289:3087–3088.
28. Blake PG, Mendelssohn DC. Quality of care in profit vs not-for-profit dialysis centers [letter]. JAMA 2003;289:3088–3089.
29. Lyons JS. Quality of care in profit vs not-for-profit dialysis centers [letter]. JAMA 2003;289:3088.
30. Kalantar-Zadeh K, Mehrotra R, Kopple JD. Quality of care in profit vs not-for-profit dialysis centers [letter]. JAMA 2003;289:3089.

4

Preparing Future Generations
of Evidence-Based Endocrinologists

Michael L. Green, MD, MSc

INTRODUCTION

There is much to recommend an increased emphasis on evidence-based medicine (EBM) training in medical education. Evidence-based practice has emerged as a national priority in efforts to improve health care quality *(1)*. Physicians are encouraged to identify, appraise, and apply the best evidence in their decision making for individual patients. However, this ideal remains far from realization. Physicians leave the majority of their clinical questions unanswered *(2,3)*, often consult nonevidence-based sources of information, watch their grasp of current information deteriorate over the years following their training *(4,5)*, and demonstrate wide practice variations for clinical maneuvers with established efficacy *(6)*. And traditional didactic continuing medical education (CME) remains of limited utility as a remedy *(7,8)*.

In response, professional organizations have called for increased training in EBM at all levels of medical education. In *Health Professions Education: A Bridge to Quality*, the Institute of Medicine identified "employ evidence-based practice" and "utilize informatics" among a set of five core competencies for all health professionals *(9)*. The American Boards of Internal Medicine (ABIM) and Medical Specialties, in their maintenance of certification, now place a premium on self-directed, practice-based learning *(10)*, taking a lesson from Canada's Maintenance of Competence program *(11)*. And various charters highlight life-long self-directed learning (LLSDL) as a central dimension of professionalism.

From: *Contemporary Endocrinology: Evidence-Based Endocrinology*
Edited by: V. M. Montori © Mayo Foundation for Medical Education and Research

In a similar reform, the Accreditation Council for Graduate Medical Education (ACGME) changed the currency of accreditation from structure and process to educational outcomes *(12)*. EBM is included within the "patient care" and "practice-based learning and improvement" general competencies, which apply to all residency and fellowship programs *(12)*. This division highlights evidence-based practice as a guide to medical decision making and a strategy for life-long self-directed learning. The general program requirements for residency education in the subspecialties of internal medicine also specify curricula related to EBM. Table 1 includes selected pertinent language from the ACGME. In short, endocrinology program directors must now document that their fellows "investigate and evaluate their patient care practices, appraise and assimilate scientific evidence, and improve their patient care practices."

As program directors strive to reform their curricula, they will find little guidance in the endocrinology (or any subspecialty fellowship) training literature. My search identified only two reports of integrating EBM training into a subspecialty fellowship program *(13,14)*. However, they can take some lessons from internal medicine and other residency programs, which have studied their residents' learning behaviors and implemented innovative curricula. In this chapter, I summarize the current curriculum in endocrinology fellowships, review the literature on EBM training in graduate medical education (including instructional strategies, effects of the hidden curriculum, and trainee evaluation), highlight the barriers to EBM training, and offer recommendations for educational reform. In addition, I provide a list of useful EBM education resources in the appendix.

I should confess, at this point, that I am not an endocrinologist. I am an academic general internist, with special interests and experience in EBM and graduate medical education. So please accept my analysis and recommendations as I offer them—with a deep commitment to grooming the next generation of physicians, an abiding passion for things metabolic, and as much humility as "chutzpah."

CURRENT CURRICULUM IN ENDOCRINOLOGY FELLOWSHIPS

To my knowledge, there are no reports of specific curricula or national surveys of endocrinology fellowships. The following description is based on a review of the ACGME requirements, interviews with program directors and other endocrinology faculty, and brief communications with Association of Program Directors in Endocrinology and Metabolism (APDEM) officials. In university-based endocrinology programs, fellows typically spend 1 "clinical" year caring for patients and 1 or 2 yr doing research. In their clinical year, fellows perform inpatient consultations, rotate through general and specialty endocrinology outpatient clinics, and follow a cadre of patients in a longitudinal endocrinology clinic. The continuity clinic often continues through their research years. Fellows attend (and sometimes present) at endocrine and interdisciplinary clinical conferences, some of which take the form of journal clubs.

EVIDENCE-BASED MEDICINE CURRICULA IN GRADUATE MEDICAL EDUCATION

Subspecialty Fellowship Training Programs

Kellum and colleagues reported their efforts to integrate EBM into critical care subspecialty training *(13)*. A didactic component included three seminars on study design,

Table 1
ACGME Requirements Related to EBM

General competencies for all GME programs[a]	Program requirements for residency education in the subspecialties of internal medicine[b]
Patient care • Make informed decisions about diagnostic and therapeutic interventions based on patient information and preferences, up-to-date scientific evidence, and clinical judgment. • Use information technology to support patient care decisions and patient education. Practice-based learning and improvement • Analyze practice experience and perform practice-based improvement activities using a systematic methodology. • Locate, appraise, and assimilate evidence from scientific studies related to their patients' health problems. • Apply knowledge of study designs and statistical methods to the appraisal of clinical studies and other information on diagnostic and therapeutic effectiveness. • Use information technology to manage information, access on-line medical information; and support their own education.	Educational program (general) • The program must emphasize scholarship, self-instruction, development of critical analysis of clinical problems, and the ability to make appropriate decisions. Medical informatics and decision-making skills • Residents should receive instruction in the critical assessment of medical literature, in clinical epidemiology, in biostatistics, and in clinical decision theory. • Each resident should have the opportunity to learn basic computer skills, including an introduction to computer capabilities and medical applications, basic techniques for electronic retrieval of medical literature, computer assisted medical instruction, and electronic information networks. Research • Residents must have experience and be productive in research. • Residents must learn the design and interpretation of research studies, responsible use of informed consent, and research methodology and interpretation of data. • The program must provide instruction in the critical assessment of new therapies and of the literature.

[a]From the ACGME outcomes project (http://www.acgme.org/outcome/comp/compFull.asp).

[b]From the ACGME program requirements for residency education in the subspecialties of internal medicine (http://www.acgme.org/acWebsite/RRC_140/140_prIndex.asp).

data analysis, and critical appraisal techniques. Each fellow, under the tutelage of a faculty member, also reviewed one report of original research, prepared a written critical appraisal, and presented a critique at journal clubs over the course of 1 yr. In a pre–post uncontrolled trial, fellows ($n = 6$) improved their scores on a critical appraisal test, which included true–false, multiple-choice, and free text questions related to two reports of therapeutic interventions for acute lung injury. Schoenfeld developed a 3-d seminar in EBM for his 24 gastroenterology fellows *(14)*. In a pre–post uncontrolled trial, fellows improved their scores—on a 14-item test—from 57 to 82% and maintained this score 6 mo later upon retesting. Neither report included information on the reliability or validity of the outcome instruments. These two remain the only reports of EBM training in a subspecialty fellowship.

Core Graduate Medical Education Residency Training Programs

Many core training programs (the majority internal medicine and family medicine) have developed innovative EBM curricula. Three systematic reviews summarized this experience specifically in graduate medical education (15–17). Additional reviews combined curricula for residents with undergraduate and other curricula (18–21). Most of these analyses included reports of both traditional journal clubs and EBM curricula. Although the two types of curricula share some features, I believe important distinctions remain. Thus, in the following, I distinguish the two in reviewing their effectiveness.

TRADITIONAL JOURNAL CLUBS

In 1995, 98% of internal medicine programs maintained traditional journal clubs (22), which generally focused on critical appraisal skills and "keeping up" with the medical literature, but neglected individual patient decision making. In the most common format, a small group of residents critically discussed articles chosen for their timeliness, clinical relevance, landmark status, or exemplification of critical appraisal teaching points. Fifteen reports of journal clubs were analyzed in a systematic review in 1999 (15). Among the six reports with a curriculum evaluation, most assessed critical appraisal skills, to the exclusion of other EBM steps. Many suffered from methodologic shortcomings, including lack of a pretest or control group, unblinded investigators, neglect of important confounding factors, or outcome instruments without established validity or reliability. In the three trials that used both a pretest and a control group, the impact of the intervention on multiple choice tests ranged from no increase to a 16% increase in scores (23–25). There was no improvement in the residents' ability to critically appraise a journal article in the one study that included this outcome (23). All of the studies that measured behaviors relied on resident self-report of hours spent reading, thoroughness of reading, attention to methods and result sections, preferred sources of medical information, or frequency of referral to original articles to answer clinical questions. However, retrospective self-reporting may underestimate physicians' information needs and overestimate their information-seeking behaviors (2).

FREESTANDING EVIDENCE-BASED MEDICINE CURRICULA

In the 1990s many programs developed EBM curricula or transformed their traditional journal clubs. From 1998 (26) to 2003 (27), the number of programs offering freestanding EBM curricula increased from 37 to 71%. These curricula still used a small group seminar format but they brought the evidence to bear on individual patient decision making (often for the residents' actual patients) and covered the "ask," "acquire," and "apply" EBM steps in addition to "appraise." In a 1998 national survey of internal medicine program EBM curricula, 68% employed small group format, 69% focused on residents' actual patients, 52% offered faculty development to preceptors, and 37% evaluated their curricula (26). Whereas 97% of the programs provided MEDLINE access, only 33% offered important electronic secondary evidence-based electronic information resources, such as *Clinical Evidence* or the *Cochrane Library*.

Several freestanding curricula have been reported, all of which used a small group seminar format (28–36). The reports that included an evaluation with a control group, pre–post study design, and an objective (nonself reported) outcome are summarized in Table 2. Three studies demonstrated improvements in residents' EBM knowledge and skills (29,34,36), which, in one study, persisted for 6 mo (34). The two studies that measured residents' EBM behaviors used residents' retrospective self-reports or the frequency of their EBM "utterances" in audiotaped teaching interactions. None of the investigators attempted to establish the "educational significance" (37) of changes attributed to the intervention. This might have been done by calculating the effect size (d), proportion of variance (Ω^2) compared to interventions with established "magnitude," or discriminating between known learner levels (38,39).

INTEGRATED EVIDENCE-BASED MEDICINE CURRICULA

Although freestanding EBM curricula represent an advance over journal clubs, residents in a "protected" and somewhat artificial seminar format do not confront the time and logistical constraints faced by clinicians in practice. Clinicians will not fully embrace EBM unless they can ask and answer most of their clinical questions as they emerge in the flow of patient care. Integrated EBM curricula represent efforts to teach and exemplify EBM in "real time" within established clinical venues. From a learning theory standpoint, this integrated EBM teaching creates conditions that may be more conducive to adult learners (40). Not only do residents direct their learning, exploit their experience, and confront actual problems, they also must link their readiness to learn to the imperatives of "real-life" clinical medicine.

In a 1998 survey, many North American internal medicine programs reported efforts to integrate EBM into attending rounds (218/261 [84%]), resident report (214/261 [82%]), continuity clinic (199/261 [76%]), bedside work rounds (177/261 [68%]), and emergency department (90/261 [35%]) (26). However, depending on the venue, only 48–64% provided on-site electronic medical information, 31–45% provided faculty development, and 10–28% tracked residents EBM behaviors.

EBM teachers have developed strategies to help faculty take advantage of the precious teaching moments that arise in the flow of patient care (41,42). In addition, several programs have described specific efforts to integrate EBM training into established educational venues, such as morning report (43,44), attending rounds (45–47), other clinical seminar curricula (48), various venues using educational prescriptions (49,50), and the activities of an entire department (51). However, with the following few exceptions, these curriculum reports lacked meaningful evaluations.

McGinn integrated EBM training into attending rounds on an internal medicine teaching service (45). Resident–student teams negotiated the ask–acquire–appraise–apply sequence for questions emerging on their patients. Twelve of sixteen (75%) questions were pursued. Effectiveness evaluation was limited to resident self-reports. Fifty percent of residents felt the process changed the management of patients on the service and 75% reported that the process would affect the care of future patients.

In a neonatal intensive care setting, Bradley provided "real-time" EBM training for medicine-pediatrics residents. On-site librarians helped residents answer clinical questions generated on bedside rounds (52) In a randomized trial, case residents formulated better questions, used limits more effectively, and improved their scores on standardized searches immediately after the intervention and further at 6 mo.

Table 2
Effectiveness Evaluations of GME Freestanding EBM Curricula[a]

Curriculum	Study design	Outcome domain	Outcome instrument			Effect
			Format	Reliability	Validity	
Green, 1997 (29) (internal med)	Pre–post controlled trial. Controls received seminars on common ambulatory topics.	Knowledge skills Behaviors	Free text critical appraisal of article and application to a case Retrospective self-report survey	Inter-rater reliability (correlation coefficient = 0.87) Not reported	Content validity by expert review Not reported	29% increase in score in cases. No change in controls. Increase in frequency of seeking original study when faced with a clinical question.
Bazarian, 1999 (35) (emergency med)	Pre–post controlled trial. Controls participated in "unstructured journal club."	Knowledge skills	Free text justification of decision to use or not use a therapy studied in a factitious journal article with "built in" flaws.	Inter-rater reliability (intra-class correlation coefficient = 0.94)	Discriminative validity (journal reviewers who recommended rejection identified more errors than those recommending acceptance)	No effect
Ross, 2003 (36) (family med)	Pre–post controlled trial	Knowledge Behavior	Multiple choice test Analysis of audiotape of resident-preceptor interactions.	Not reported Not reported	Content validity by expert review Not reported	36% increase in score in cases. No change in controls. Increase in resident EBM phrases from 0.21 to 2.9 events/h. Control group phrases decreased.
Smith, 2002 (34) (internal med)	Pre–post controlled trial with long term follow up	Knowledge skills	Case-based test. Follow up versions had different cases and wording of questions.	Not reported	Not reported	60% increase in scores in cases. No change in controls. Improved performance was sustained for 9 mo.
Akl, 2004 (113)	Pre–post controlled trial	Knowledge skills	Berlin Questionnaire (59)	Internal consistency (Cronbach's α 0.75–0.82)	Discriminative validity (experts vs novices) and responsiveness to educational intervention.	14% nonsignificant increase in score in cases. 20% decrease in score in controls.

[a]Reports that included an evaluation with a control group, pre–post study design, and an objective (nonself reported) outcome.

Several programs write "educational prescriptions" for their trainees *(49,50)*. This document specifies the clinical problem that generated the question, states the question (in all of its key elements), specifies who is responsible for answering it, and reminds everyone of the deadline for answering it. Some variations have the trainee articulate foreground questions in the PICO format, grade the level of evidence, or document what he or she learned from the process. Several examples of educational prescriptions are available in print *(50)* and on the Internet (*see* the appendix). In our internal medicine residency program, we are experimenting with a more structured format, which constrains responses to easily coded choices, in anticipation of transition to an Internet-based version (available on request).

Effects of the Hidden Curriculum on Evidence-Based Medicine Training

One could argue that a large part of graduate medical education training experience already involves EBM, even if not explicitly stated in specific curricula. That is, the prevailing model of giving trainees graduated responsibility for patients creates frequent and strong EBM triggers. They care for patients, encounter uncertainty, experience a pressing "need to know," seek new information or skills, apply them to the current problem, incorporate them into future scenarios, and, ideally, reflect on the process. As much as we believe that trainees acculturate to these socializing influences, EBM remains part of the hidden curriculum.

What, then, is the impact of the hidden curriculum on trainees' EBM attitudes and behaviors? Before entering residency, the undergraduate "hidden curriculum" helps students acknowledge and accept uncertainty in medicine and begin to discriminate between their personal knowledge deficits and gaps in the current state of medical science *(53)*. The medical sociologist Renee Fox called this process "training for uncertainty."

To consider subspecialty fellowship programs, we must, once again, extrapolate from studies in graduate medical education (GME) core programs. Faculty behavior, team dynamics, and hospital institutional culture can greatly influence resident EBM behaviors during residency training. For example, in one qualitative study, residents were more inclined to pursue their clinical questions when working with attending physicians who cultivated an atmosphere of collaborative learning and granted them a degree of decision-making autonomy to act on the answers *(54)*. In addition, while rotating at a community hospital, they encountered a perception that computers in clinical areas were reserved for managing patient data (rather than for looking up medical information) and felt under suspicion for inappropriate use of computers, such as personal correspondence or "surfing" the Internet. Residents from several surgery programs at one institution approached EBM with trepidation, fearing reprisal from a highly skeptical faculty *(55)*.

EVALUATING EVIDENCE-BASED MEDICINE COMPETENCIES

Much of the research relevant to evaluating EBM involves the development of instruments to evaluate EBM skills, including *ASKING* clinical questions, *ACQUIRING* the best evidence, *APPRAISING* the evidence, *APPLYING* the evidence to individual patient decision making, and *ASSESSING* one's performance. The Society of General Internal Medicine (SGIM) EBM task force recently developed a conceptual framework for EBM evaluation, which accounts for different types of learners, educational interventions, and outcomes *(56)*. This model acknowledges, for instance, that many practitioners prefer to "use" evidence-based summaries rather than "do" direct critical appraisal *(57)* and, thus, should be evaluated accordingly. Taking a different perspective than EBM researchers, educational psychologists have developed instruments to measure the closely related construct of self-directed learning "readiness." This "readiness" might be considered a combination of EBM attitudes, skills, and learning style or preference. Herein I review the psychometric properties and feasibility of extant approaches to evaluate trainees' EBM knowledge, skills (or competence), behaviors (or performance), attitudes, and overall EBM "effectiveness" via global ratings. I also consider the possibility of collecting patient level data, either clinical outcomes or resident performance of evidence-based maneuvers, as a measure of EBM performance.

EVIDENCE-BASED MEDICINE KNOWLEDGE AND SKILLS

The last few years have witnessed the development of psychometrically robust written instruments *(34,58–60)* and promising reports of Objective Structured Clinical Exams (OSCEs), with standardized patients (SPs) *(61,62)* or computer stations *(63)*, to evaluate EBM knowledge and skills. Among the written examinations, I highlight the Fresno Test *(58)*, which was developed for family practice residents and based on two pediatric cases. This instrument probes underlying thinking processes and assesses multiple EBM competencies, including formulating questions, identifying appropriate study designs, knowledge of electronic database searching, considering the relevance and validity of articles, and assessing the magnitude and importance of results. Many of the questions require free text responses, so the investigators provide a rubric for grading. Psychometric testing demonstrated excellent inter-rater reliability, content validity (confirmed by experts), discriminative construct validity (confirmed by comparing scores of family practice interns and EBM experts), and responsive construct validity (confirmed by pre–post testing). The test must be scored by "experts" exercising their best judgment, and implementation may not therefore be feasible in some settings. The actual instrument, grading rubric, and psychometric data are available on the Internet (*see* the appendix).

In an EBM OSCE station for medical students, a standardized patient asks a question that prompts an EBM "moment *(62)*." The student (1) poses a question, (2) searches for articles, (3) appraises and chooses the best evidence, and (4) returns for a subsequent encounter with the SP to make a decision. A physician-educator graded steps 1, 3, and 4 and step 2 was graded by a librarian using a 5-point Likert-like scale. Two hundred and twenty-four students took the EBM OSCE (1 of 16 different variations) 6 mo after an extensive EBM course. The students generally performed well, with mean scores of 3.96, 4.10, 3.92, and 3.73 on steps 1–4, respectively. For grading step 4, there was good inter-rater reliability between the "station author" and course director ($n = 0.6$ [$p < 0.0001$]). The students' EBM OSCE scores did not correlate with grade point average, class rank, or United States Medical Licensing Examination (USMLE) step 1 scores.

In a case-based computer station OSCE, students (1) articulated a question in the Patient-Intervention-Comparison-Outcome format *(64)*, (2) generated "appropriate" search terms, and (3) selected and justified the one "appropriate" abstract from a group of 3 *(63)*. Based on predetermined grading criteria, 71, 81, and 49% of 140 students "passed" the three components respectively (29% passed all three). The grading process showed good inter-rater reliability ($n = 0.64$, 0.82, and 0.94 for the components). The investigators did not report validity data or the students' level of EBM expertise or prior training.

Evidence-Based Medicine Behaviors (Performance)

Evaluating EBM behaviors remains the most challenging. In the past, investigators relied on trainees' retrospective self-reports (which suffer from bias) and direct debriefing and follow up after patient encounters *(2,65)* (which, although more valid, remains unfeasible outside of the research setting). More recently, researchers have analyzed audiotapes of resident–faculty interactions, looking for phrases related to literature searching, clinical epidemiology, or critical appraisal *(36,66)*. In a family practice program, residents' "EBM utterances" increased from 0.21 to 2.9/h after an educational intervention (*see* Table 2) *(36)*. In my view, however, this outcome lacks face validity as a surrogate for EBM behaviors.

Another approach is to have residents catalogue their EBM learning "moments" in portfolios, which can range from a collection of EBM seminar presentations or "educational prescriptions" (*see* EBM Curriculum) on paper to sophisticated Internet-based learning logs *(67,68)*. Rucker tracked the use of "educational prescriptions" in his program *(49)*. Of 125 prescriptions written for 54 residents and 31 medical students, 105 (83%) were completed and 82 (65%) were completed on time. Of these, 76 (60%) included appropriate references and 37 (29%) affected patient care decisions. A teacher's positive EBM attitude predicted the number of prescriptions written and the likelihood of completion.

Obstetrics and gynecology faculty in Canada implemented a "Computerized Obstetrics and Gynecology Automated Learning Analysis (KOALA™)" at several programs *(68)*. This Internet-based portfolio allowed residents to record their obstetrical, surgical, ultrasound, and ambulatory patient encounters; directly link to information resources; and document critical incidents of learning that arose during these encounters. During a 4-mo pilot at four programs, 41 residents recorded 7049 patient encounters and 1460 critical learning incidents. Residents at one of the programs, which had a prior 1-yr experience with KOALA, had a higher perception of their self-directed learning (measured by SDLRS, *see* Evidence-Based Medicine's Readiness or Attitudes) and believed their future learning was less likely to be from continuing medical education, textbooks, and didactic lectures and more likely from a learning portfolio with online resources.

Emergency medicine and obstetrics and gynecology residents in the United Kingdom, documented critical learning incidents in a written portfolio *(69)*. In a controlled study, there was no difference in specialty-specific knowledge (by multiple-choice test) and confidence between the two groups, but adherence with the log system was low. Finally, internal medicine residents on inpatient rotations at one American program entered their clinical questions, MEDLINE reference links, and validated article summaries into an Internet-based compendium *(67)*. Over 10 mo they entered 625 patient-based questions and obtained "useful information" for 82% of them (77% from MEDLINE searches). The residents reported that, for 47% of the questions (39% of total questions), obtaining medical information altered patient management. The compendium itself, as it accumulated questions, became a useful information resource in the program.

One could argue, however, that all of these behaviors (using EBM jargon in discussions, pursuing clinical questions, documenting learning episodes) represent intermediate outcomes. That is, we *assume* that physicians who pursue EBM behaviors will provide more evidence-based care, which, in turn, will lead to better patient outcomes. But our *clinical* experience reminds us that intermediate outcomes may fail to guarantee the ultimate outcomes of interest. For example, perimenopausal hormone replacement therapy had favorable effects on serum lipid levels (intermediate outcome) *(70)* but did not reduce the risk of recurrent coronary heart disease (CHD) events (ultimate outcome) *(71)*. Accordingly, EBM investigators have turned their attention to the ultimate outcome of quality of care delivered by practicing physicians following an educational intervention *(72–74)*. For example, Langham measured physicians' attention to cardiovascular risk factors, including documentation, clinical interventions, and actual improvements *(72)*.

Should endocrinology fellowship program evaluators, then, bypass fellows' "intermediate" learning outcomes" and just focus on the clinical care they deliver? I believe that programs should strive to document both measures of EBM behavior. Certainly, fellows' practice profiles (presented in the context of evidence-based guidelines or local or national practice patterns) may incline them to improve their performance. However, easily collected administrative practice data is a blunt instrument. A fellow's final clinical decision, such as prescribing an angiotensin-converting enzyme (ACE) inhibitor for a patient with diabetes and microalbulinuria, represents the end result of myriad inputs in addition to "learning," some of which may be outside of his or her control. Furthermore, "neglect" of this evidence-based guideline in a particular case, which would be detected as a quality "miss" as an ultimate outcome, may actually reflect a careful consideration of a patient's preferences, actions, and clinical context, rather than a failed learning episode *(75,76)*. And finally, we should ensure fellows' inclination toward EBM, in anticipation that they will direct it to the unforeseeable clinical problems they will encounter after leaving training programs.

EVIDENCE-BASED MEDICINE'S READINESS OR ATTITUDES

Although many EBM instruments include a few questions about attitudes, few explore this domain in depth. Three investigators studied practicing physicians with surveys exploring attitudes, beliefs, practices, and barriers to EBM *(57,77,78)*. And a brief Likert scale questionnaire was used in a pre–post trial of an EBM curriculum for internal medicine residents *(30)*. The Self-Directed Learning Readiness Scale (SDLRS) *(79)* is the most widely used instrument for assessing SDL "readiness," which has been defined as "the degree [to which] the individual possesses the attitudes, abilities, and personality characteristics necessary for SDL *(80)*." This instrument includes 58 statements with Likert-style responses ranging from 1 (almost never true of me; I hardly ever feel this way) to 5 (almost always true of me; there are very few times when I don't feel this way). Subjects receive a single score, ranging from 58 (indicating a low level of readiness to direct one's learning) to 290. The national norm for general adult learners is 214. A self-scoring format is available as the Learning Preference Assessment.

Factor analysis of SDLRS responses revealed eight separate constructs, including openness to learning opportunities, self-concept as an effective learner, initiative and independence in learning, acceptance of responsibility for one's own learning, love of learning, creativity, positive orientation to the future, and problem-solving skills. Psychometric testing showed excellent inter-item consistency and test-retest reliability. Several studies have confirmed convergent validity (correlation with andragogy [adult learning] on the Student's Orientation Questionnaire) *(81)*, divergent validity (inverse correlation with preference for structure) *(82)*, and criterion validity (correlations with learning projects, SDL time, and SDL behaviors) *(83)*. I found no studies of the SDLRS's ability to predict future behaviors.

The SDLRS has been widely used in business, industry, and higher education. Within medical education, investigators have used the SDLRS primarily to evaluate undergraduate medical and nursing students in PBL curricula *(84–86)*. In a cross-sectional study at a single medical school, there was no increase in SDLRS score by curriculum year *(84)*. Shokar administered the SDLRS to beginning third-year students after completing 2 yr of a PBL curriculum *(85)*. Their SDLRS scores correlated with their final grade and all of its components in two clerkships, but only the association with the faculty preceptor evaluation achieved statistical significance. In the only GME experience with the SDLRS, obstetrics-gynecology residents using an Internet-based learning portfolio for a longer period of time scored higher than residents with a shorter exposure *(68)*.

Other SDL instruments include the Continual Learning Inventory *(87)*, Ryan's questionnaire *(88)*, which assesses perceptions of the importance of SDL, and Knowles' instrument, which assesses self-directed skills through self-rating *(89)*.

GENERAL COMPUTER AND TECHNOLOGY SKILLS, ATTITUDES, AND USE

Several instruments have been developed to evaluate general computer and Internet skills, attitudes, and behaviors. The Computers in Medical Care Survey is a written instrument that assesses self-reported computer uses, computer knowledge, computer feature demand (for functionality and usability), and computer "optimism" of academic physicians *(90)*. It has demonstrated good inter-item consistency, with Cronbach's α of 0.69–0.86 for different scales. The Information Technology in Family Practice Scale assesses opinions about computers and self-reported computer use *(91)* Basic Internet competencies for physicians have been articulated *(92)*, but I found no specific evaluation instruments.

GLOBAL RATINGS

Since the American Board of Medicine revised its rating form to reflect the six new ACGME competencies, programs are gaining experience with faculty's global rating of residents' "practice-based learning and improvement," which includes EBM and quality improvement. In this evaluation, a faculty member rates each resident's overall competence (encompassing knowledge, skills, behaviors, and attitudes) on a 9-point scale. A recent factor analysis of rating forms including all six competencies demonstrated that faculty raters actually discriminated only between two broad dimensions (medical knowledge and interpersonal skills)—the same "halo effect" seen on the original rating forms *(93)*.

BARRIERS TO EVIDENCE-BASED MEDICINE TRAINING

Many of the barriers to evidence-based practice challenge EBM teachers. Practicing physicians, in several studies *(57,75–77,94–96)*, identified lack of time as the primary barrier to answering their clinical questions. In addition, they reported difficulty phrasing clinical questions, not knowing when to stop searching, and their lack of awareness, access, and skills in searching medical information resources. Of note, while some physicians expressed negative perceptions of EBM, most did not identify skepticism of the idea as a barrier.

Medical residents face the same pragmatic barriers of insufficient time, limited access to information resources, and poorly developed skills *(54,65,97)*. They also frequently forget their clinical questions, lacking an effective system to track the ones they fail to pursue at the time of the patient encounter. Somewhat in contrast to practicing physicians, residents may encounter several attitudinal or cultural barriers, including variable learning climates, authoritarian attending physicians, multiple learner levels, and inhospitable hospital institutional culture *(54)*. And surgery residents in several programs at one institution lamented widespread resistance (and even hostility) to EBM among their faculty *(55)*.

RECOMMENDATIONS

Given the deficiencies previously described, I believe that EBM deserves much more explicit emphasis at all levels of medical education. In endocrinology fellowships (as in all subspecialty training programs) trainees can build on the skills they learned as medical residents, apply them in their care of patients with endocrine disorders, and further develop life-long learning habits to sustain them in their practices. If endocrinology program directors take one general recommendation from this essay, it would be to develop or adapt curricula that help fellows capitalize on the fertile moments of uncertainty that arise in their care of patients. All lines of evidence converge on the power of these moments, variously labeled as "questions," "breakdowns" *(98)*, "surprises" *(99)*, or "problems" *(100)*.

Learning Infrastructure

Fellows should have rapid, reliable, and continuously available access to electronic medical information resources at the point of care in every clinical setting. The Internal Medicine Residency Review Committee would give program directors more leverage in their budgetary negotiations with sponsoring hospitals if it strengthened this "institutional requirement."

Newer generation electronic medical record (EMR) systems have the capability to support direct linkages between patient-specific data and evidence-based knowledge resources in a manner that integrates clinical decision support with documentation processes and provides a data infrastructure to automatically generate trainee performance evaluations. Fellows should also have access to population data from their continuity clinic practices and hospital catchment areas, another deliverable well within the capability of robust EMR systems.

Curriculum

All curricula, like politics, are local, because they must attend to "contextual variables" *(101)*, such as local values, resources, and expertise. Thus, I offer general recommendations that program directors can adapt to their own institutions *(37)*.

FREESTANDING EVIDENCE-BASED MEDICINE CURRICULA

Programs should supplement their "traditional" journal clubs with freestanding EBM curricula, which provide the "tools" for EBM. Successful curricula include case-based, learner-centered seminars that cover all five steps of evidence-based decision making *(29,34,36)*. Table 3 shows a possible format for a freestanding EBM seminar.

Table 3
Freestanding EBM Seminar Format[a]

1. Presentation of case and clinical question (5 min).
2. Description of literature search (5–10 min).
   The resident projects his or her Medline search, describing the effectiveness of certain strategies and search terms. He or she may also demonstrate the usefulness of searching secondary electronic medical information resources such as Clinical Evidence or the Cochrane Library.
3. Summary of study's main methods and results (10 min).
   The resident summarizes the study's main methods and results, including the research protocol, statistical techniques, main measure of effect, and data presentation.
4. Critical appraisal questions (20 min).
   The resident poses the corresponding "User's Guide" or other critical appraisal questions to the group. For each question he or she asks whether or not the investigator satisfied the particular criterion and the implications of failing to do so.
5. Interpretation of results for this patient (20 min).
   The resident leads a discussion about ho to consider the results in the decision making for the patient. After entertaining opinions from the participants, he or she declares what he or she did (or will do) regarding the patient's evaluation, management, or counseling.

[a]Reprinted from ref. *29* with permission from Blackstone Publishing. Faculty facilitating techniques are described in the article.

For example, a fellow assigned to present at such a seminar recalls a patient with type 2 diabetes mellitus and compensated ischemic cardiomyopathy, whose glycemic control worsens after taking a sulfonourea for 2 yr. She considers adding a thiazolidenedione (TZD), but is concerned that it may cause fluid retention and worsen the patient's congestive heart failure. She meets once or twice with an assigned faculty preceptor to help her frame the clinical question in the PICO format, seek the best evidence, appraise the evidence, and integrate the evidence into her decision making for the patient. In advance of the seminar, the other fellows review the case, the clinical question, the journal article or evidence-summary, and a critical appraisal guide related to a therapy question (from a syllabus). She recapitulates the EBM decision-making process at an interactive seminar, inviting responses from the group at each step. The faculty preceptor participates by highlighting key points, clarifying areas of confusion, redirecting an off-track discussion, and ensuring time for a substantial discussion of the decision making for *this particular patient*. Such programs can equip fellows with the basic "tools" of EBM. In particular, this setting remains suited for teaching critical appraisal, which often requires detailed scrutiny of reports of original research studies.

INTEGRATED EVIDENCE-BASED MEDICINE CURRICULA

In addition, program directors should link these freestanding EBM sessions to efforts to integrate EBM into existing educational and clinical venues. In this setting, harried clinical activities allow only brief (but potentially crystalline) teaching moments. Examples of specific integrated EBM curricula are described above. In addition, the Evidence-Based Medicine Teaching Tips Working Group has just launched a series

Table 4
Integrated EBM Teaching Strategies[a]

General	ASK questions	ACQUIRE the evidence	APPLY the evidence
Splint 'em where they lay	Seize the moment	Match the need with the source	reCast the evidence
Bite off less than you can chew	Stay alert for "unrecognized information needs"	Save MEDLINE for last	Customize the evidence
Carry a bag of tricks	Offer the "right question"	Stay in real time, if possible	Consider the evidence (decision-making frameworks)
Close the loop	Specify type and clinical task	Write and fill "educational prescriptions"	Communicate the evidence
Do as I say and as I do	Formulate "well-built" questions		
Lead "the examined medical life"	Don't feign ignorance		

[a]Reprinted from ref. *41* with permission from Blackstone Publishing.

of articles in the *Canadian Medical Association Journal (102–104)* (*see* the appendix for URL). Each piece focuses on a small chunk of EBM and includes a version for the learner, an online companion article for the teacher (organized by "teaching scripts"), and additional Internet-based features. Finally, I have collected a number of "real time" EBM teaching strategies that can be deployed in these brief encounters, including general tactics and those specific to individual steps in evidence-based decision making (Table 4) *(41)*. I have gleaned these strategies from workshops, colleagues, collaborators, study of adult learning theory, and years of trial and error.

General Strategies

Adult learners' readiness peaks at the moment they are faced with a real life problem that requires learning new skills. As these moments arise in the course of clinical activities, faculty can seize them to teach EBM. The medical-military metaphor *"splint 'em where they lay"* captures this approach. In this context, teachers must maintain facility in EBM and in case-based teaching. In particular, they cannot rely on "canned" vignettes that perfectly illustrate EBM concepts. Instead, they must improvise with real life clinical scenarios with all of their warts, including conflicting clinical data, a dearth of directly applicable evidence, and complex decision making. It may be messy but these are the situations, after all, faced by clinicians everyday.

Teachers must not succumb to the quixotic urge to illustrate all of EBM that applies to a particular scenario. Instead, he or she must focus on the fellow's momentary learning agenda, whether this is appreciating information needs, formulating a question, searching for the evidence, or considering the evidence in decision making. I glibly refer to this restraint as *biting off less than you can chew*. Similarly, Scott Richardson recommends teaching EBM "by the slice" (as opposed the whole pie) *(42)*. To prepare themselves for these unanticipated EBM moments, teachers should *carry a bag of tricks*, filling their white-coat pockets (or personal digital assistants) with quick references, data, formulae, and calculators (*see* the appendix). Thus, when the moment arises, they can, for example, estimate a pretest probability with a clinical prediction rule or determine a number needed to treat from two event rates.

Of course, even with the best-laid plans, time constraints may preclude complete resolution of an EBM moment. Faculty then should make specific plans with the fellow to *close the loop* in the near future, lest the opportunity vanish from memory. And finally, EBM teachers should *do as I say* and *as I do* and *lead the examined medical life*, role modeling EBM behaviors in their own practice and fostering a spirit of inquiry in their program.

ASKING Fruitful Clinical Questions

Here again, faculty must remain prepared to *seize the moment*, highlighting clinical questions at the moment uncertainty arises in trainees' presentations. There should be no shortage of these moments as internal medicine residents, for example, encountered two new questions for every three patients they saw in continuity clinic, even after exhausting their preceptors' wisdom *(65)*. Additionally, faculty must *stay alert for unrecognized information needs*. A fellow may "not know what he or she does not know." For example, she suggests, this time without hesitation, starting rosiglitazone for our patient with worsening glycemic control, unaware of its adverse effect of fluid retention. We encounter this frequently in our undergraduate EBM curriculum, in which many students cannot think of a single moment of uncertainty over a month-long rotation in a community internal medicine office.

A fellow, when prompted, may identify the wrong question. Perhaps she asks whether loop diuretics or thiazides would be more effective for this patient's cardiomyopathy. The teacher, in this case, should *offer the right question*, which queries the effectiveness of ACE inhibitors in reducing mortality, in this euvolemic patient.

Once the question is identified, the teacher should help the fellow *specify the type* (background vs foreground) *and the clinical task*. Because she is *deciding* whether or not to start a therapeutic agent, she may think that her question about rosiglitazone represents a *therapy* question. However, she already knows the effectiveness of rosiglitazone in improving glycemic control. The fellow really needs information relating to the drugs potential *harm* in causing edema. An accurate classification will help direct the fellow to a more fruitful search strategy and an easier recognition when she finds "the answer" *(105)*. The additional time required to *reformulate* a vague foreground question into the four-part structure of a *well-built question (64)* will also be well spent. Questions with a clearly specified Patient (New York Heart Association [NYHA] class II congestive heart failure [CHF]), Intervention (rosiglitazone), Comparison (no intervention, insulin), and Outcome (fluid retention and worsening CHF) avoid frustrating searches or confused decision making.

And finally, when confronted with a clinical question to which you know the answer, *don't feign ignorance* just to exemplify the EBM process. As an endocrinology section faculty member, you are, of course, already familiar with the TZD and CHF literature and recommendation. Our own real uncertainty provides more than enough opportunities.

ACQUIRING the Evidence

Trainees often succumb to a sense of futility upon reaching this step, especially in the context of "real-time" EBM. As previously described, they encounter many barriers to answering their clinical questions. Nonetheless, Sackett's group in Oxford demonstrated that "real time" EBM can be done. Using an "EBM cart" equipped with various medical information sources, his inpatient team answered 90% of their emerging questions within a few moments during "team rounds" *(106)*. Of course, the program must have robust electronic resources at the point of care.

When a fellow identifies, classifies, and reformulates a clinical question, the teacher can then help him or her *match the need with the source*, choosing initially among secondary evidence-based information resources. For example, for a foreground therapy question, one can first quickly search *American College of Physicians (ACP) Journal Club, Cochrane Library*, and *DARE* (often grouped for simultaneous searching by vendors like OVID®) for a clinical trial or a meta-analysis of trials. In addition, some institutions maintain a local database of questions and the corresponding appraised and digested evidence *(67,107,108)*, which might assume an even earlier position in a searching algorithm. The *United States Preventive Services Task Force's Guide to Preventive Services, Third Edition: Periodic Updates (109)* remains the best source for prevention questions related to screening, immunizations, counseling, and chemoprophylaxis. The Rational Clinical Exam *(110)* series in the *Journal of the American Medical Association* also includes excellent systematic reviews of *clinical examination* maneuvers. One can then *save MEDLINE for last*, reserving it for more obscure questions that elude the more clinician-friendly sources.

If at all possible, teachers should encourage trainees to *stay in real time*, asking and answering their clinical question before the patient leaves. This demonstration goes a long way to assuage the trainee's sense of futility. Furthermore, trainees are much less likely to pursue postponed questions. To increase the pursuit rate of the remaining questions, teachers can *write and fill* education prescriptions *(see* Evidence-Based Medicine Curriculum*)*. This gives the fellow an assignment to seek "the evidence" and discuss it with the preceptor at a specified date. In addition to helping trainees keep track of their questions, faculty can use educational prescriptions to make brief teaching points many aspects of evidence-based decision making. Finally, fellows can collect the prescriptions into a portfolio to provide documentation of the practice-based learning and improvement performance *(see* Evaluating Evidence-Based Medicine Competencies*)*.

APPLYING the Evidence

If the teacher perceives the educational need, he or she can use the "EBM moment" to help residents integrate the evidence into their decision making for individual patients. This step presents the greatest challenge for teachers but it remains the most critical. First, the trainee often must *recast the evidence* originally reported in a format not conducive to individual patient decision making. For example, while investigators often report relative risk reduction in trials of therapies, the clinician needs to know the absolute risk reduction or number needed to treat, which account for the baseline untreated risk. For diagnosis questions, fellows may need to determine the likelihood ratios for a diagnostic test to determine if the posttest probabilities will cross their decision thresholds.

The fellow's patient, however, usually does not resemble the patients in the best available study. In this case, the teacher can demonstrate the importance of *customizing the evidence*. For our harm question, the fellow should attempt to determine the risk of edema and CHF for her patient with NYHA class II CHF, taking a diuretic and ACE inhibitor, and not on insulin. With some provisos, she might examine a pre-hoc study subgroup of similar patients. (In the TZD studies, of note, patients not on insulin had a lower incidence of edema.) For a therapy question, the trainee can recast the number needed to treat in a study to account for the patient's individual baseline risk.

To ultimately make a decision, the trainee must then *consider the evidence*, once customized, with other important considerations, including the particular clinical circumstances and the patient's preferences and actions *(76)*. (In many scenarios, these "other considerations" dominate the decision making and, if considered up front, obviate the need for a detailed review of the evidence.) Trainees may be able to better process all of the inputs if we make the implicit explicit using *decision-making frameworks*. Table 5 lists the issues in considering the harm of rosiglitazone in the fellow's patient. Explicitly and simultaneously embracing all of the considerations may point to a decision that would seem counterintuitive based on just one. After weighing the considerations, faculty might use a brief EBM moment to invite the patient into the decision-making process, demonstrating emerging techniques of *communicating the evidence* (risk communication and elicitation of health state utilities or values).

FACULTY DEVELOPMENT

As trainees engage these EBM episodes, we hope they develop the skills and inclinations that foster a lifelong habit of pursuing and reflecting upon important clinical questions that arise in clinical practice. The challenge for their faculty educators will be to observe, assist, mentor, role-model, document, offer formative feedback, and evaluate residents as they "perform" these "procedures," which carry no less consequence than technical maneuvers. Faculty development, then, should accompany implementation of EBM training, because this effort will involve the faculty at large rather than a small group of experts. The Societal of General Internal Medicine EBM Task Force regularly convenes regional and national workshops. In addition, McMaster University in Hamilton Ontario conducts intensive week-long courses in "how to teach evidence-based clinical practice" (*see* the appendix).

THE HIDDEN CURRICULUM

The hidden curriculum deserves much attention. Programs should cultivate reflection and evidence-based practice among faculty and remain sensitive to the program and hospital institutional cultures. In this endeavor, directors can look to emerging research about how to affect the hidden curriculum *(111)*. For example, Frankford proposes a model of administration that might foster, "institutionalized reflection" *(112)*.

Evaluation

Programs will continue to use the ABIM rating form to evaluate fellows' practice-based learning and improvement. However, the rating form alone remains insufficient for this purpose, because of its psychometric limitations and, as currently configured, it lumps EBM with other constructs, such as quality improvement. Thus, program directors should consider additional evaluation approaches for this important competency.

Table 5
Decision-Making Framework for a Harm Question

	Consideration	Rosiglitazone/fluid retention and CHF
The Evidence[a]	Strength of association	Strong (RCTs and other controlled trials)
	Magnitude of effect (Customized if possible)	Edema: NNH[b] = 29
		New onset or worsening CHF = less common
	Tolerability of harm	Worsening edema and CHF
Clinical state and circumstances[a]	Reversibility of harm	Yes, upon stopping medication or increasing diuretics
	Benefit of exposure OR possible consequences of stopping exposure already in effect	Improved glycemic control
		Other favorable cardiovascular effects
		Decreased risk of microvascular disease
		Possible decreased risk of coronary artery and other macrovascular disease?
	Availability, effectiveness and risks of alternatives	Insulin
		(Metformin contraindicated in this patient with CHF requiring pharmacologic therapy)
Patient preferences and actions[a]	Risk aversion	?
	Preferences	?
	Adherence with monitoring for adverse effects	?

[a]Three decision-making considerations from ref. 76.
[b]Trials of rosiglitazone in patients not on insulin (excluded NYHA III, IV).
Control event rate = 1.3%.
Experimental event rate = 4.8%.
Absolute risk increase = 4.8–1.3 = 3.5%.
Number needed to harm (NNH) = 1/0.035 = 29.

Instruments like the Fresno test and EBM OSCEs can be used to evaluate knowledge and skills. The utility of determining fellows' self-directed learning "readiness," via the SDLRS, deserves further exploration. This information may inform program development, assist with individual fellow remediation, or serve as a barometer of the hidden curriculum in this area.

Portfolios represent the most promising technology for fellows to document EBM performance. Internet-based systems with trainee entry of some information and tracking of information-seeking behavior may make this approach more feasible. Program directors (or regulatory bodies) might also consider requiring documentation of a minimum number of "EBM episodes," much in the same way the ABIM does for technical procedures. The educational value of these could be enhanced if faculty could review a portion of these and provide formative feedback.

Recognizing the caveats discussed earlier, emerging technology will permit educators to profile fellows' performance as a measure of the ultimate outcome of their evidence-based practice performance. Interoperable EMR systems can link fellows' behaviors (reviewing information, ordering tests, using decision-support tools, selecting therapies) to the corresponding ACGME competencies and the standards for demonstrating proficiency. Michael Zaroukian at the Michigan State College of Human Medicine coined the term "automated nonstop competency assessment" (ANCA) to describe this ability to automatically and continuously capture, analyze, and report resident competence-related behaviors. ANCA represents a promising alternative (or compliment) to recording individual "direct observation" of trainees, which, for all of their richness, remain time intensive and inefficient. The current capabilities of advanced EMR systems can support ANCA. However, before its full realization, further psychometric studies must identify the best "competency indicators" among the potential EMR data.

Appendix
EBM Education Resources

EBM Centers

Centre for EBM (Oxford)	http://www.cebm.net/
Centre for EBM (Toronto)	http://www.cebm.utoronto.ca/
Centre for Health Evidence (Alberta)	http://www.cche.net/che/home.asp

Other EBM Education Sites

Teaching evidence-based clinical practice workshop (McMaster)	http://www.cche.net/ebcp/default.asp
Society of General Internal Medicine EBM Task Force	http://www.sgim.org/ebm.cfm
The Fresno EBM Test	http://bmj.bmjjournals.com/cgi/content/full/ 326/7384/319/DC1
Educational prescription (Oxford Centre for EBM)	http://www.cebm.net/downloads/ educational_prescription.rtf
Educational prescription (Toronto Centre for EBM)	http://www.cebm.utoronto.ca/practise/formulate/ eduprescript.htm
EBM Tips electronic resources	http://www.ebmtips.net/risk001.asp

TEXTBOOKS

Sackett DL, Straus SE, Richardson WS, Rosenberg W, Haynes RB. Evidence-based medicine: how to practice and teach EBM Churchill Livingstone, Edinburgh, 2000.

Guyatt G, Rennie D (eds.). User's guides to the medical literature: A manual for evidence-based clinical practice. AMA Press, Chicago, 2002. Available at: http://www.usersguides.org/).

Greenhalgh T. How to read a paper: The basics of evidence-based medicine. BMJ Press, London, 2001.

Black ER, Bordley DR, Tape TG, Panzer RG (eds). Diagnostic strategies for common medical problems, second edition. American College of Physicians, Philadelphia, 1999.

Sackett DL, Haynes RB, Tugwell P, Guyatt GH. Clinical epidemiology: a basic science for clinical medicine. Lippincott, Williams, and Wilkins, Philadelphia, 1991.

Fletcher RH, Fletcher SW, Wagner EH. Clinical epidemiology: The essentials. Lippincott, Williams, & Wilkins, Philadelphia, 1996.

REFERENCES

1. Institute of Medicine. Crossing the Quality Chasm: A New Health System for the 21st Century. National Academy Press, Washington, DC, 2001.
2. Covell DG, Uman GC, Manning PR. Information needs in office practice: are they being met? Ann Intern Med 1985;103:596–599.
3. Gorman PN, Helfand M. Information seeking in primary care: how physicians choose which clinical questions to pursue and which to leave unanswered. Med Decis Making 1995;15:113–119.
4. Ramsey PG, Carline JD, Inui TS, et al. Changes over time in the knowledge base of practicing internists. JAMA1991;266:1103–1107.
5. van Leeuwen YD, Mol SS, Pollemans MC, Drop MJ, Grol R, van der Vleuten CP. Change in knowledge of general practitioners during their professional careers. Fam Pract 1995;12:313–317.
6. McGlynn EA, Asch SM, Adams J, et al. The quality of health care delivered to adults in the United States. N Engl J Med 2003;348:2635–2645.
7. Davis DA, Thomson MA, Oxman AD, Haynes RB. Changing physician performance. A systematic review of the effect of continuing medical education strategies. JAMA 1995;274:700–705.
8. Davis D, O'Brien MA, Freemantle N, Wolf FM, Mazmanian P, Taylor-Vaisey A. Impact of formal continuing medical education: do conferences, workshops, rounds, and other traditional continuing education activities change physician behavior or health care outcomes? JAMA 1999;282:867–874.
9. Institute of Medicine. Health Professions Education: A Bridge to Quality. National Academies Press, Washington, DC, 2003.
10. ABIM Program for Continuous Professional Development, 2004. Available at: www.abim.org/cpd/cpdhome/index.htm. Accessed January 2004.
11. Parboosingh JT, Gondocz ST. The Maintenance of Competence Program of the Royal College of Physicians and Surgeons of Canada. JAMA 1993;270:1093.
12. Accreditation Council for Graduate Medical Education. Outcomes project: general competencies, 2004. Available at http://www.acgme.org/outcome/comp/compFull.asp, 2004. Accessed January 2004.
13. Kellum JA, Rieker JP, Power M, Powner DJ. Teaching critical appraisal during critical care fellowship training: a foundation for evidence-based critical care medicine. Crit Care Med. 2000;28:3067–3070.
14. Schoenfeld P, Cruess D, Peterson W. Effect of an evidence-based medicine seminar on participants' interpretations of clinical trials: a pilot study. Acad Med 2000;75:1212–1214.
15. Green ML. Graduate medical education training in clinical epidemiology, critical appraisal, and evidence-based medicine: a critical review of curricula. Acad Med 1999;74:686–694.
16. Coomarasamy A, Taylor R, Khan KS. A systematic review of postgraduate teaching in evidence-based medicine and critical appraisal. Med Teach Jan 2003;25:77–81.
17. Alguire PC. A review of journal clubs in postgraduate medical education. J Gen Intern Med 1998;13: 347–353.
18. Parkes J, Hyde C, Deeks J, Milne R. Teaching critical appraisal skills in health care settings. Cochrane Database of Systematic Reviews 2001:CD001270.
19. Ebbert JO, Montori VM, Schultz HJ. The journal club in postgraduate medical education: a systematic review. Med Teach. 2001;23:455–461.
20. Taylor R, Reeves B, Ewings P, Binns S, Keast J, Mears R. A systematic review of the effectiveness of critical appraisal skills training for clinicians. Med Educ 2000;34:120–125.

21. Norman GR, Shannon SI. Effectiveness of instruction in critical appraisal (evidence-based medicine) skills: a critical appraisal. CMAJ 1998;158(2):177–181.

22. Sidorov J. How are internal medicine residency journal clubs organized, and what makes them successful? Arch Intern Med 1995;155:1193–1197.

23. Linzer M, Brown JT, Frazier LM, DeLong ER, Siegel WC. Impact of a medical journal club on house-staff reading habits, knowledge, and critical appraisal skills. A randomized control trial. JAMA 1988;260:2537–2541.

24. Langkamp DL, Pascoe JM, Nelson DB. The effect of a medical journal club on residents' knowledge of clinical epidemiology and biostatistics [see comments]. Fam Med 1992;24:528–530.

25. Kitchens JM, Pfeifer MP. Teaching residents to read the medical literature: a controlled trial of a curriculum in critical appraisal/clinical epidemiology. J Gen Intern Med 1989;4:384–387.

26. Green ML. Evidence-based medicine training in internal medicine residency programs a national survey. J Gen Intern Med 2000;15:129–133.

27. Dellavalle RP, Stegner DL, Deas AM, et al. Assessing evidence-based dermatology and evidence-based internal medicine curricula in US residency training programs: a national survey. Arch Dermatol 2003;139:369-372.

28. Grad R, Macaulay AC, Warner M. Teaching evidence-based medical care: description and evaluation. Fam Med 2001;33:602–606.

29. Green ML, Ellis PJ. Impact of an evidence-based medicine curriculum based on adult learning theory. J Gen Intern Med 1997;12:742–750.

30. Baum KD. The impact of an evidence-based medicine workshop on residents attitudes towards and self-reported ability in evidence-based practice. Med Educ Online 2003;8:4–10.

31. Cramer JS, Mahoney MC. Introducing evidence based medicine to the journal club, using a structured pre and post test: a cohort study. BMC Medical Education 2001;1:6.

32. Edwards KS, Woolf PK, Hetzler T. Pediatric residents as learners and teachers of evidence-based medicine. Acad Med 2002;77:748.

33. Elnicki DM, Halperin AK, Shockcor WT, Aronoff SC. Multidisciplinary evidence-based medicine journal clubs: curriculum design and participants' reactions. Am J Med Sci 1999;317:243–246.

34. Smith CA, Ganschow PS, Reilly BM, et al. Teaching residents evidence-based medicine skills: a controlled trial of effectiveness and assessment of durability. J Gen Intern Med 2000;15:710–715.

35. Bazarian JJ, Davis CO, Spillane LL, Blumstein H, Schneider SM. Teaching emergency medicine residents evidence-based critical appraisal skills: a controlled trial. Ann Emerg Med 1999;34:148–154.

36. Ross R, Verdieck A. Introducing an evidence-based medicine curriculum into a family practice residency: is it effective? Acad Med 2003;78:412–417.

37. Green ML. Identifying, appraising, and implementing medical education curricula: a guide for medical educators. Ann Intern Med Nov 20 2001;135:889–896.

38. Colliver JA, Robbs RS. Evaluating the effectiveness of major educational interventions. Acad Med 1999;74:859–860.

39. Hojat M, Xu G. A visitor's guide to effect sizes: statistical significance versus practical (clinical) importance of research findings. Adv Health Sci Educ Theory Pract 2004;9:241–249.

40. Knowles MS, Holton EF, Swanson RA. The Adult Learner. Butterworth-Heinemann, Woburn, MA, 1998.

41. Green ML. Evidence-based medicine training in graduate medical education: past, present and future. J Eval Clin Pract 2000;6:121–138.

42. Richardson WS. One slice or the whole pie? Evidence-based health care newsletter. 2001;21:17–18.

43. Reilly B, Lemon M. Evidence-based morning report: a popular new format in a large teaching hospital. Am J Med 1997;103:419–426.

44. Ozuah PO, Orbe J, Sharif I. Ambulatory rounds: a venue for evidence-based medicine. Acad Med 2002;77:740–741.

45. McGinn T, Seltz M, Korenstein D. A method for real-time, evidence-based general medical attending rounds. Acad Med 2002;77:1150–1152.

46. Schneeweiss R. Morning rounds and the search for evidence-based answers to clinical questions. J Am Board Fam Pract 1997;10:298–300.

47. Lovett PC, Sommers PS, Draisin JA. A learner-centered evidence-based medicine rotation in a family practice residency. Acad Med 2001;76:539–540.

48. Korenstein D, Dunn A, McGinn T. Mixing it up: integrating evidence-based medicine and patient care. Acad Med 2002;77:741–742.

49. Rucker L, Morrison E. The "EBM Rx": an initial experience with an evidence-based learning prescription. Acad Med 2000;75:527–528.
50. Khunti K. Teaching evidence-based medicine using educational prescriptions. Med Teach 1998;20: 380–381.
51. Grimes DA. Introducing evidence-based medicine into a department of obstetrics and gynecology [see comments]. Obstet Gynecol 1995;86:451–457.
52. Bradley DR, Rana GK, Martin PW, Schumacher RE. Real-time, evidence-based medicine instruction: a randomized controlled trial in a neonatal intensive care unit. J Med Libr Assoc 2002;90:194–201.
53. Fox RD. Training for uncertainty. In: Merton R, Reader GC, Kendell PL, eds. The Student Physician. Harvard University Press, Cambridge, MA, 1957, pp. 207–241.
54. Green ML, Ruff TR. Why do residents fail to answer their clinical questions? A qualitative study of barriers to evidence-based medicine. Acad Med 2005;80:176–182.
55. Bhandari M, Montori V, Devereaux PJ, Dosanjh S, Sprague S, Guyatt GH. Challenges to the practice of evidence-based medicine during residents' surgical training: a qualitative study using grounded theory. Acad Med 2003;78:1183–1190.
56. Straus SE, Green ML, Bell DS, et al. Evaluating the teaching of evidence based medicine: conceptual framework. BMJ 2004;329:1029–1032.
57. McColl A, Smith H, White P, Field J. General practitioner's perceptions of the route to evidence based medicine: a questionnaire survey. BMJ 1998;316:361–365.
58. Ramos KD, Schafer S, Tracz SM. Validation of the Fresno test of competence in evidence based medicine. BMJ 2003;326:319–321.
59. Fritsche L, Greenhalgh T, Falck-Ytter Y, Neumayer HH, Kunz R. Do short courses in evidence-based medicine improve knowledge and skills? Validation of Berlin questionnaire and before and after study of courses in evidence based medicine. BMJ 2002;325:1338–1341.
60. Taylor R, Reeves B, Mears R, et al. Development and validation of a questionnaire to evaluate the effectiveness of evidence-based practice teaching. Med Educ 2001;35:544–547.
61. Bradley P, Humphris G. Assessing the ability of medical students to apply evidence in practice: the potential of the OSCE. Med Educ 1999;33:815–817.
62. Davidson RA, Duerson M, Romrell L, Pauly R, Watson RT. Evaluating evidence-based medicine skills during a performance-based examination. Acad Med 2004;79:272–275.
63. Fliegel JE, Frohna JG, Mangrulkar RS. A computer-based OSCE station to measure competence in evidence-based medicine skills in medical students. Acad Med 2002;77:1157–1158.
64. Richardson WS, Wilson MC, Nishikawa J, Hayward RS. The well-built clinical question: a key to evidence-based decisions [editorial]. ACP Journal Club 1995;123:A12–A13.
65. Green ML, Ciampi MA, Ellis PJ. Residents' medical information needs in clinic: are they being met? Am J Med 2000;109:218–223.
66. Flynn C, Helwig A. Evaluating an evidence-based medicine curriculum. Acad Med 1997;72:454–455.
67. Crowley SD, Owens TA, Schardt CM, et al. A web-based compendium of clinical questions and medical evidence to educate internal medicine residents. Acad Med 2003;78:270–274.
68. Fung MF, Walker M, Fung KF, et al. An internet-based learning portfolio in resident education: the KOALA multicentre programme. Med Educ 2000;34:474–479.
69. Kelly DR, Murray TS. The development and evaluation of a personal learning log for senior house officers. Med Educ1999;33:260–266.
70. The Writing Group for the PEPI Trial. Effects of estrogen or estrogen/progestin regimens on heart disease risk factors in postmenopausal women. The Postmenopausal Estrogen/Progestin Interventions (PEPI) Trial. JAMA 1995;273:199–208.
71. Hulley S, Grady D, Bush T, et al. Randomized trial of estrogen plus progestin for secondary prevention of coronary heart disease in postmenopausal women. Heart and Estrogen/progestin Replacement Study (HERS) Research Group. JAMA 1998;280:605-613.
72. Langham J, Tucker H, Sloan D, Pettifer J, Thom S, Hemingway H. Secondary prevention of cardiovascular disease: a randomised trial of training in information management, evidence-based medicine, both or neither: the PIER trial. Br J Gen Pract 2002;52:818–824.
73. Forsetlund L, Bradley P, Forsen L, Nordheim L, Jamtvedt G, Bjorndal A. Randomised controlled trial of a theoretically grounded tailored intervention to diffuse evidence-based public health practice [ISRCTN23257060]. BMC Med Educ 2003;3:2.
74. Lucas BP, Evans AT, Reilly BM, et al. The impact of evidence on physicians' inpatient treatment decisions. J Gen Intern Med 2004;19:402–409.

75. Oswald N, Bateman H. Treating individuals according to evidence: why do primary care practitioners do what they do? J Eval Clin Pract 2000;6:139–148.
76. Haynes RB, Devereaux PJ, Guyatt GH. Clinical expertise in the era of evidence-based medicine and patient choice. ACP Journal Club 2002;136:A11–14.
77. Young JM, Ward JE. Evidence-based medicine in general practice: beliefs and barriers among Australian GPs. J Eval Clin Pract 2001;7:201–210.
78. McAlister FA, Graham I, Karr GW, Laupacis A. Evidence-based medicine and the practicing clinician. J Gen Intern Med 1999;14:236–242.
79. Guglielmino LM. Development of the self-directed learning readiness scale (doctoral dissertation, University of Georgia). Diss Abstr Int 1997;38:6467A.
80. Wiley K. Effects of a self-directed learning project and preference for structure on self-directed learning readiness. Nurs Res 1983;32:181–185.
81. Delahaye BL, Smith HE. The validity of the Learning Preference Assessment. Adult Education Quarterly 1995;45:159–173.
82. Russell JW. Learner preference for structure, self-directed learning readiness, and instructional methods (Doctoral Dissertation, University of Missouri). Diss Abstr Int 1988;49:1689.
83. Hall-Johnson K. The relationship between readiness for self-directed learning and participation in self-directed learning (Doctoral dissertation, Iowa State University). Diss Abstr Int 1981;46:7A.
84. Harvey BJ, Rothman AI, Frecker RC. Effect of an undergraduate medical curriculum on students' self-directed learning. Acad Med 2003;78:1259–1265.
85. Shokar GS, Shokar NK, Romero CM, Bulik RJ. Self-directed learning: looking at outcomes with medical students. Fam Med 2002;34:197–200.
86. Williams B. Self direction in a problem based learning program. Nurse Educ Today 2004;24:277–285.
87. Oddi LF, Ellis AJ, Roberson JA. Construct validation of the Oddi Continuing Learning Inventory. Adult Education Quarterly 1990;40:139–145.
88. Ryan G. Student perceptions about self-directed learning in a professional course implementing problem-based learning. Stud Higher Educ 1993;18:53–63.
89. Knowles MS. Self-directed learning. Follett, Chicago, 1975.
90. Cork RD, Detmer WM, Friedman CP. Development and initial validation of an instrument to measure physicians' use of, knowledge about, and attitudes toward computers. J Am Med Inform Assoc 1998;5:164–176.
91. Dixon DR, Stewart M. Exploring information technology adoption by family physicians: survey instrument valuation. Paper presented at: Proceedings of the American Medical Informatics Association Annual Symposium, 2000; Los Angeles, CA.
92. McGowan JJ, Berner ES. Proposed curricular objectives to teach physicians competence in using the World Wide Web. Acad Med 2004;79:236–240.
93. Silber CG, Nasca TJ, Paskin DL, Eiger G, Robeson M, Veloski JJ. Do global rating forms enable program directors to assess the ACGME competencies? Acad Med 2004;79:549–556.
94. Putnam W, Twohig PL, Burge FI, Jackson LA, Cox JL. A qualitative study of evidence in primary care: what the practitioners are saying. CMAJ 2002;166:1525–1530.
95. Freeman AC, Sweeney K. Why general practitioners do not implement evidence: qualitative study. BMJ 2001;323:1100–1102.
96. Ely JW, Osheroff JA, Ebell MH, et al. Obstacles to answering doctors' questions about patient care with evidence: qualitative study. BMJ 2002;324:710.
97. Montori VM, Tabini CC, Ebbert JO. A qualitative assessment of 1st-year internal medicine residents' perceptions of evidence-based clinical decision-making. Teach Learn Med 2001;14:114–118.
98. Smith CS, Morris M, Francovich C, Hill W, Gielselman F. A qualitative study of resident learning in ambulatory clinic. Adv Health Sci Educ Theory Pract 2004;9:93–105.
99. Schon DA. Educating the Reflective Practitioner. Jossey-Bass, San Francisco, 1987.
100. Slotnick HB. How doctors learn: physicians' self-directed learning episodes. Acad Med 1999;74:1106–1117.
101. Stenhouse L. An introduction to curriculum research and development. Helnemann, London, 1975.
102. Wyer PC, Keitz S, Hatala R, et al. Tips for learning and teaching evidence-based medicine: introduction to the series. CMAJ 2004;171:347–348.
103. Barratt A, Wyer PC, Hatala R, et al. Tips for learners of evidence-based medicine: 1. Relative risk reduction, absolute risk reduction and number needed to treat. CMAJ 2004;171:353–358.

104. Montori VM, Kleinbart J, Newman TB, et al. Tips for learners of evidence-based medicine: 2. Measures of precision (confidence intervals). CMAJ 2004;171:611–615.
105. Richardson WS, Wilson MC. On questions background and foreground. Evidence-based Healthcare Newsletter Nov 6 1997:6.
106. Sackett DL, Straus SE. Finding and applying evidence during clinical rounds: the "evidence cart." JAMA 1998;280:1336–1338.
107. Ely JW, Osheroff JA, Ferguson KJ, Chambliss ML, Vinson DC, Moore JL. Lifelong self-directed learning using a computer database of clinical questions. J Fam Pract 1997;45:382–388.
108. Sauve S, Lee HN, Meade MO, et al. The critically appraised topic: a practical approach to learning critical appraisal. Annals CRMCC 1995;28:396–398.
109. The United States Preventive Services Task Force. Guide to Preventive Services, Third Edition: Periodic Updates. Available at http://www.ahrq.gov/clinic/cps3dix.htm, 2004. Aaccessed November 2004.
110. Rational Clinical Exam series. JAMA. Available at http://jama.ama-assn.org/cgi/collection/physical_examination, 2004. Accessed November 2004.
111. Suchman AL, Williamson PR, Litzelman DK, Frankel RM, Mossbarger DL, Inui TS. Toward an informal curriculum that teaches professionalism. J Gen Intern Med 2004;19:501–504.
112. Frankford DM, Patterson MA, Konrad TR. Transforming practice organizations to foster lifelong learning and commitment to medical professionalism. Acad Med 2000;75:708–717.
113. Akl EA, Izuchukwu IS, El-Dika S, Fritsche L, Kunz R, Schunemann HJ. Integrating an evidence-based medicine rotation into an internal medicine residency program. Acad Med 2004;79:897–904.

II PRACTICING EVIDENCE-BASED ENDOCRINOLOGY

5 Finding Current Best Evidence in Endocrinology

R. Brian Haynes, MD, PhD
and Cynthia J. Walker-Dilks, MLS

CONTENTS

INTRODUCTION
SYSTEMS
SYNOPSES
SYNTHESES
STUDIES
SUMMARY
REFERENCES

INTRODUCTION

Two years ago we presented various resources likely to provide the best research evidence concerning endocrine disorders *(1)*. At the time, an already overwhelming array of resources existed and have since grown. Clinicians are bombarded by information arriving by regular mail and e-mail, in educational rounds and seminars, and through countless other avenues. Many resources make claims to be "evidence-based" or "the only resource you need," and quite often they are free. With such an onslaught of information, how can you pay attention to any of them, let alone summon the time and energy to sort through all of them to find resources truly useful to your own clinical practice? Indeed, a recent study of primary care literature indicated that 627.5 h of physician effort would be required to evaluate the 7287 articles published per month in five primary care journal review services *(2)*. The plethora of evidence-based resources now available means that more than ever, clinicians must be discriminating about how to make best use of them.

In this chapter, we update our previous discourse *(1)*, highlighting new resources we believe will be helpful to the practice of endocrinology. As before, we follow the "4S" hierarchy of resources, in descending order of importance *(3)*:

- Information systems in which studies, syntheses, and synopses are organized around clinical topics (e.g., *Clinical Evidence* and *Physicians' Information and Education Resource* [PIER] or, ultimately, integrated into electronic medical records [e.g., Infobuttons]).

From: *Contemporary Endocrinology: Evidence-Based Endocrinology*
Edited by: V. M. Montori © Mayo Foundation for Medical Education and Research

- Synopses of the original studies or reviews (e.g., *American College of Physicians [ACP] Journal Club*).
- Syntheses or systematic reviews of the studies (e.g., the *Cochrane Database of Systematic Reviews*).
- Databases of studies themselves (e.g., *Medline*).

This hierarchy of systems, synopses, syntheses, and studies has been labeled the "4S" evolution of services for finding current best evidence *(3,4)*.

SYSTEMS

The ideal system for endocrinology would be an integrated decision-support system that summarizes important research evidence about endocrinology problems and links to a specific patient's circumstances. Electronic medical record systems with computerized decision support have been shown in randomized trials to improve the process and outcome of care *(5)*. We are unaware of such an integrated system for endocrinology in usual practice settings, but progress is being made in this area. For example, researchers at Columbia University have developed "Infobuttons" to link contextual information, such as patient data, to Web-based information resources *(6)*. Such a system provides a standardized method for matching user contexts to information.

Whereas integrated systems are still under development, electronic textbooks are still very useful to practitioners because they integrate evidence-based information around specific clinical problems and provide regular updating. The key is to use textbooks that are explicitly evidence-based *(7)*. *Clinical Evidence* (www.clinicalevidence.com), from the BMJ Publishing Group, is based on systematic reviews and original articles and integrates evidence about therapy for a broad range of clinical problems in a question and answer format. It is available in print and electronic versions (including personal digital assistant [PDA]) formats and the electronic versions have monthly updates.

Whereas Clinical Evidence provides summaries of evidence and leaves management decisions up to the reader, PIER (http://pier.acponline.org/index.html?hp) provides specific guidance to readers, with the evidence "behind the scenes."

Both publications target primary care clinicians, and include a number of important endocrinology topics. PIER topics cover diseases, screening and prevention, complementary and alternative medicine, ethical and legal issues, procedures, and drugs. Modules are written by academic authors and are updated continually with supporting medical literature searches performed with quality filtering. PIER is also designed to integrate with electronic medical records, order entry systems, hospital information systems, and practice management systems.

UpToDate (www.uptodate.com) is a leading evidence-based textbook for general internal medicine with a comprehensive section on endocrinology and diabetes mellitus, but it is just in the process of developing an explicit approach to finding and summarizing evidence. *ACP Medicine* (formerly *WebMD*) (www.acpmedicine.com) has a continually updated web version in addition to monthly updated print and quarterly CD-ROM versions, with chapters written by academic physicians. Again, it is just in the process of developing an explicit approach to evidence updating and quality assessment.

In addition to electronic textbooks, several web-based "one-stop shopping" search engines are tuned for primary and secondary evidence sources. Although not interfaced with patient information systems, these "meta-search" services offer links to information further down the 4S pyramid, are easy to navigate, and many are free—or at least parts of them are free. InfoRetriever (www.infopoems.com) is a point-of-care tool that is updated at least three times a year and is available in PDA, Windows, and web formats. The content is based on the *Patient-Oriented Evidence that Matters* (POEMs) database and the *Cochrane Database of Systematic Reviews*. It is supplemented with guideline summaries, clinical decision rules, clinical calculators, and the *5-Minute Clinical Consult (8)*.

Turning Research into Practice (TRIP) (www.tripdatabase.com) is a database of Internet links to high-quality health care resources. The resources are updated and expanded regularly, and criteria for quality include clinical relevance, coverage, and rigor of product. TRIP has an annual subscription fee, although nonsubscribers may use it if making less than five searches/wk.

The *National Electronic Library of Health* (www.nelh.nhs.uk) is another web-based meta-resource from the United Kingdom. It is free, but some sites, such as clinical databases, are only available to registered National Health Service health providers. It links to several evidence-based resources, particularly UK initiatives.

NLM Gateway is a one-stop searching interface for the US National Library of Medicine. It allows users to search simultaneously in several databases from one search window. Results are grouped into five categories: journal citations, books/ serials/audiovisual, consumer health, meeting abstracts, and other collections. *Gateway* (http://gateway.nlm.nih.gov/gw/Cmd) is useful for searchers who wish to perform an overall search intending to pull information from as many *NLM* and other US government resources as possible. It is also useful for searchers who are unfamiliar with *NLM* resources or are unsure about the best place to look for information on a given question.

MedlinePlus (medlineplus.gov) is a web-based resource targeted to health care consumers as well as providers. The *NLM* maintains links to information resources that it evaluates for quality according to selection guidelines. Many links are to National Institutes of Health (NIH) sites. Users can search by general health topics or perform a search with text words in the search window. Results are grouped by health topics, drug information, medical encyclopedia, news, and other. Drug prescribing and patient information is most directly retrieved by searching *MedlinePlus* and the generic drug name—or US or Canadian brand name—on the Google search line (e.g., *MedlinePlus* metformin). This is particularly useful for discussions with patients when you prescribe a new medication for them, as it provides useful background information about the medication and a balanced description of adverse effects. *MedlinePlus* also provides general information about disease conditions for patients and consumers, with links to many additional resources.

Using these meta-resources can help save a practitioner time, given that the systems search a broad array of information and perform quality filtering. Nevertheless, it is still imperative that the user start with a clear and answerable question, understand evidence-based principles, and be able to choose the most appropriate source for their question.

SYNOPSES

When an answer for a clinical question cannot be found from one of the current evidence-based information systems, the next best resource is a synopsis of a systematic review or an individual study. When systematic reviews or individual studies are presented in a one-page structured abstract format, even better. *ACP Journal Club* (www.acpjc.org), *Evidence-Based Medicine* (ebm.bmjjournals.com), and *Evidence-Based Obstetrics and Gynecology* (www.elsevier.com/wps/find/journaldescription. cws_home/623029/description#description) all provide structured abstracts with accompanying clinical commentaries of original studies and systematic reviews that have "passed muster" for methodological soundness and clinical relevance, including studies with relevance to endocrinology. The particular strength of these resources is a complex quality-filtering procedure that allows the reader to relax their "doubt factor" when reading the material. The producers of these evidence-based abstract journals scan a broad array of clinical journals using strict methodological criteria. These methodologically sound articles are further reviewed by clinicians who rate the articles for relevance and newsworthiness. Only those that warrant "prime time attention" are abstracted. By reading resources of this synoptic nature, practitioners can keep up to date with the current best evidence.

Bandolier (www.ebandolier.com) is another secondary publication aimed at primary care. It presents summaries of evidence drawn from systematic reviews and original studies with the results presented as simple bullet points. It is published monthly in print and has an online version. Two other synopses that present evidence in "bite sized" portions are *POEMs* (www.infopoems) and *Critically Appraised Topics* (CATs). POEMs, which are included in the InfoRetriever POEMs database (discussed in the Systems section), are summaries of valid studies that are deemed to have the potential to change practice. They also are published in some clinical journals, including the *British Medical Journal*.

CATs were developed at McMaster University and perfected at Oxford. They are evidence bites emanating from clinical encounters. They tend to follow the question and answer theme seen in *Clinical Evidence*, but on a much smaller scale being based on individual patients. Because they are individual and specific, they lack broad application, but the creation of CAT "banks" provides an increasing collection of individual items of evidence on real-life clinical topics presented in an easily digestible format. CATS are usually local journal club efforts, but some groups, such as the Oxford Centre for Evidence-Based Medicine (http://www.cebm.net/cats.asp) and the University of North Carolina (www.med.unc.edu/medicine/edursrc/!catlist.htm), post their CATs on the Internet. Although more renowned as educational and teaching tools, as short summaries of high-quality evidence, they fit in our synopsis category.

SYNTHESES

When more detail is needed than is provided in a synopsis, or no synopsis is at hand, then a database of systematic reviews ("syntheses") should be sought. The leading example is the Cochrane Library, available on CD-ROM, the Web (www.thecochranelibrary. com), *Aries Knowledge Finder* (www.kfinder.com), and *Ovid's Evidence-Based Medicine Reviews Service*. There is a Cochrane metabolic and endocrine disorders group as well as a Cochrane menstrual disorders and subfertility group. Numerous reviews from these and other review groups in the *Cochrane Database of Systematic Reviews* are of interest to endocrinologists. The success of the Cochrane Collaboration has stimulated substantial growth in systematic reviews in the medical literature. Indeed, systematic reviews occupy a growing fraction of the high-quality medical literature *(9)*. If a

Cochrane review cannot be located, *PubMed* can be easily searched to retrieve systematic reviews through use of clinical queries in *PubMed* (www.ncbi.nlm.nih.gov/entrez/query/static/clinical.html). OVID also provides a systematic review search strategy on its "limits" page (click on the limits "target" after you enter search terms for the topic you are interested in).

STUDIES

If searches in systems, synopses, or syntheses fail then original studies should be sought. These studies can be retrieved on the Web in several ways, and some of these web-based services are attuned to evidence-based principles. *SUMSearch* (http://sumsearch.uthscsa.edu/) searches in several locations from one entry search and attempts to provide the highest quality resources first. With the use of "focus" buttons, a user can tailor the content of their search to such aspects as intervention, screening and prevention, etiology, or prognosis. Search results are presented in two sections: broad, easy to read discussions such as reviews, editorials, and practice guidelines, and as more up to date answers to specific questions such as systematic reviews and original research. The user still must appraise individual items identified.

The *Medline* clinical queries screen (www.ncbi.nlm.nih.gov/entrez/query/static/clinical.html) provides detailed search strategies that augment the retrieval of studies that are clinically relevant and sound in the areas of treatment, prognosis, diagnosis, and etiology. The clinical queries search strategies have recently been updated based on new research *(10)*, and are also being tested in Embase, PsycINFO, and Cinahl to expand the usefulness of methodological search strategies beyond *Medline*.

Alerting systems targeted to individual practitioners are also being developed. The McMaster MORE project (hiru.mcmaster.ca/more) invites front-line clinicians to become "sentinel readers" to rate articles online for relevance and newsworthiness. Clinicians can indicate the medical disciplines in which they are interested and then only articles matching those disciplines are sent to them.

If all else fails, a general search on the Web is worth a try. Google (www.google.com) is still one of the most effective, and certainly the most used, search engines. No single search engine searches more than 30–40% of the current Web content, so a combination of search approaches may be warranted. Google's search function lets you type in words, or concepts of interest, and then retrieves Web sites that contain these terms ranked in the order of how many other sites have linked to the original site, sort of a quality indicator. Google searches are typically fast and can pull up a product monograph for a new drug or a disease Web site in a few seconds. As previously mentioned, going through *MedlinePlus* provides some assurance of quality.

Problem-Based Exercises

PROBLEM 1

Ms. Jones is a 63-yr-old woman with severe osteoporosis. Despite regular weight-bearing exercise, vitamin D, calcium, and alendronate, she continues to experience vertebral fractures and recently broke her left wrist in a minor fall. She has a strong family history of breast cancer, and hormonal replacement therapy seems relatively contraindicated for this reason. Unfortunately, she developed intolerable adverse effects on raloxifene. You are aware of a recent trial of parathyroid hormone, but can't recall the details and don't know if parathyroid hormone could be combined with her current therapy or be substituted for it.

A search for evidence begins with a properly formulated question. The elements of a question relevant to this situation include the patient's features, the intervention of interest and alternatives (if applicable), and the clinical outcome(s) of most importance. For Ms. Jones, the search question could be formulated as follows: for a 63-yr-old post-menopausal woman with severe osteoporosis, who is failing on conventional treatment, does parathyroid hormone, alone or in combination with other treatments, reduce the incidence of fractures? In keeping with the "4S" structure above, we'll look in *Clinical Evidence* for an answer. Searching on the term "osteoporosis" quickly leads to a summary of treatment alternatives for fracture prevention in post-menopausal women, but parathyroid hormone isn't listed.

Undeterred, you head for OVID's *Evidence-Based Medicine Reviews*, providing one-stop access to the *Cochrane Database of Systematic Reviews, ACP Journal Club*, and the *Database of Abstracts of Reviews of Evidence*. There, entering the terms "parathyroid hormone AND osteoporosis AND postmenopausal" yields seven citations, the third and fourth of which are *ACP Journal Club* reviews of two studies comparing parathyroid hormone alone and in combination with alendronate in men *(11)* and postmenopausal women *(12)*. Both studies show no benefit of combining parathyroid hormone with alendronate. Going back to *Clinical Evidence*, you review the effective options for your patient.

Problem 2

You've been meaning to shape up the prevention of foot ulcers in patients with diabetes in your clinic for some time. A 57-yr-old man with diabetes for 20 yr and persistent ulcers on both feet leading to amputation, spurs you to take action. You vow to set up a screening and management program for foot problems so that you can intervene earlier.

The questions that might lead off this search could be as follows: what are the most important risk factors for diabetic foot ulcers in patients with longstanding diabetes mellitus? What is the efficacy and cost-effectiveness of early intervention for preventing foot ulcers and amputations in such patients?

A search in *Clinical Evidence* with the term "diabetic foot" leads to a summary of prevention interventions and treatment options, categorized according to evidence concerning their effectiveness. As noted at the top of the chapter, the literature searches for this topic were last run in September 2003, so you venture out to *Medline* to determine if anything new has come up. Searching from the clinical queries screen, you click on Therapy, choosing a "sensitive" search, and enter the terms "diabetes AND ulcer." This yields 622 citations, but only 41 of these were published since September 2003, and only one of these catches your eye, a randomized trial of home monitoring of foot temperature (with a simple infrared heat detector) for high-risk patients *(13)*. Added to close follow-up and regular podiatric review, this yielded an impressive reduction in foot complications.

UpToDate also has a chapter on diabetic foot care, but it's not obvious how systematic the review of evidence was for this chapter and there is very little information about effective preventive measures.

Problem 3

Mr. Addams, a 57-yr-old patient of yours with longstanding Zollinger Ellison Syndrome as part of multiple endocrine neoplasia-type (MEN) 1, begins to complain of flushing episodes. His gastrinoma has been managed medically on omeprazole, with minimal symptoms. A 24-h urinary 5-hydroxy-indoleacetic acid test was normal. You are aware of the increased risk for carcinoid in patients with hypergastrinemia but not clear on the current best way to determine whether Mr. Addams has developed a gastric carcinoid.

A search in an evidence-based database is unlikely to be productive in this situation, as these databases are not usually produced for such uncommon clinical problems. A general medical textbook is also unlikely to be helpful. An endocrine tumor text might be best, but the slow production cycle of such books often means that they will be out of date. This is a situation in which a MEDLINE search may be the best route to look for evidence concerning incidence and diagnosis.

A search in PubMed using the terms "gastrinoma AND carcinoid AND diagnosis" yields 132 citations, a few too many to work though. Switching the search to the clinical queries screen, putting in just the terms "gastrinoma and carcinoid," and clicking the terms "diagnosis" AND "specificity," leads to nine citations, several of which seem pertinent. The first of these provides details of a study of 145 consecutive referrals with Zollinger-Ellison syndrome to the NIH, who were assessed by various tests and gastric biopsy for gastric carcinoid *(14)*.

SUMMARY

New medical information is accumulating at an astonishing rate. It is available in many forms and flavors and information seekers will benefit from being discriminating in searches for answers to clinical problems. Very few problems can be satisfactorily addressed by simply entering some relevant content terms into MEDLINE. Such a search, unless the problem is extremely rare, usually results in a flood of citations with no arrangement according to quality, and the user must painstakingly determine which citations are relevant and clinically useful. Fortunately, evidence-based information services are catching up with the growth of the medical literature. Such services organize and provide access to the current best evidence at the point of need.

We have described a "4S" hierarchy of evidence-based resources to help focus a practitioner's information seeking strategies, with systems at the highest level of organization, followed by synopses, syntheses, and studies. Practitioners should become familiar with the best access routes for regularly updated services of relevance to their interests, and direct their inquiries initially to the highest level of organization of information that exists for their interests. Evidence-based resources continue to be created and evolve, so keeping an eye out for new resources, and examining their pedigrees according to the "4S" approach, will permit practitioners to assemble and organize an ever improving personal evidence-based library for endocrinology.

REFERENCES

1. Haynes RB, Walker-Dilks CJ. Evidence-based endocrinology. Finding the current best research evidence for practice in endocrinology. Endocrinol Metab Clin North Am 2002;31:527–535.
2. Alper BS, Hand JA, Elliott SG, et al. How much effort is needed to keep up with the literature relevant for primary care? J Med Libr Assoc 2004;92:429–437.
3. Haynes RB. Of studies, syntheses, synopses, and systems: the "4S" evolution of services for finding current best evidence. ACP J Club 2001;134:A11–A13.
4. Booth A. Finding current best evidence: putting the 4Ss into searching. Diabet Med 2002;19:1–3.

5. Hunt DL, Haynes RB, Hanna SE, et al. Effects of computer based clinical decision support systems on physician performance and patient outcomes: a systematic review. JAMA 1998;280:1339–1346.

6. Cimino JJ, Li J. Sharing infobuttons to resolve clinicians' information needs. AMIA Annu Symp Proc 2003;815.

7. Richardson WS, Wilson MC. Textbook descriptions of disease—where's the beef? ACP Journal Club 2002;137:A11–A12.

8. Damro MR, ed. Griffith's 5-minute clinical consult. 12th edition. Lippincott Williams and Wilkins, Philadelphia, PA, 2003.

9. Walker-Dilks C. Contribution of the Cochrane Library to the evidence-based journals. ACP Journal Club 2004;141:A11.

10. Haynes RB, Wilczynski NL. Optimal search strategies for retrieving scientifically strong studies of diagnosis from Medline: analytical survey. BMJ 2004;328:1040.

11. Finkelstein JS, Hayes A, Hunzelman JL, et al. The effects of parathyroid hormone, alendronate, or both in men with osteoporosis. N Engl J Med 2003;349:1216–1226.

12. Black DM, Greenspan SL, Ensrud KE, et al. The effects of parathyroid hormone and alendronate alone or in combination in postmenopausal osteoporosis. N Engl J Med 2003;349:1207–1215.

13. Lavery LA, Higgins KR, Lanctot DR, et al. Home monitoring of foot skin temperatures to prevent ulceration. Diabetes Care 2004;27:2642–2647.

14. Bashir S, Gibril F, Ojeaburu JV, et al. Prospective study of the ability of histamine, serotonin or serum chromogranin A levels to identify gastric carcinoids in patients with gastrinomas. Aliment Pharmacol Ther2002;16:1367–1382.

6   Integrating Evidence
Into Clinical Diagnosis

W. Scott Richardson, MD

CONTENTS

INTRODUCTION

In busy clinical practice, diagnosis is our daily bread. All day, every day, we confront patients' predicaments in which both of us want to know what is the matter. Many diagnostic tests are already available to help us, with more being developed all the time. Increasingly, diagnostic tests are undergoing rigorous evaluations of their accuracy and usefulness, with the results published as clinical care research *(1)*. How can the results of this clinical care research be incorporated into our diagnostic decision making? This chapter addresses this topic, by starting with some illustrative cases, considering different modes of diagnostic thought, and then examining how evidence can be integrated into clinical diagnosis.

ILLUSTRATIVE CASES

1. As soon as you enter the room, you recognize this patient has acromegaly, as he is almost 8-ft tall, has an enormous overall head size, very large supraorbital ridges, mouth, and tongue, and gigantic hands. Testing confirms growth hormone excess and pituitary enlargement.

From: *Contemporary Endocrinology: Evidence-Based Endocrinology*
Edited by: V. M. Montori © Mayo Foundation for Medical Education and Research

2. You've been asked to see a young woman with known type 1 diabetes mellitus in the emergency department. As you enter the cubicle, several sensations reach you quickly—the fruity smell of ketones, the speed and depth of her breathing, the sick look on her face, the clammy feel of her skin, and the hair standing on end on your own neck. Her blood tests confirm what you already know—she has diabetic ketoacidosis.

3. You're asked to see an older woman who was hospitalized yesterday with new atrial fibrillation. The hospital's protocol for this condition includes a thyroid stimulating hormone (TSH) measurement, and this patient's result came back very low, surprising the patient's doctors and prompting your consultation. The patient has no history of thyroid disease, yet further testing confirms hyperthyroidism.

4. A long-standing patient of yours returns for follow-up, but with a new problem. You've seen him for hypothyroidism, well controlled on hormone supplements. He has also been found to have chondrocalcinosis of several joints on prior radiographs. Today he describes 4 d of increasing right knee pain and swelling, limiting his walking. His knee appears inflamed with a definite effusion and reduced range of motion. His radiograph shows soft tissue swelling and no fracture. To confirm Calcium Pyrohosphate Deposition Disease (CPPD) crystal-associated arthritis and exclude other causes, an arthrocentesis is done, yielding a white cell count over 100,000 and Gram-positive cocci in clusters on Gram stain. Later, cultures confirm staphylococcal infectious arthritis.

5. You are asked to see an older man hospitalized with hypercalcemia. After the presumed malignancy could not be found, they turn to you to sort things out. A detailed review of the patient data so far turns up few clues. The patient's calcium levels remain high, yet the parathyroid hormone (PTH) levels are repeatedly low and the urinary calcium excretion is repeatedly high, leading you to suspect a cause not mediated via PTH. Looking back, you recall the patient's subtle headaches, so even though the chest radiograph is normal you order an magnetic resonance (MR) of the head, which shows neurosarcoidosis.

6. You are consulted on a young woman with suspected fasting hypoglycemia. Evaluation so far has excluded alcoholism, malnutrition, and liver disease. It takes several visits and many tests to identify that the patient has become adrenally insufficient, and she recovers fully on hormone replacement.

MODES OF DIAGNOSTIC THINKING

In these cases, we see the clinicians appear to engage in different types of diagnostic thinking, depending on the particular circumstances (Table 1). In the first two cases, the clinicians recognize the correct diagnoses rapidly, within less than a second, and quite easily and automatically, like recognizing a family member. These features have suggested to cognitive scientists that such diagnoses are made during the perceptual stage of thinking—the clinical cues are perceived and the pattern is recognized before the conscious mind has had a chance for deliberate processing—hence its name (2,3). This mode of diagnostic thinking relies heavily on the implicit or tacit knowledge from our past experience, stored in our memories as libraries of prior cases we've seen with this disorder (4–6). We update these case libraries automatically as we go, and they are always available and are as quick as our thoughts. Yet if we've not seen and stored instances of the target disorder in our memories, we cannot use this mode of diagnostic thinking.

The third and fourth cases illustrate the middle mode of diagnostic thinking in Table 1, wherein a rule for diagnostic action is applied to a particular case, yielding the diagnosis. In the third case, the rule is embedded in the preprinted orders of a hospital's condition-specific protocol. In the fourth case, the clinician may or may not consciously

Table 1
Modes of Diagnostic Thinking

	Perceptual	*Aphorismic*	*Analytic*
Other terms	"Skill-based" Intuitive Pattern recognition	"Rule-based" Maxims Protocols	"Knowledge-based" Deductive Systematic approach
Relative speed	Faster	Medium	Slower
Knowledge used	Patterns of illness	Rules for diagnostic action	Knowledge that supports diagnostic inference
Knowledge for excellence	Vast case library "Compiled" Mostly tacit	Recommendations, reminders, rules, and previously stored diagnostic solutions "Compiled" Mixture of tacit and explicit	Numerous, well organized structures of "background" and "foreground" knowledge "Elaborated" Mostly explicit
Cognitive activity	Rapidly recognize this patient's illness as an instance of a specific disorder	Recall a rule or previously derived diagnostic solution to apply to this patient's illness	Recall knowledge and use it to make inferences and derive a deliberate diagnostic solution for this patient's illness
Uses of patient's clinical features	As a whole, both to recognize the presenting clinical problem and to recognize the specific disorder	As a whole to recognize the presenting clinical problem Sometimes, as individual findings if used by the rule	As a whole to recognize the presenting clinical problem As individual findings, focusing on discriminatory power
Main use of diagnostic tests	To confirm the already-recognized disorder	To confirm or exclude a specific disorder by the rule	To discriminate between competing "active alternatives," aiming to confirm one and exclude the others
Main use of evidence from clinical care research	If implicitly embedded in memories of cases	Encapsulated in rules and recommendations	Explicit use in deducing cause of patient's illness
Examples of evidence that may be used	Clinical manifestations of disease	Practice guidelines Clinical decision rules	Disease probability Accuracy of tests or clinical findings

remember the sources of the rules acted upon, although we can sometimes still hear our teachers' voices when thinking of their admonitions, such as "a hot joint isn't gout or pseudogout until the Gram stain is negative." In this mode of thinking, diagnostic action is guided by tersely phrased statements of fact and opinion, or aphorisms, hence its name. These aphorisms can summarize the rules and recommendations of past or current experts, the admonitions of our teachers, and our own lessons from, and solutions to, previous diagnostic problems *(7–9)*. Medical teachers from Hippocrates to Osler have written diagnostic aphorisms, and they are still being taught today *(10)*. Using this mode of diagnostic thinking requires that we have an applicable aphorism, that we recall it when appropriate (or we are prompted externally to do so), and that we act accordingly. Without access to an appropriate aphorism, we can't use this mode of thinking.

By contrast, in the fifth and sixth cases the clinicians are engaging in a more or less analytic mode of diagnostic thought, as described in the right-hand column of Table 1. In this slower, more deliberate process, the case details stimulate us to recall specific chunks of knowledge from memory, which we use to make inferences about the patient's findings and deduce the correct diagnosis *(7,11–13)*. This analytic mode of thought relies more heavily on our fund of explicit knowledge than either the skill-based perceptual mode or the rule-based aphorismic mode *(14,15)*. If we don't have access to the relevant knowledge, or if it is available but we cannot reason well with it, we won't be able to use this analytic approach to clinical diagnosis.

These modes of diagnostic thinking differ on more than speed. One of the main distinctions is in the relative importance of tacit knowledge from experience for the perceptual mode compared to the relative importance of explicit knowledge for the analytic approach, while the aphorismic mode draws upon both forms. Another key distinction is the nature of the cognition involved, from the automatic pattern recognition of the perceptual mode, to the "semi-automatic" use of rules in the aphorismic mode, and to the deliberate inferences of the analytic mode.

This characterization of three modes of diagnostic thinking is supported in part by studies of problem solving and decision making in the cognitive sciences, including the recognition of "skill-based," "rule-based," and "knowledge-based" types of cognition *(16,17)*. A full explication on the current state of this science, including the areas of congruence and of controversy, is beyond the scope of this chapter, so we refer interested readers elsewhere *(18–28)*. Although some commentators emphasize only one of these modes, to the exclusion of the others, we find these three modes complementary, not contradictory, and we aspire toward excellence in all. The best diagnosticians we've seen or read about appear to use all three modes well, moving from one to the next to fit the specific diagnostic situation.

DIAGNOSTIC TRADITIONS FOR ANALYTIC THINKING

Within the analytic mode of diagnostic thinking, we can identify several fairly distinct diagnostic traditions, as noted in Table 2 *(7)*. The first is a collection of separate belief systems about disease causation that employ these beliefs in a similar fashion, using fairly circular logic. The next two, descriptive and criteria-based, rely on our detailed, centuries-old-yet-still-evolving taxonomy of all diseases, with the latter approach adding explicit diagnostic criteria. The next two, anatomic and pathophysiological, allow the clinician to apply the results of almost two centuries of inquiry into the biology of human health and disease and into how tests work. The probabilistic tradition enables the clinician to apply the results of several decades of clinical care research into *how well* tests work *(29)*. Finally, the biopsychosocial tradition seeks to integrate the biological, psychological, and social dimensions into a more complete understanding of human illness *(30)*.

Except for the first, these traditions differ primarily on the knowledge substrate used for making inferences about patient data and for deducing diagnoses. The best diagnosticians we have seen or read about appear to draw upon several of these traditions (except the belief-based) when pursuing diagnoses in an analytic mode, moving from one to the next depending on the specific circumstances and the availability of the different types of knowledge. Whereas we are advocates *for* the optimal use of evidence in the probabilistic tradition, we are not advocates *against* using other traditions such as the pathophysiologic and biopsychosocial, when they are appropriate. Rather, we think it wise to employ any diagnostic tradition that can help us serve our patients with better diagnoses and reduced diagnostic error. In the following sections, we highlight the probabilistic tradition in order to show how research evidence can be integrated into diagnostic decisions.

CLINICAL CARE RESEARCH EVIDENCE USEFUL FOR CLINICAL DIAGNOSIS

What types of clinical care research can yield evidence of potential use in clinical diagnosis? We think there are quite a few types, and we've listed 15 of them in Table 3. The first listed may be the only type of research that some will expect—cross-sectional studies of the accuracy and precision of individual diagnostic tests. Yet increasingly, these are being collected and appraised in the form of systematic reviews, listed as the second type *(1,31–33)*. Taking a wide view of the available clinical care research, we count at least 13 other types of studies that can inform a broad range of diagnostic decisions, as shown in Table 3.

As is explained elsewhere in this book, deciding whether and how to integrate research evidence into diagnostic decision making goes beyond considerations of access and availability. After asking questions about diagnostic issues in answerable ways (look again at the right-hand column of Table 3) and acquiring relevant evidence, the next step would be to carry out a critical appraisal of this evidence. Because explaining the details of full critical appraisal for each of the 15 types of evidence in Table 3 is beyond the scope of this chapter, we have cited the relevant appraisal guides for each type of evidence. The three main decisions involved in critical appraisal of all 15 types of evidence are: (1) Are the results of the study sufficiently valid they should inform your practice? (2) Are the results of the study important enough to yield a substantial impact if used? (3) Are the results of the study sufficiently applicable to the patients you see and the diagnostic decisions you face *(34,35)*?

A careful look at Table 3 shows that many of the results of the 15 types of research will be quantitative in nature. For instance, studies of the frequency of underlying diseases in those with a defined clinical problem will yield results that can be expressed as probabilities. Similarly, studies of how well tests discriminate a target disorder from the remaining conditions yield results that can be expressed in likelihood ratios, which are used to revise disease probabilities. In short, evidence from clinical care research provides knowledge that supports the inferences made within the probabilistic tradition of diagnostic analysis.

(text continued on p. 79)

Table 2
Some Diagnostic Traditions

Tradition	Description	Example	What's involved
Belief-based	The clinician's beliefs about the general causes of human illness are used to pronounce the specific cause of an individual person's illness.	"Because toxins in the blood cause all disease, and you are sick, therefore you have toxins in the blood."	Involves strong belief in the theory of illness causation. No proof of diagnosis is usually needed.
Descriptive	Starting with a detailed description of human illnesses as a taxonomy of disease, the clinician identifies which class of disease best fits the features of an individual person's illness.	"Your painful eruption of grouped vesicles in a single dermatome means you have shingles, or the reactivation of Herpes Zoster infection."	Involves judging how well a person's illness fits the diseases in the taxonomy, and the "best fit wins." No proof of diagnosis is usually needed.
Criteria-based	Starting with an explicit set of diagnostic criteria for each disease, the clinician identifies which disorders criteria are best met by the features of an individuals illness.	"This patient's illness has all four of the major criteria in the DSM-IV-TR for acute delirium."	Requires an explicit set of criteria for each diagnosis, along with a scoring rule (e.g., needs 4 or more of these 11 criteria to qualify). Proof of the diagnosis involves the match of the patient's features to disease criteria, while disproof involves the lack of matching.
Anatomic	Examination of the patient (alive or dead) or of patient specimens yields the presence or absence of anatomic features, from which is deduced the specific cause of an individual person's illness.	"The biopsy of this patient's thyroid nodule showed follicular adenocarcinoma."	Requires that the target disorder manifest some anatomic abnormality, whether at the gross, the microscopic, or the molecular level. Proof of the diagnosis involves demonstration of the particular anatomic features in the patient, while disproof involves showing their absence.

Table 2 *(continued)*

Tradition	Description	Example	What's involved
Pathophysiological	Testing of the patient or of patient specimens yields the presence or absence of pathophysiologic states, from which is deduced the specific cause of an individual person's illness.	"The metabolic acidosis with increased anion gap, the high serum ketones and the hyperglycemia confirm this patient has diabetic ketoacidosis."	Requires that the target disorder manifest some detectable pathophysiological derangement. Proof of the diagnosis involves demonstration of the particular pathophysiological state in the patient, while disproof involves showing its absence.
Probabilistic	Clinical findings and test results, either individually or in clusters, are used to revise the probability of disease, either upward toward certainty (confirming the diagnosis) or downward toward zero (excluding the diagnosis).	"The very large likelihood ratio of this very low TSH level raises the probability of hyperthyroidism in this patient to well over 98%, which is above our threshold for treatment."	Involves quantifying the uncertainty in diagnosis and the discriminatory power of findings or tests. Proof of a target disorder involves raising the probability of disease above the threshold close to certain, whereas disproof involves lowering the disease probability below a threshold close to zero.
Biopsychosocial	Medical interview, nonverbal behavior, and life contexts are examined for health of psychological and sociological dimensions, which are then integrated with biological considerations when deducing the causes of the patient's illness.	"This episode of acute environmental hypothermia has occurred along with acute alcohol intoxication, in the setting of chronic alcohol dependence and homelessness since his discharge from military combat duty."	Aims to integrate the biological, the psychological, and the sociological dimensions into a more complete understanding of the nature of the patients suffering. Proof involves identifying disruptions in the patient's psychological or sociological health when ill, and finding the patient improves if and when these disruptions leave. Disproof involves finding the absence of psychological or sociological troubles.

Table 3
Some Forms of Evidence From Clinical Care Research Evidence
That Can Be Useful for Diagnostic Decisions

Type of research	Output of research	Guides to critical appraisal	Diagnostic decisions
1. Cross-sectional studies of test accuracy	Accuracy and discriminatory power of tests	Users' guides IIIA and IIIB (49,50)	Which tests should be ordered? How should these test results be interpreted?
2. Systematic reviews of cross-sectional studies of test accuracy	Pooled test accuracy Summary levels of evidence supporting test use	Users' guides VI, IX, IIIA, and IIIB (49–52)	Which tests should be ordered? How should these test results be interpreted?
3. Consecutive case series or cohort studies of defined clinical problems	Frequency of underlying disorders that cause this clinical problem	Users' guide XV (40)	What is the starting probability of this target disorder? Is this disorder likely enough that it should be pursued in all with this clinical problem?
4. Derivation or validation studies of clinical decision rules	Probability of the target disorder in different patient groups, divided by the decision rule	Users' guide XXII (53)	What is the revised pretest probability of the target disorder (after using the decision rule)?
5. Consecutive case series or cohort studies of the clinical manifestations of disease.	Frequency of clinical findings in those proved to have the target disorder	Users' guide XXIV (48)	Should this finding cue this diagnostic hypothesis? Does the absence of this finding allow us to safely discard this diagnostic hypothesis? Do the known manifestations of this target disorder adequately explain all the findings of this patient's illness?
6. Case–control or cohort studies of risk factors for disease	Strength of association between risk factor and target disorder	Users' guide IV (54)	Does this factor place the patient at particular risk of the target disorder?

Table 3 *(continued)*

Type of research	Output of research	Guides to critical appraisal	Diagnostic decisions
7. Cohort studies of prognosis and prognostic factors	Range and likelihood over time of disease outcomes	Users' guide V *(55)*	How serious is the target disorder if left undiagnosed and untreated? Therefore, how vigorously should this diagnosis be pursued?
			Could the known course over time of the target disorder explain this individual person's illness trajectory so far?
8. Randomized trials of treatments for the target disorder	Effectiveness of treatments for this disorder	Users' guides IIA and IIB *(56,57)*	How responsive is the target disorder to treatment? Therefore, how vigorously should this diagnosis be pursued?
9. Clinical decision analyses of diagnostic or screening strategies	Expected impact on outcomes if strategies are used	Users' guides VIIA and VIIB *(58,59)*	When formulating diagnostic or screening policy, what impact on clinical outcomes can be expected from each strategy?
10. Economic analyses of diagnostic or screening strategies	Expected impact on resource use if strategies are used	Users' guides XIIIA and XIIIB *(60,61)*	When formulating diagnostic or screening policy, what impact will each strategy have on resource use? Is this diagnostic or screening program worth doing?

(continued)

Table 3 *(continued)*

Type of research	Output of research	Guides to critical appraisal	Diagnostic decisions
11. Randomized trials of diagnostic or screening strategies	Effectiveness and impact of these strategies	Users' guides IIA, IIB, and XVII *(56,57,62)*	When considering this target disorder, which diagnostic strategy yields the greatest impact? Should screening for this target disorder be undertaken?
12. Utilization review or observational "outcomes" studies of the impact of diagnostic policies, or of the occurrence of diagnostic errors	Observed impact of diagnostic policy in real world settings Frequency and determinants of diagnostic error	Users' guides X, XI *(63,64)*	How well do these diagnostic strategies hold up in real-world clinical settings? For which target disorders are errors most likely? Under which conditions are we most prone to diagnostic error?
13. Studies of use of computerized clinical decision support systems (CDSS) for diagnosis	Impact of CDSS on diagnostic outcomes	Users' guides XVIII *(65)*	Should we implement this CDSS to improve our clinical diagnoses and reduce diagnostic error?
14. Randomized trials of interventions to reduce diagnostic errors	Effectiveness of interventions on errors	Users' guides IIA and IIB *(56,57)*	By what methods can we most effectively reduce our chances of diagnostic error?
15. Evidence-based practice guidelines of diagnostic or screening strategies	Summary levels of evidence supporting use of strategies Graded recommendations for diagnosis or screening	Users' guides VIIIA, VIIIB, IX, and XVII *(52,62,66,67)*	What are the recommended strategies for diagnosis or screening for this target disorder? When should and when shouldn't these recommendations be followed?

INTEGRATING EVIDENCE INTO ANALYTIC
DIAGNOSTIC THINKING

How specifically can these forms of evidence be integrated into clinical diagnosis? To consider this question, we'll divide the tasks of diagnosis into five steps, gathering clinical findings, selecting a differential diagnosis, choosing diagnostic tests, interpreting test results, and verifying final diagnoses (36). In Table 4, we list how research evidence can be integrated into each of these steps, and we illustrate using a case from the beginning of this chapter.

In the third scenario, hyperthyroidism was found in an older woman with atrial fibrillation after the surprise finding of a very low TSH. How could evidence help us in gathering clinical findings? To start with, since the frequency of atrial fibrillation as a manifestation of hyperthyroidism is greater than zero (i.e., it does occur), the patient's atrial fibrillation could cue us to actually consider the hypothesis of hyperthyroidism while we're examining her. Evidence about the accuracy of individual clinical findings could guide our selection of which parts of the history and physical examination are worth gathering (37,38). Evidence about the discriminating power of a cluster of findings in a clinical decision rule such as Crook's index could also be used in deciding which findings will help us either confirm or exclude hyperthyroidism (39).

When selecting the differential diagnosis, it'd be wise to consider not only how likely a given diagnosis is (probabilistic considerations), but also how serious it is if left undiagnosed and untreated (prognostic considerations) and how responsive it is to treatment if diagnosed (pragmatic concerns) (40–43). In this scenario, evidence about the frequency of hyperthyroidism among those who present with atrial fibrillation could guide our probabilistic judgments, whereas evidence about the prognosis of hyperthyroidism and its responsiveness to treatment could guide our judgments about the other matters. For instance, in series of patients presenting with atrial fibrillation, hyperthyroidism has been found in between about 1 and 2.5% of patients (44), so we might estimate a starting pretest probability of 2%. Turn to Fig. 1 and locate 2% on the left-hand vertical line for pretest probability.

When choosing tests, in the probabilistic tradition we would want to pick the test that provides the largest change in disease probability. In evidence about test accuracy, this strength of probability revision is expressed as the likelihood ratio. The farther away from one the test result's likelihood ratio is, in either direction, the greater that test result can change the probability of disease. For instance, the likelihood ratio found for sensitive TSH levels below 0.1 is estimated to be about 99 for ambulatory patients and about 20 for sick inpatients (45). Let's see the effect of using both values—in Fig. 1, find the values of 20 and 99 (close to 100) on the middle vertical line for likelihood ratios.

Because the TSH result was very low, we can estimate the post-test probability using Fig. 1 by simply placing a straight edge beginning at the 2% point on the pretest probability scale, connecting through the 100 mark on the likelihood ratio (for the second try, connect through the 20 mark), and following the straight edge across to the point where it intersects the post-test probability line, about 67% (or 30%, when using the likelihood ratio of 20). How do we interpret these post-test probabilities? Note that compared to the pretest probability, these post-test probabilities are substantially higher, raising the probability of the diagnosis of hyperthyroidism. Next, we could compare the resulting post-test probability to our thresholds for further action, such as

Table 4
Integrating Research Evidence Into Analytic Diagnostic Thinking

Diagnostic task	Useful research evidence (relevant users guides, as appropriate)
1. Gathering clinical findings	*Cueing diagnostic hypotheses:* Frequency of manifestations in patients proved to have disease (XXIV) *(48)* Choosing findings to gather: Accuracy and precision of individual findings for target disorder (IIIA and B) *(49,50)* Discriminatory power of clusters of findings in clinical decision rules (XXII) *(53)*
2. Selecting a differential diagnosis	*Probabilistic considerations:* Probability of disease in patients with defined clinical problem (XV) *(61)* Revised probability of disease with clinical decision rule (XXII) *(53)* *Prognostic considerations:* Seriousness of target disorder if left undiagnosed and untreated (V) *(55)* *Pragmatic considerations:* Responsiveness of target disorder to treatment if diagnosed (IIA and B) *(56,57)*
3. Choosing diagnostic tests	*Test accuracy considerations:* Individual studies (IIIA and B) *(49,50)* Systematic reviews (VI) *(51)* *Impact of testing strategies:* Randomized trials (IIA and B) *(56,57)* Clinical decision analyses (VIIA and B) *(58,59)* Economic analyses (XIIIA and B) *(60,61)* Observational studies (X, XI) *(63,64)* *Recommended test strategies:* Practice guidelines (VIIIA and B) *(66,67)*
4. Interpreting test results	*Deriving post-test probabilities:* Starting pretest probabilities (XV) *(40)* Revised pretest probabilities (XXII) *(53)* Likelihood ratios (IIIA and B) *(49,50)* *Comparing post-test probability to action thresholds:* Clinical decision analysis (VIIA and B) *(58,59)* Economic analysis (XIIIA and B) *(60,61)* Practice Guidelines (VIIIA and B) *(66,67)*
5. Verifying the diagnosis	*Explicit use of "Six Tests of a Diagnosis" when verifying a diagnosis:* Frequency of clinical manifestations of the target disorder (XXIV) *(48)* Clinical course of the target disorder (V) *(55)*

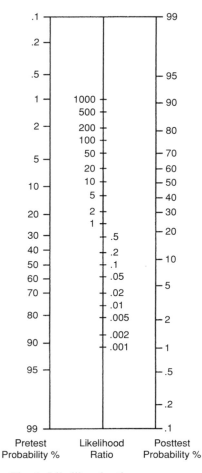

Fig. 1. Likelihood ratio nomogram.

starting initial treatment, undertaking further testing, and counseling patients and family. The setting of these thresholds can be done through formal analysis *(46,47)*, or be embedded in evidence-based recommendations from other types of evidence listed in Table 4, such as practice guidelines.

For many diagnostic situations, we may approach diagnostic verification implicitly. Yet it can be done explicitly, using the "Six Tests of a Diagnosis" *(48)*: does the diagnosis adequately explain all the patient's findings? Is the diagnosis coherent with the pathophysiologic state found in the patient? Is the diagnosis the best fit among the alternatives? Is the diagnosis the simplest explanation, within reason? Is the diagnosis robust to attempts to disprove it? Does this diagnosis predict the subsequent clinical course better than the alternatives *(48)*? Note that evidence about the frequency of clinical manifestations of disease and about the prognosis of the condition can help us make these decisions. Doing this explicitly can help us troubleshoot at times of residual diagnostic uncertainty, and can give us a shared language to untangle disagreements we may have with our colleagues in a particular patient's case.

INTEGRATING EVIDENCE INTO APHORISMIC DIAGNOSTIC THINKING

Can evidence be integrated into diagnostic thinking in the aphorismic mode? We think so, as long as the evidence is purposefully included when the rules for diagnostic action are derived and recommended. When well-made, evidence-based practice guidelines have the potential to function this way, in that the aphorismic recommendations should comprise explicitly weighed evidence integrated with explicitly weighed values of the decision stakeholders. Similarly, the rules for diagnostic action that can come from well-studied clinical decision rules could become tersely stated rules or aphorisms to guide us. In the future, computerized decision support systems for diagnosis might incorporate evidence more explicitly and consistently, and these systems could in turn mediate the use of evidence for clinicians operating in the aphorismic mode.

INTEGRATING EVIDENCE INTO PERCEPTUAL DIAGNOSTIC THINKING

Can evidence be integrated into diagnostic thinking in the perceptual mode? Not directly, because this mode occurs at the preconscious, perceptual stage of thought. Yet evidence might be incorporated indirectly, for as we go about diagnostic tasks using evidence in the analytic or aphorismic modes, this explicit knowledge could become embedded along with other memories in the case libraries we draw upon to recognize patterns of disease. In particular, knowledge from studies of the frequency of clinical manifestations of disease could be learned when we experience of first several cases of each disorder, so that our memories store more accurate 'theme and variation' patterns of disease for later retrieval.

CONCLUSION

In conclusion, we have examined three different modes of diagnostic thought: perceptual, aphorismic, and analytic. Within the analytic mode, we have considered seven different diagnostic traditions, including the probabilistic tradition for which much knowledge can be derived from clinical care research. We then examined how the evidence from 15 types of clinical care research can inform many diagnostic decisions within this probabilistic tradition. We illustrated the integration of evidence into five tasks of clinical diagnosis. Figure 1 shows that it is already feasible to integrate evidence into diagnostic decision making now. Yet we look forward to advances in research, synopsis, and retrieval systems that should make it even easier, even better, and even faster to use evidence in clinical diagnosis in the future.

REFERENCES

1. Knottnerus JA, ed. The Evidence Base of Clinical Diagnosis, BMJ Books, London, 2002.
2. Norman GR, Brooks LR. The non-analytical basis of clinical reasoning. Adv Health Sci Educ 1997;2:173–184.
3. Cox K. Perceiving clinical evidence. Med Educ 2002;36:1189–1195.
4. Goldman GM. The tacit dimension of clinical judgment. Yale J Biol Med 1990;63:47–61.
5. Peters RM. The role of intuitive thinking in the diagnostic process. Arch Fam Med 1995;4: 939–941.
6. Round A. Introduction to clinical reasoning. J Eval Clin Pract 2001;7:109–117.

7. Kassirer JP. Diagnostic reasoning. Ann Intern Med 1989;110:893–900.
8. Mellers BA, Schwartz A, Cooke AD. Judgment and decision making. Annu Rev Psychol 1998;49: 447–477.
9. Hunter K. "Don't think zebras": uncertainty, interpretation, and the place of paradox in clinical education. Theor Med 1996;17:225–241.
10. Mangrulkar RS, Saint S, Chu S, Tierney LM. What is the role of the clinical pearl? Am J Med 2002; 113:617–624.
11. Kassirer JP, Kopelman RI. Learning Clinical Reasoning. Williams and Wilkins, Baltimore, MD, 1991.
12. Barondess JA, Carpenter CCJ, eds. Differential Diagnosis. Lea and Febiger, Philadelphia, PA, 1994.
13. Glass RD. Diagnosis: A Brief Introduction. Oxford University Press, Melbourne, Australia, 1996.
14. Bordage G. Elaborated knowledge: a key to successful diagnostic thinking. Acad Med 1994;69: 883–885.
15. Eva KW, Neville AJ, Norman GR. Exploring the etiology of content specificity: Factors influencing analogic transfer and problem solving. Acad Med 1998;73:S1–S5.
16. Goodstein LP, Andersen HB, Olsen SE. Tasks, Errors, and Mental Models. Taylor and Francis, London, UK, 1988.
17. Wickens CD, Gordon SE, Liu Y, eds. An Introduction to Human Factors Engineering. Addison-Wesley-Longman, New York, 1998.
18. Elstein AS, Shulman L, Sprafka S. Medical Problem Solving: An Analysis of Clinical Reasoning. Harvard University Press, Cambridge, MA, 1978.
19. Dawson NV, Arkes HR. Systematic errors in medical decision making: judgment limitations. J Gen Intern Med 1987;2:183–187.
20. Schmidt HG, Norman GR, Boshuizen HPA. A cognitive perspective on medical expertise: theory and implications. Acad Med 1990;65:611–621.
21. Custers EJ, Regehr G, Norman GR. Mental representations of medical diagnostic knowledge: a review. Acad Med 1996:71:S55–S61.
22. Hammond KR. How convergence of research paradigms can improve research on diagnostic judgment. Med Decis Making 1996;16:281–287.
23. Higgs J, Jones M, eds. Clinical Reasoning in the Health Professions. Butterworth-Heinemann, Oxford, UK, 1996.
24. Cox K. Doctor and Patient: Exploring Clinical Thinking. UNSW Press, Sydney, Australia, 1999.
25. Norman GR. The epistemology of clinical reasoning: perspectives from philosophy, psychology, and neuroscience. Acad Med 2000;75:S127–S136.
26. Bornstein BH, Emler AC. Rationality in medical decision making: a review of the literature on doctors' decision-making biases. J Eval Clin Pract 2001;7:97–107.
27. Redelmeier DA, Ferris LE, Tu JV, Hux JE, Schull MJ. Problems for clinical judgment: introducing cognitive psychology as one more basic science. CMAJ 2001;164:358–360.
28. Patel VL, Kaufman DR, Arocha JF. Emerging paradigms of cognition in medical decision making. J Biomed Inform 2002;35:52–75.
29. Jaeschke R, Guyatt GH, Montori VM. Evidence-based diagnosis in endocrinology. Endocrinol Metab Clin North Am 2002;31:567–581.
30. Engel GL. The need for a new medical model: a challenge for biomedicine. Science 1977;196: 129–136.
31. Irwig L, Tosteson ANA, Gatsonis C, et al. Guidelines for meta-analysis evaluating diagnostic tests. Ann Intern Med 1994;120:667–676.
32. Deeks JJ. Systematic reviews of evaluations of diagnostic and screening tests. In: Egger M, Smith GD, Altman DG, eds. Systematic Reviews in Health Care: Meta-analyses in Context. BMJ Books, London, UK, 2001.
33. Montori VM, Guyatt GH. Summarizing studies of diagnostic test performance. Clin Chem 2003;49: 1783–1784.
34. Guyatt GH, Rennie DR, eds. Users' Guides to the Medical Literature: A Manual for Evidence-Based Clinical Practice. AMA Press, Chicago, IL, 2002.
35. Straus SE, Richardson WS, Glasziou P, Haynes RB, eds. Evidence-Based Medicine: How to Practice and Teach EBM, 3/e. Churchill-Livingstone, Edinburgh, UK, 2005.
36. Richardson WS. Evidence-based diagnosis: More is needed [EBM Note] Evidence-Based Medicine 1997;v:70–71.

37. Sackett DL. A primer on the precision and accuracy of the clinical examination. JAMA 1992;267: 2638–2644.

38. Simel DL, Rennie DR. The clinical examination—an agenda to make if more rational [Editorial]. JAMA 1997;277:572–574.

39. Crooks J, Murray IPC, Wayne EJ. Statistical methods applied to the clinical diagnosis of thyrotoxicosis. Q J Med 1959;28:211–234.

40. Richardson WS, Wilson MC, Guyatt GH, Cook DJ, Nishikawa J, for the Evidence-Based Medicine Working Group. Users' guides to the medical literature. XV. How to use an article about disease probability for differential diagnosis. JAMA 1999;281:1214–1219.

41. Richardson WS. Where do pretest probabilities come from? Evidence Based Medicine 1999;4:67–68.

42. Richardson WS, Glasziou P, Polashenski WA, Wilson MC. A new arrival—evidence about differential diagnosis. ACP J Club 2000;133:A11–A12.

43. Richardson WS. Five uneasy pieces about pretest probability. J Gen Intern Med 2002;17:882–883.

44. Attia J, Margetts P, Guyatt G. Diagnosis of thyroid disease in hospitalized patients: a systematic review. Arch Intern Med 1999;159:658–665.

45. Dolan JG, Wittlin SD. Hyperthyroidism and hypothyroidism. In: Black ER, Bordley DR, Tape TG, Panzer RJ, eds. Diagnostic Strategies for Common Medical Problems, 2nd edition. ACP, Philadelphia, PA, 1999, pp. 473–483.

46. Pauker SG, Kassirer JP. The threshold approach to clinical decision making. N Engl J Med 1980;302: 1109–1117.

47. Gross R. Making Medical Decisions: An Approach to Clinical Decision Making for Practicing Physicians. ACP, Philadelphia, PA, 1999.

48. Richardson WS, Wilson MC, Williams JW Jr, Moyer VA, Naylor CD, for the Evidence-Based Medicine Working Group. Users' guides to the medical literature. XXIV. How to use an article on the clinical manifestations of disease. JAMA 2000;284:869–875.

49. Jaeschke R, Guyatt GH, Sackett DL, for the Evidence-Based Medicine Working Group. Users' guides to the medical literature. III. How to use an article about a diagnostic test. A. Are the results of the study valid? JAMA 1994;271:389–391.

50. Jaeschke R, Guyatt GH, Sackett DL, for the Evidence-Based Medicine Working Group. Users' guides to the medical literature. III. How to use an article about a diagnostic test. B. What are the results and will they help me in caring for my patients? JAMA 1994;271:59–63.

51. Oxman AD, Cook DJ, Guyatt GH, for the Evidence-Based Medicine Working Group. Users' guides to the medical literature. VI. How to use an overview. JAMA 1994;272:1367–1371.

52. Guyatt GH, Sackett DL, Sinclair JC, Hayward R, Cook DJ, Cook RJ, for the Evidence-Based Medicine Working Group. Users' guides to the medical literature. IX. A method for grading health care recommendations. JAMA 1995;274:1800–1804.

53. McGinn TG, Guyatt GH, Wyer PC, Naylor CD, Stiell IG, Richardson WS, for the Evidence-Based Medicine Working Group. Users' guides to the medical literature. XXII. How to use articles about clinical decision rules. JAMA 2000;284:79–84.

54. Levine M, Walter S, Lee HN, Haines T, Holbrook A, Moyer V, for the Evidence-Based Medicine Working Group. Users' guides to the medical literature. IV. How to use an article about harm. JAMA 1994;271:1615–1619.

55. Laupacis A, Wells G, Richardson WS, Tugwell P, for the Evidence-Based Medicine Working Group. Users' guides to the medical literature. V. How to use an article about prognosis. JAMA 1994;272: 234–237.

56. Guyatt GH, Sackett DL, Cook DJ, for the Evidence-Based Medicine Working Group. Users' guides to the medical literature. II How to use an article about therapy or prevention. A. Are the results of the study valid? JAMA 1993;270:2598–2601.

57. Guyatt GH, Sackett DL, Cook DJ, for the Evidence-Based Medicine Working Group. Users' guides to the medical literature. II. How to use an article about therapy or prevention. B. What are the results and will they help me in caring for my patients? JAMA 1994;271:59–63.

58. Richardson WS, Detsky AS, for the Evidence-Based Medicine Working Group. Users' guides to the medical literature. VII. How to use a clinical decision analysis. A. Are the results of the study valid? JAMA 1995;273:1292–1295.

59. Richardson WS, Detsky AS, for the Evidence-Based Medicine Working Group. Users' guides to the medical literature. VII. How to use a clinical decision analysis. B. What are the results and will they help me in caring for my patients? JAMA 1995;273:1610–1613.

60. Drummond MF, Richardson WS, O'Brien BJ, Levine M, Heyland DK, for the Evidence-Based Medicine Working Group. Users' guides to the medical literature. XIII. How to use an article on economic analysis of clinical practice. A. Are the results of the study valid? JAMA 1997;277:1552–1557.
61. O'Brien BJ, Heyland DK, Richardson WS, Levine M, Drummond MF, for the Evidence-Based Medicine Working Group. Users' guides to the medical literature. XIII. How to use an article on economic analysis of clinical practice. B. What are the results and will they help me in caring for my patients? JAMA 1997;277:1802–1806.
62. Barratt A, Irwig L, Glasziou P, et al, for the Evidence-Based Medicine Working Group. Users' guides to the medical literature. XVII. How to use guidelines and recommendations about screening. JAMA 1999;281:2029–2034.
63. Naylor CD, Guyatt GH, for the Evidence-Based Medicine Working Group. Users' guides to the medical literature. X. How to use an article reporting variations in the outcomes of health services. JAMA 1996;275:554–558.
64. Naylor CD, Guyatt GH, for the Evidence-Based Medicine Working Group. Users' guides to the medical literature. XI. How to use an article about a clinical utilization review. JAMA 1996;275:1435–1439.
65. Randolph AG, Haynes RB, Wyatt JC, Cook DJ, Guyatt GH, for the Evidence-Based Medicine Working Group. Users' guides to the medical literature. XVIII. How to use an article evaluating the clinical impact of a computer-based clinical decision support system. JAMA 1999;282:67–74.
66. Hayward RS, Wilson MC, Tunis SR, Bass EB, Guyatt GH, for the Evidence-Based Medicine Working Group. Users' guides to the medical literature. VIII. How to use clinical practice guidelines. A. Are the recommendations valid? JAMA 1995;274:570–574.
67. Wilson MC, Hayward RS, Tunis SR, Bass EB, Guyatt GH, for the Evidence-Based Medicine Working Group. Users' guides to the medical literature. VIII. How to use clinical practice guidelines. B. What are the recommendations and will they help you in caring for your patients? JAMA 1995;274:1630–1632.

7 Supporting Evidence-Based Endocrine Practice

Steven A. Smith, MD
and Geoffrey S. Gates, MD

CONTENTS

INTRODUCTION
INFORMATION FOR THE PHYSICIAN
INFORMATION FOR THE PATIENT
IMPROVING THE UTILITY OF INFORMATION FOR THE PROVIDER
IMPROVING THE UTILITY OF INFORMATION FOR THE PATIENT
BARRIERS IN IMPLEMENTATION
SYSTEM IMPLEMENTATION SOLUTIONS
CONCLUSIONS
REFERENCES

INTRODUCTION

The increasing prevalence and complications of endocrine and metabolic disorders such as diabetes *(1)* places a tremendous burden on affected individuals and will continue to strain the resources of health care systems and effective national health policy planning unless there are significant changes in health care delivery strategies. As such, diabetes serves as the quintessential model for demonstrating the value of evidence-based clinical practice. Large, well-designed clinical trials have provided convincing evidence that the risks of diabetes can be altered by appropriate treatment *(2–9)*, and based on these trials the goals of treatment have been expanded from glycemic control to include lipid and blood pressure outcomes. At the same time that professional societies are calling for lower and lower targets *(10–12)*, the complexity of medical decision making has increased for both the patient and health care team. Informed treatment decision making will require that the physician, health care team, and patients are fully informed *(13)*.

Outcomes in diabetes are dependent on the patient's health behavior, guided by the primary-care team. Integrating self-management support for the patient and intensification of treatment appears necessary to improve metabolic outcomes *(14–16)*. Therefore, systems are needed that support both the patient's self-management as well as the

From: *Contemporary Endocrinology: Evidence-Based Endocrinology*
Edited by: V. M. Montori © Mayo Foundation for Medical Education and Research

primary-care team's guidance. Developments in information technology and the principles of evidence-based practice present an opportunity to improve care provided to patients with diabetes. The goal of evidence-based medicine (EBM) is to use the best available evidence in clinical decision making. The promise of information technology has been to improve the efficiency of clinical decision for the physician by organizing the available data from the individual patient and linking this data to the knowledge derived from the critical assessment of medical evidence. Information technology and EBM are hypothesized to facilitate knowledge, inform choice, and support patient self-management and training.

Using diabetes as a model, we will first describe what is known about how physicians and patients seek and acquire information and knowledge. We will give examples of practice redesign efforts ongoing in our institution for the effective implementation of decision-support systems to increase the utility of information in clinical decision making for both providers and patients. Finally, we will define barriers to effective implementation and possible solutions for overcoming these barriers.

INFORMATION FOR THE PHYSICIAN

A number of diverse physician learning strategies have been found to be effective *(17)* and these processes are enhanced if there is an opportunity to ask questions that are directly applicable to the patient. Because physicians appear to learn best during the patient-care encounter, decision-support systems at the point of care are much more likely to influence practice patterns than traditional didactic lectures *(18)*. The need for knowledge at the point of care is increased by the proliferation of clinically relevant treatment goals and pharmaceutical choices for reaching these goals. Contrary to the Adult Learning Theory, where an individual is presumed to be self-directed and can identify what they need to know *(19)*, physicians often have difficulty with self assessment *(20,21)* or formulating the right questions and taking corrective action when necessary *(22–24)*. Depending on level of experience, clinicians ask an average of 0.6–1.5 questions per patient *(25,26)* and are more likely to ask and pursue answers if the questions are important and are easily accessible *(27)*. Up to two-thirds of questions remain unanswered because of lack of time, skills to formulate answerable questions, and access to the necessary information at the point of care *(25,28)*. The most commonly used resources for primary-care physicians have been consultations with colleagues (formal or informal), books, and journals *(29)*.

It has been said that practice based education should consider the learning environment and learner (e.g., physician and health care team) as more important than the information *(30,31)*. However, it is presumed that information in support of the clinical encounter will be valued if it is specific to the patient and provided in a format that is concise but flexible enough to permit a more in-depth review. Information and its presentation at the point of care needs to be able to adapt to time constraints of the clinical encounter as well as the dynamic stages of the learner that is either dependent, interested, involved, or self-directed *(32,33)*.

INFORMATION FOR THE PATIENT

Patients are felt to learn best when they need to know; they will gain knowledge when it relates to their everyday life. The conditions for optimal learning are multiple, and are influenced by the patient's own pre-existing knowledge and experiences *(34)*. The patient may have pre-existing positive or negative feelings for treatment and this will influence their acceptance and use of health information. In addition to life experiences, other factors such as age, maturity, locus of control, self-efficacy, goal-setting and problem-solving skills, and a desire to contribute also influence patient decision making and are attributes that may determine the best format and presentation of information by the health care team *(34,35)*.

Traditionally, patient education has been one way that the physician or health care team member provides expert knowledge and skills to the patient in support of self-management. Patients, however, are increasingly seeking more active involvement in medical decision making and in a horizontal relationship, attempting to provide "expert" insight into their own acceptance and ability to adhere to treatment advice. The pharmaceutical industry has increasingly recognized this, as is reflected in their direct to consumer (DTC) advertising, which approached $7.5 billion in spending in 2005 *(36)*. Oral diabetes medications account for 3% of all DTC ads, whereas 14% target lifestyle interventions such as smoking. Effectiveness, symptom control, innovativeness, and convenience are perceived to be important issues in DTC approaches for people with diabetes *(36)*. Framing of information and visual cues are important, and are used to emphasize the patient's identification with the clinical situation, motivators, and the value of adherence in treatment *(37–40)*. Incentives are common and for diabetes these have been most often informational.

IMPROVING THE UTILITY OF INFORMATION FOR THE PROVIDER

Evidence-Based Medicine at the Point of Care

Similar to other chronic disease management, diabetes care has evolved from an acute medical model to a planned chronic care model that is based on regularly scheduled visits using a team approach *(41,42)*. In this setting, the encounter ideally provides time for patient concerns and integrates six interrelated aspects: (1) self-management support, (2) clinical information systems, (3) delivery system redesign, (4) decision support, (5) health care organization, and (6) community resources. Health care organization is fundamentally important in the success of the planned chronic care and, because of the time constraints, efficient information and knowledge systems in support of EBM play a critical role. In the context of the chronic care model, small group sessions *(43,44)*, outreach *(45–50)*, academic detailing *(51)*, audits and feedback *(52)*, disease registries *(53–56)*, and electronic management systems *(57,58)* are all formats that have been used with variable success.

Asking relevant clinical questions during the course of a patient encounter has become easier as access to online information resources has increased, but the integration and use of such technologies into clinical practice has been slow for a number of reasons. Physicians who see more patients per hour ask fewer questions *(59)* and those health care providers who are skilled in the processes of asking questions and searching the literature *(60)* do so less than 1% of the time *(25)*. If physicians find answers, they do not always feel comfortable critically assessing the quality of the studies or their appropriateness for a specific patient *(61)*. A set of criteria has been published to help users assess the validity of evidence *(62)*. In addition, a number of publications offer critically appraised articles (e.g., *ACP Journal Club, Evidence-based Medicine, Clinical Evidence, Cochrane Collaboration of Systematic Reviews, Critically-appraised topics* [CAT]-banks) and a number of web-based searchable knowledge resources (e.g., *Clineguide, Pier, UpToDate*) are available to physicians. To date, there is little evidence to critically assess how the busy clinician uses a systematic framework of assessment or use of these tools.

Point-of-Care Evidenced-Based Medicine and the Value of Information Technology

The purpose of continuing medical education (CME) is to provide current medical knowledge in the context of specialty-specific learning needs with the goal of just-in-time information to effectively answer questions arising in practice *(63)*. The traditional role of the endocrinologist in chronic illness care has been based on conventional advice and support through requested consultation or traditional CME. Just-in-time or point-of-care CME, as in other CME, should include a needs assessment, preferably a problem-based primary interactive intervention, and secondary interventions that enable and reinforce the initial intervention. In this respect, an understanding of physicians' prescribing and the counseling efforts of the health care team (e.g., a limited clinical data set) would help target continuing education interventions to improve intensification of treatment *(64,65)*.

To support appropriate intensification of treatment and to overcome the barriers of point-of-care CME, we have created a system of early detection of performance gaps for individual patients from a limited data set derived from the health care team's use of a diabetes management system *(66)*. When an individual patient's clinical data suggests an outcome gap defined by evidence-based treatment guidelines, this triggers the delivery of pre-appraised up-to-date evidence-based messages (EBMs) just in time to the point-of-care. Because of the risks of cardiovascular disease in diabetes *(67)*, we have focused on EBMs for cardiovascular risk reduction as it relates to therapy *(60)*. We feel that the crucial step in converting evidence into action is the EBM (*see* Fig. 1). Because our objective is to promote action, we have used positive framing and relative measures of risk *(68)*. In addition, the format of the messages has been developed to incorporate local circumstances or constraints and preferences of the members of the health care team (brief and fully referenced).

Using information systems and the delivery of EBMs and specialty advice in the setting of planned chronic care (what we refer to as Using Networks, Information Technology, and Education in Planned Care [UNITED Planned Care]), we provide a level of decision support for the primary-care team targeting a patient's performance and outcome gaps. In a pilot study of 205 clinical encounters involving 81 patients and 16 primary-care providers, UNITED Planned Care was well accepted and lead to significant improvement in metabolic outcomes when action was taken *(69)*. We believe this model of an adult-learning cycle provides a potentially new CME paradigm of continuous "medical evidence" at the point of care, which links directly to outcomes of care. This paradigm incorporates the most effective conceptual elements of CME—audit with feedback, preplanned and personalized feedback of prescribing behaviors, and feedback from peers *(70,71)*.

Evidence-based Message		ACE Inhibition & Diabetes
	In patients with diabetes, ACE inhibition over 5 years can lower the risk of combined vascular outcomes by 25%	
Study type:	Randomized Controlled Trial	**Article:** HOPE Study Investigators. Lancet v355 p255, 2000
Intervention control:	Ramipril 10 mgm/d vs Placebo	**National Guidelines:** ADA
Outcome:	Combined vascular outcome Relative Risk Reduction 0.25	**Local Guidelines:** ICSI
Patient Population:	3577 people with diabetes (55+ years, mean age 65.4 years), with prior cardiovascular event or at least one other cardiovascular risk factor, no clinical proteinuria, heart failure, or low ejection fraction.	
Evidens Summary:	Randomized (concealed allocation), blinded (patients, health care team, and outcome assessors), controlled 2x2 factorial design (ACE inhibition and use of Vitamin E) trial. Intervention and control group were equal with regards to a large number of patient demographic characteristics at the time of randomization and aside for the intervention, it is presumed that the each group was treated equally. Intention to treat analysis was used and follow-up was complete. Subgroup analysis noted the beneficial effects of ACE inhibition irrespective of a history of cardiovascular event, hypertension, microalbuminuria, type of diabetes, or current treatment for hyperglycemia.	

Fig. 1. Evidence-based message regarding the use of angiotensin receptor blocking agents in diabetes.

IMPROVING THE UTILITY OF INFORMATION FOR THE PATIENT

Health Information and Patient Access to Medical Evidence

Patients have increasing expectations for general and personal health information. Similar to CME goals for health care providers, the purpose of patient education is to provide current medical information in the context of patient's specific learning needs in a timely and effective way in order to provide knowledge and skills, as well as to answer questions arising in support of patient's self-management. No matter what the format, the content of patient health education should fit the individual patient's need for information that is simple or comprehensive, concrete or abstract *(72)*.

Pamphlets, brochures, books, and videos have been used to reinforce information discussed within health care encounters and their use have had inconsistent effects in the retention (more than 1 yr) of knowledge *(14,73–76)*. Touch-screen or other stand-alone computer-based information systems have had success in the transfer of knowledge with mixed results in improvement of metabolic control *(77–79)*. A significant fraction of Internet users have searched for health information on-line. A Harris Interactive study in 2002 found that 66% of the population in the United States used the Internet, with 80% of these users having searched for health care information at least once *(80)*. The percent of the population with on-line access is somewhat lower in Europe and Japan, but is increasing rapidly with a majority of people using the Internet as one source of health care information. Sixty-one percent of people who seek health information on-line believe the Internet has improved their ability to self-manage their chronic illnesses *(81)*.

Despite the wealth of information available to the individual patient, a gap exists between the goals recommended for diabetes care and the care patients actually receive *(82)*.

A systematic review of self-management education and support has concluded that behavior-change strategies are more effective than didactic patient education in improving metabolic control *(83,84)*. In addition to knowledge, intensification of treatment and changes in attitude-motivation are needed to affect change *(15,85,86)*. Confidence in one's abilities in self-management, and the belief that this will translate into positive outcomes (e.g., self-efficacy), is the theoretical construct for a collaborative model of diabetes care *(87)*. Lifestyle interventions in support of self-efficacy targeting weight loss *(88–92)*, glycemic control *(91–93)*, and diet-medication adherence have used individual and group sessions as well as telecare *(94–98)*. Small studies, heterogeneity of studies, and short-term interventions using telecare, including modem transmission of self-monitoring parameters (e.g., glycemia, blood pressure) *(99,100)*, telephonic counseling *(101–103)*, proctored web sites *(104–107)*, and e-mail *(108–112)* have yet to suggest that these interventions are associated with a significant effect.

Patient Care and Telecare

MAYO TRACK

Guide to Good Care is an example of an on-line personalized course of 35 articles that cover the full range of topics suggested by the American Diabetes Association (ADA) for a comprehensive diabetes self-management program. The articles are written at a level that can be understood by most adult users of the Internet and at an educational level that is higher than that typical of printed brochures distributed in the clinical setting. Illustrations and animations enhance the content in the text. The articles are chosen based on a 15-item registration questionnaire. Some of the items are objective questions about health status, whereas others elicit responses about lifestyle and attitudes. Adapting the course to the individual is important to maintain interest and motivation. For example, the patient without retinopathy needs an article on how to prevent this complication, whereas the patient requiring laser treatment for retinopathy would find an article on preventing retinopathy inappropriate and discouraging. Most topics that comprise the course are written from several perspectives. There are almost 250,000 unique combinations of articles based on responses to the registration questionnaire.

To further improve the utility of the information provided to the patients, there are questions at the end of each article in the Mayo Track course that test comprehension and also register the completion of that topic. Patients can track their own progress through the course and are aware that their diabetes educator is following along with them. Alerts are automatically sent to the diabetes educator by the program's software if the patient is inactive for a number of weeks or answers too many questions incorrectly. This feature allows the diabetes educator to identify patients who may be having difficulty and to offer these patients extra encouragement and assistance as necessary.

A Personal Scorecard in MayoTrack allows the individual patient to compare their current results to the guidelines of the ADA. Goals for the patient are set with the patient's physician that are appropriate for the individual and may differ from the guidelines for reasons such as hypoglycemic unawareness. The selected outcome measures include recommended frequency of physician appointments, body mass index, blood pressure, and foot exam, as well as the laboratory measures of HbA1c, cholesterol profile, and urine albumin. Each of these measures is explained for the patient on the same web page as their personal data and goals.

The final concept, and one we feel is critical in demonstrating value in patient decision support systems, is effective communication with the primary-care team. Issues of importance to the patient can be discussed with the diabetes educator using the *Message Center* feature of MayoTrack. The tracking features of the MayoTrack program also allow the diabetes educator to send appropriate reminders to the patient to encourage participation in self-management training and behaviors to reach diabetes care goals. MayoTrack differs from standard e-mail by using the encryption features of web-browsers to secure the messages that are exchanged. Diabetes self-management support, provided by nonphysician clinicians using evidence based protocols and telecare, can reinforce goals set during the traditional clinical encounter as well as free up resources (e.g., clinical encounter appointments) to deliver more intensive advice and support to patients requiring face to face encounters *(113)*.

Evidence in Support of Telecare

Clinical trials of on-line interventions to change diet or physical activity patterns, although limited, have reported encouraging results for a subset of participants *(114,115)*. The success of these programs has been limited by high dropout rates and declining intensity of participation with duration of enrollment. These barriers may be overcome by linking the on-line self-management programs to the participant's medical care in the clinic with support by allied health professionals who are known to the patient. For example, MayoTrack and NovoTrack are identical on-line diabetes self-management training programs for patients. NovoTrack is available in the United States direct to Internet users without support by a diabetes educator or a connection to the patient's clinic. In a recent evaluation, almost half of registered NovoTrack users returned to the site. Of those who completed at least 1 article, 35% completed more than 5 articles, but only 9% completed more than 30 of the 35 articles in the course. In contrast to NovoTrack, MayoTrack is an integral part of the participant's medical care and is supported by a nurse who is known to the participant from clinic visits. Adding the connection to the clinic encourages a high level of participation. Of the participants in the MayoTrack clinical trial who completed at least 1 article, 58% completed more than 30 articles. The high proportion of course completion persisted across differences in age, gender, educational achievement, and diabetes treatment *(116)*.

BARRIERS IN IMPLEMENTATION

Information systems that can define performance and outcome gaps for patients are essential elements in the support of EBMs and the UNITED Planned Care model *(56,66,117)*. We, along with others, have reported that use of these systems can improve compliance with the process of care delivery by providers in both primary and specialty settings *(57,58,69)*. Despite this, the current use of such systems in care delivery by physicians is less than 15% *(118)*. A variety of barriers explain the lack of incorporation of information systems into the clinical work flow, but the time and expense of data entry into management systems or registries is felt to be the single biggest obstacle for cost-effective solutions *(118)*.

Patient-interactive decision-support systems such as MayoTrack (that effectively interface with the health care team) also require additional time in proctoring. To date in the MayoTrack Clinical Trial, more than 69% of participants have sent at least one message to the diabetes educator. Of those participants sending messages, the average number was 3.0 with an average text of 78 words each. The diabetes educator sent an average of 3.7 messages with an average text of 92 words each. Assuming 10 min per message, the time required of the diabetes educator to support the typical participant was 37 min over 6 mo. Whereas at present not a reimbursable activity, if this type of decision support for patients can be demonstrated to have value, then it has the potential to provide cost-effective educational support to a broader range of patients than are currently served by accredited diabetes self-management training programs.

SYSTEM IMPLEMENTATION SOLUTIONS

Provider

In response to the barriers of data entry, some solutions in the use of information systems have included the collection of a more limited data-set in disease registries (119), the retrospective targeted data retrieval of automated administrative data-sets (120), linking automated administrative data-sets (121), and XML identification, capture, and creation of concept-oriented views of clinical text with mapping to knowledge-based systems (122). Alternatively, a design element of the Diabetes Electronic Management System (DEMS) emphasizes the point-of-care capture, documentation, and reporting of information while de-emphasizing the need for traditional provider dictation and transcription and the time and costs associated with this activity (66,123). Data entry by the user is primarily by predefined data responses using pick lists, drop-down boxes, and radial buttons. Through a companion DEMS Transcription Tool, the provider can dictate via modular transcription or keyboard, free text entries to supplement the systematic capture of clinical information prompted by DEMS (66).

The successful implementation of DEMS into primary care has required clinical practice redesign in support of three key concepts: (1) pre-evaluation sessions occurring prior to the clinical encounter for providers using DEMS (124), (2) decentralized diabetes education that occurs in primary care (125), and (3) audit encounters (126). Cost analysis during a pilot of this practice redesign and use of DEMS, revealed a reduction in relative cost of 20%, because of appropriate work assignment to a clinical assistant, guided through the pre-evaluation session by the management system, the lack of physician dictation (and transcription of that dictation), and a positive impact on coding revenue based on appropriate documentation of the clinical encounter. Additional cost savings resulted from the amount of clinical and laboratory information that was available to an auditor when using the management system and an audit encounter for the provision of performance metrics to accrediting organizations. Finally, the use of DEMS by the diabetes educator in documentation of their clinical activity served to create and enhance the primary-care team's use of DEMS as a disease management registry and facilitated the effective delivery of EBMs and specialty advice in the UNITED Planned Care model. This appears to positively impact on the processes of care and metabolic outcomes, which would be expected to translate into additional cost savings.

Patient

There are significant gaps in our knowledge of effective strategies in support of diabetes care. Additional studies are needed to identify the predictors of metabolic control, and it seems clear that behavioral theory will have an explicit role in improving the self-management of chronic illness. As an example, in a clinical trial with 123 participants using MayoTrack completed in October 2003, participants who were randomly assigned to immediate access to the program had a statistically significant decrease in A1c of 0.6%. Participants in this group with an A1c greater than 8% had a greater decrease in A1c of 1.6%. Participants whose access to the program was delayed by 6 mo also had a decrease in A1c of 0.3% for the full group and 0.6% for the subgroup with baseline A1c values greater than 8%. The difference between the immediate and the delayed access groups was not statistically significant. When the delayed access group was given access to the program there was no further improvement in the A1c values, though the initial gains were maintained.

Patient interventions will need to be practical, feasible, low cost, and cost effective in a variety of settings for large patient populations. The MayoTrack program is now being offered to patients at the Mayo Clinic in Jacksonville, Florida as a subscription service that is not covered by insurance. The charge for the program is similar to on-line weight-loss programs, such as Weight Watchers, and is just sufficient to cover the services of the diabetes educator who preceptors the program.

CONCLUSIONS

To bring clinical practice closer to the diabetes care recommendations will require changes in health care delivery. More frequent and longer appointments with the physician in the clinic are not viable options. Practice redesign in support of specialty electronic management systems in the clinical setting can permit the physician to spend more time in review and counseling with the patient and less time in documentation. The short-term cost savings in data collection can support the significant challenge in creation of a clinical data set to support the effective management of chronic disease. Information systems that demonstrate the ability to offer continuous medical information and evidence at the point of care, and extend care from the clinic into the patient's home, may provide an opportunity to reduce the long-term costs (e.g., complications and health care dollar) of diabetes. The lessons we learn in system re-design in support of diabetes will have wide application to other chronic disease.

ACKNOWLEDGMENT

According to Mayo Foundation policy, Dr. Smith is 1 of 16 inventors of DEMS for which all royalties will support education and clinical research in the care of people with diabetes mellitus.

REFERENCES

1. Engelgau MM, Geiss LS, Saaddine JB, et al. The evolving diabetes burden in the United States. Ann Intern Med, 2004;140:945–950.
2. Group, DR. The effect of intensive treatment of diabetes on the development and progression of long-term complications insulin-dependent diabetes mellitus. N Engl J Med 1993;329:977–986.

3. UK Prospective Diabetes Study (UKPDS) Group. Effect of intensive blood-glucose control with metformin on complications in overweight patients with type 2 diabetes (UKPDS 34). Lancet 1998;352: 854–865.

4. UK Prospective Diabetes Study (UKPDS) Group. Intensive blood-glucose control with sulfonylureas or insulin compared with conventional treatment and risk of complications in patients with type 2 diabetes (UKPDS 33). Lancet 1998;352:837–853.

5. UK Prospective Diabetes Study (UKPDS) Group. Tight blood pressure control and risk of macrovascular and microvascular complications in type 2 diabetes: UKPDS 38. BMJ 1998;317:703–713.

6. UK Prospective Diabetes Study (UKPDS) Group. Efficacy of atenolol and captopril in reducing risk of macrovascular and microvascular complications in type 2 diabetes: UKPDS 39. BMJ 1998;317: 713–720.

7. Pyorala K, Pedersen TR, Kjekshus J, Faergeman O, Olsson AG, Thorgeirsson G. Cholesterol lowering with simvastatin improves prognosis of diabetic patients with coronary heart disease. A subgroup analysis of the Scandinavian Simvastatin Survival Study (4S). Diabetes Care 1997 20:614–620.

8. Heart Outcomes Prevention Evaluation Study Investigators. Effects of ramipril on cardiovascular and microvascular outcomes in people with diabetes mellitus: results of the HOPE study and MICRO-HOPE substudy. Lancet 2000;355:253–259.

9. Collins R, Armitage J, Parish S, Sleigh P, Peto R; Heart Protection Study Collaborative Group. MRC/BHF Heart Protection Study of cholesterol-lowering with simvastatin in 5963 people with diabetes: a randomised placebo-controlled trial. Lancet 2003;361:2005–2016.

10. Fleming BB, Greenfield S, Engelgau MM, Pogach LM, Clauser SB, Parrott MA. The Diabetes Quality Improvement Project: Moving science into health policy to gain an edge on the diabetes epidemic. Diabetes Care 2001;24:1815–1820.

11. American Diabetes Association. Standards of medical care for patients with diabetes mellitus. Diabetes Care 2004;27:S15–S35.

12. Grundy SM, Cleeman JI, Merz CN, et al., for the Coordinating Committee of the National Cholesterol Education Program. Implications of recent clinical trials for the National Cholesterol Education Program Adult Treatment Panel III guidelines. Circulation 2004;110:227–239.

13. Charles C, Gafni A, Whelan T. Shared decision-making in the medical encounter: What does it mean? (Or, it takes at least two to tango). Soc Sci Med 1997;44:681–692.

14. Bloomgarden ZT, Karmally W, Metzger MJ, et al. Randomized, controlled trial of diabetic patient education: improved knowledge without improved metabolic status. Diabetes Care 1987;10:263–272.

15. de Weerdt I, Visser AP, Kok GJ, de Weerdt O, van der Veen EA. Randomized controlled multicentre evaluation of an education programme for insulin-treated diabetic patients: effects on metabolic control, quality of life, and costs of therapy. Diabet Med 1991;8:338–345.

16. Phillips LS, Branch WT, Cook CB, et al. Clinical inertia. Ann Intern Med 2001;135:825–834.

17. Oxman AD, Thomson MA, Davis DA, Haynes RB. No magic bullets: a systematic review of 102 trials of interventions to improve professional practice. CMAJ 1995;153:1423–1431.

18. Davis D, O'Brien MA, Freemantle N, Wolf FM, Mazmanian P, Taylor-Vaisey A. Impact of formal continuing medical education: do conferences, workshops, rounds, and other traditional continuing education activities change physician behavior or health care outcomes? JAMA 1999;282:867–874.

19. Shannon, S. Adult learning and CME. Lancet 2003;361:266.

20. Reiter HI, Eva KW, Hatala RM, Norman GR. Self and peer assessment in tutorials: application of a relative-ranking model. Acad Med 2002;77:1134–1139.

21. Rudy DW, Fejfar MC, Griffith CH 3rd, Wilson JF. Self- and peer assessment in a first-year communication and interviewing course. Eval Health Prof 2001;24:436–445.

22. Crilly M. General practitioners' self assessment of knowledge. Knowledge gaps were identified by general practitioners. BMJ 1998;316:1610.

23. Sibley JC, Sackett DL, Neufeld V, Gerrard B, Rudnick KV, Fraser W. A randomized trial of continuing medical education. N Engl J Med 1982;306:511–515.

24. Tracey JM, Arroll B, Richmond DE, Barham PM. The validity of general practitioners' self assessment of knowledge: cross sectional study. BMJ 1997;315:1426–1428.

25. Ramos K, Linscheid R, Schafer S. Real-time information-seeking behavior of residency physicians. Fam Med 2003;35:257–260.

26. Barrie AR, Ward AM. Questioning behaviour in general practice: a pragmatic study. BMJ 1997;315: 1512–1515.

27. Smith R. What clinical information do doctors need? BMJ 1996;313:1062–1068.

28. Covell DG, Uman, GC, Manning PR. Information needs in office practice: are they being met? Ann Intern Med 1985;103:596–599.

29. Verhoeven AA, Boerma EJ, Meyboom-de Jong B. Use of information sources by family physicians: a literature survey. Bull Med Libr Assoc 1995;83:85–90.

30. Mowatt G, Grimshaw JM, Davis DA, Mazmanian PE. Getting evidence into practice: the work of the Cochrane Effective Practice and Organization of Care Group (EPOC). J Contin Educ Health Prof 2001;21:55–60.

31. Shannon S. Practice-based CME. Lancet 2003;361:618.

32. Newman P, Peile E. Valuing learners' experience and supporting further growth: educational models to help experienced adult learners in medicine. BMJ 2002;325:200–202.

33. Grow G. Teaching learners to be self-directed. Adult Educ Q 1991;41:125–149.

34. Trento M, Passera P, Borgo E, et al. A 5-year randomized controlled study of learning, problem solving ability, and quality of life modifications in people with type 2 diabetes managed by group care. Diabetes Care 2004;27:670–675.

35. Hunt LM, Arar NH, Larme AC. Contrasting patient and practitioner perspectives in type 2 diabetes management. West J Nurs Res 1998;20:656–676.

36. Bell RA, Kravitz RL, Wilkes MS. Direct-to-consumer prescription drug advertising, 1989–1998. A content analysis of conditions, targets, inducements, and appeals. J Fam Prac 2000;49:329–335.

37. Fortin JM, Hirota LK, Bond BE, O'Connor AM, Col NF. Identifying patient preferences for communicating risk estimates: a descriptive pilot study. BMC Med Inform Decis Mak 2001;1:2.

38. Welch Cline RJ, Young HN. Marketing drugs, marketing health care relationships: a content analysis of visual cues in direct-to-consumer prescription drug advertising. Health Commun 2004;16:131–157.

39. Holmer AF. Direct-to-consumer prescription drug advertising builds bridges between patients and physicians. JAMA 1999;281:380–382.

40. Bell RA, Kravitz RL, Wilkes MS. Direct-to-consumer prescription drug advertising and the public. J Gen Intern Med 1999;14:651–657.

41. Bodenheimer T, Wagner EH, Grumbach K. Improving primary care for patients with chronic illness: the chronic care model, Part 2. JAMA 2002;288:1775–1779.

42. Bodenheimer T, Wagner EH, Grumbach K. Improving primary care for patients with chronic illness. JAMA 2002;288:1909–1914.

43. Pereles L, Lockyer J, Fidler H. Permanent small groups: group dynamics, learning, and change. J Contin Educ Health Prof 2002;22:205–213.

44. Premi J, Shannon S, Hartwick K, Lamb S, Wakefield J, Williams J. Practice-based small-group CME. Acad Med 1994;69:800–802.

45. Ricordeau P, Durieux P, Weill A, et al. Effect of a nationwide program of educational outreach visits to improve the processes of care for patients with type 2 diabetes. Int J Technol Assess Health Care 2003;19:705–710.

46. Bernal-Delgado E, Galeote-Mayor M, Pradas-Arnal F, Peiro-Moreno S. Evidence based educational outreach visits: effects on prescriptions of non-steroidal anti-inflammatory drugs. J Epidemiol Community Health 2002;56:653–658.

47. Tan KM. Influence of educational outreach visits on behavioral change in health professionals. J Contin Educ Health Prof 2002;22:122–124.

48. Watson M, Gunnell D, Peters T, Brookes S, Sharp D. Guidelines and educational outreach visits from community pharmacists to improve prescribing in general practice: a randomised controlled trial. J Health Serv Res Policy 2001;6:207–213.

49. New JP, Mason JM, Freemantle N, et al. Educational outreach in diabetes to encourage practice nurses to use primary care hypertension and hyperlipidaemia guidelines (EDEN): a randomized controlled trial. Diab Med 2004;21:599–603.

50. Thomson O'Brien MA, Oxman AD, Davis DA, Haynes RB, Freemantle N, Harvey EL. Educational outreach visits: effects on professional practice and health care outcomes. Cochrane Database Syst Rev 2000;(2):CD000409.

51. Thomson O'Brien MA, Oxman AD, Haynes RB, Davis DA, Freemantle N, Harvey EL. Local opinion leaders: effects on professional practice and health care outcomes. Cochrane Database Syst Rev 2000;(2):CD000125.

52. Thomson O'Brien MA, Oxman AD, Davis DA, Haynes RB, Freemantle N, Harvey EL. Audit and feedback: effects on professional practice and health care outcomes. Cochrane Database Syst Rev 2000;(2):CD000259.

53. Dugas M, Hoffmann E, Janko S, et al. Complexity of biomedical data models in cardiology: the Intranet-based AF registry. Comput Methods Programs Biomed 2002;68:49–61.

54. Stroebel RJ, Scheitel SM, Fitz JS, et al. A randomized trial of three diabetes registry implementation strategies in a community internal medicine practice. Jt Comm J Qual Improv 2002;28:441–450.

55. Metzger J, Haughton J, Smithson K. Improvement-focused information technology for the clinical office practice: a patient registry for disease management. Manag Care Q 1999;7:67–74.

56. Dinneen SF, Bjornsen SS, Bryant SC, et al. Towards an optimal model for community-based diabetes care: design and basline data from the Mayo Health System Diabetes Translation Project. J Eval Clin Pract, 2000;6:421–429.

57. Montori VM, Dinneen SF, Gorman CA, et al. for the Translation Project Investigator Group. The impact of planned care and a diabetes electronic management system on community-based diabetes care. The Mayo Health System Diabetes Translation Project. Diabetes Care 2002;25:1952–1957.

58. Smith SA, Murphy ME, Huschka TR, et al. Impact of a diabetes electronic management system on the care of patients seen in a subspecialty diabetes clinic. Diabetes Care 1998;21:972–976.

59. Ely JW, Burch, RJ, Vinson DC. The information needs of family physicians: case-specific clinical questions. J Fam Pract 1992;35:265–269.

60. Ely JW, Osheroff JA, Ebell MH, et al. Analysis of questions asked by family doctors regarding patient care. BMJ 1999;19:358–361.

61. McAlister FA, Graham I, Karr GW, Laupacis A. Evidence-based medicine and the practicing clinician. J Gen Intern Med 1999;14:236–242.

62. Oxman AD, Sackett, DL, Guyatt, G. Users' guides to the medical literature: I. How to get started. JAMA 1993;270:2093–2095.

63. Manning P, DeBakey L. Continuing medical education: the paradigm is changing. J Contin Educ Health Prof 2001;21:46–54.

64. Beaulieu MD, Dufresne L, LeBlanc D. Treating hypertension. Are the right drugs given to the right patients? Can Fam Physician 1998;44:294–298.

65. Boissel JP, Cucherat M, Amsallem E, et al. Getting evidence to prescribers and patients or how to make EBM a reality. Stud Health Technol Inform 2003;95:554–559.

66. Gorman CA, Zimmerman BR, Smith SA, et al. DEMS- a second generation diabetes electronic management system. Comput Methods Programs Biomed 2000;62:127–140.

67. Geiss L, Herman W, Smith P. Mortality in non-insulin dependent diabetes. In: Harris MD, ed., Diabetes in America. National Institutes of Health, Bethesda, MD, 1995, pp. 233–255.

68. McGettigan P, Sly K, O'Connell D, Hill S, Henry D. The effects of information framing on the practices of physicians. J Gen Intern Med 1999;14:633–642.

69. Montori VM, Smith SA. Information Systems in diabetes: in search of the Holy Grail in the era of evidence-based diabetes care. Exp Clin Endocrinol Diabetes 2001;109:S358–S372.

70. Cantillon P, Jones R. Does continuing medical education in general practice make a difference? BMJ 1999;318:1276–1279.

71. Kiefe CI, Allison JJ, Williams OD, Person SD, Weaver MT, Weissman NW. Improving quality improvement using achievable benchmarks for physician feedback: a randomized controlled trial. JAMA 2001;285:2871–2879.

72. Selander S, Troein M, Finnegan J Jr, Rastam L. The discursive formation of health. A study of printed health education material used in primary care. Patient Educ Couns 1997;31:181–189.

73. Mulrow C, Bailey S, Sonksen PH, Slavin B. Evaluation of an Audiovisual Diabetes Education Program: negative results of a randomized trial of patients with non-insulin-dependent diabetes mellitus. J Gen Intern Med 1987;2:215–219.

74. McCulloch DK, Mitchell RD, Ambler J, Tattersall RB. Influence of imaginative teaching of diet on compliance and metabolic control in insulin dependent diabetes. Br Med J (Clin Res Ed) 1983;287:1858–1861.

75. Boundouki G, Humphris G, Field A. Knowledge of oral cancer, distress and screening intentions: longer term effects of a patient information leaflet. Patient Educ Couns 2004;53:71–77.

76. Boekeloo BO, Jerry J, Lee-Ougo WI, et al. Randomized trial of brief office-based interventions to reduce adolescent alcohol use. Arch Pediatr Adolesc Med 2004;158:635–642.

77. Wise PH, Dowlatshahi DC, Farrant S, Fromson S, Meadows KA. Effect of computer-based learning on diabetes knowledge and control. Diabetes Care 1986;9:504–508.

78. Turnin MC, Beddok RH, Clottes JP, et al. Telematic expert system Diabeto. New tool for diet self-monitoring for diabetic patients. Diabetes Care 1992;15:204–212.

79. Glasgow RE, Toobert DJ, Hampson SE. Effects of a brief office-based intervention to facilitate diabetes dietary self-management. Diabetes Care 1996;19:835–842.

80. The Harris Poll. Four nation survey shows widespread but different levels of Internet use for health purposes. Harris Interactive Health Care News, 2002;2:1–4.

81. Fox SF, Rainie L. How Internet users decide what information to trust when they or their loved ones are sick. In: Vital Decisions. Pew Internet and American Life Project: Washington, DC, 2002.

82. Saaddine JB, Engelgau MM, Beckles GL, Gregg EW, Thompson TJ, Narayan KM. A diabetes report care for the United States: quality of care in the 1990s. Ann Intern Med 2002;136:565–574.

83. Norris SL, Nichols PJ, Caspersen CJ, et al. Increasing diabetes self-management education in community settings. A systematic review. Am J Prev Med 2002;22:39–66.

84. Clement S. Diabetes self-management education. Diabetes Care 1995;18:1204–1214.

85. Korhonen T, Huttunen JK, Aro A, et al. A controlled trial on the effects of patient education in the treatment of insulin-dependent diabetes. Diabetes Care 1983;6:256–261.

86. Lockington TJ, Farrant S, Meadows KA, Dowlatshahi D, Wise PH. Knowledge profile and control in diabetic patients. Diabet Med 1988;5:381–386.

87. Glasgow RE, Anderson RM. In diabetes care, moving from compliance to adherence is not enough. Something entirely different is needed. Diabetes Care 1999;22:2090–2092.

88. Hillier TA, Pedula KL. Characteristics of an adult population with newly diagnosed type 2 diabetes: the relation of obesity and age of onset. Diabetes Care 2001;24:1522–1527.

89. D'Eramo-Melkus GA, Wylie-Rosett J, Hagan JA. Metabolic impact of education in NIDDM. Diabetes Care 1992;15:864–869.

90. Glasgow RE, Toobert DJ, Mitchell DL, Donnelly JE, Calder D. Nutrition education and social learning interventions for type II diabetes. Diabetes Care 1989;12:150–152.

91. Agurs-Collins TD, Kumanyika SK, Ten Have TR, Adams-Campbell LL. A randomized controlled trial of weight reduction and exercise for diabetes management in older African-American subjects. Diabetes Care 1997;20:1503–1511.

92. Kaplan RM, Hartwell SL, Wilson DK, Wallace JP. Effects of diet and exercise interventions on control and quality of life in non-insulin-dependent diabetes mellitus. J Gen Intern Med 1987;2: 220–228.

93. Raz I, Soskolne V, Stein P. Influence of small-group education sessions on glucose homeostasis in NIDDM. Diabetes Care 1988;11:67–71.

94. DeMolles DA, Sparrow D, Gottlieb DJ, Friedman R.A pilot trial of a telecommunications system in sleep apnea management. Med Care 2004;42:764–769.

95. Akerblad AC, Bengtsson F, Ekselius L, von Knorring L. Effects of an educational compliance enhancement programme and therapeutic drug monitoring on treatment adherence in depressed patients managed by general practitioners. Int Clin Psychopharmacol 2003;18:347–354.

96. Kennedy A, Nelson E, Reeves D, et al. A randomised controlled trial to assess the impact of a package comprising a patient-orientated, evidence-based self-help guidebook and patient-centred consultations on disease management and satisfaction in inflammatory bowel disease. Health Technol Assess 2003;7:1–113.

97. Krueger KP, Felkey BG, Berger BA. Improving adherence and persistence: a review and assessment of interventions and description of steps toward a national adherence initiative. JAMA 2003;43: 668–678.

98. Peterson AM, Takiya L, Finley R. Meta-analysis of interventions to improve drug adherence in patients with hyperlipidemia. Pharmacotherapy 2003;23:80–87.

99. Chase HP, Pearson JA, Wightman C, Roberts MD, Oderberg AD, Garg SK. Modem transmission of glucose values reduces the costs and need for clinic visits. Diabetes Care 2003;26:1475–1479.

100. Montori VM, Helgemoe PK, Guyatt GH, et al. Telecare for patients with type 1 diabetes and inadequate glycemic control—A randomized controlled trial and meta-analysis. Diabetes Care 2004;27: 1088–1094.

101. King AC, Friedman R, Marcus B, et al. Harnessing motivational forces in the promotion of physical activity: the Community Health Advice by Telephone (CHAT) project. Health Educ Res 2002;17: 627–636.

102. Strecher V, Wang C, Derry H, Wildenhaus K, Johnson C. Tailored interventions for multiple risk behaviors. Health Educ Res 2002;17:619–626.

103. Dietrich AJ. The telephone as a new weapon in the battle against depression. Eff Clin Pract 2000;3: 191–193.

104. Umefjord G, Petersson G, Hamberg K. Reasons for consulting a doctor on the Internet: Web survey of users of an Ask the Doctor service. J Med Internet Res 2003;5:22.
105. Abbott KC, Boocks CE, Sun Z, Boal TR, Poropatich RK. Walter Reed Army Medical Center's Internet-based electronic health portal. Mil Med 2003;168:986–991.
106. Bhavnani SK, Bichakjian CK, Schwartz JL, et al. Getting patients to the right healthcare sources: from real-world questions to strategy hubs. Proc AMIA Symp 2002:51–55.
107. Labiris G, Coertzen I, Katsikas A, Karydis A, Petounis A. An eight-year study of internet-based remote medical counselling. J Telemed Telecare 2002;8:222–225.
108. Perlemuter L, Yomtov B. Modem transmission of glucose values reduces the costs of and need for clinic visits: response to Chase et al. Diabetes Care 2003;26:2969–70.
109. Hobbs J, Wald J, Jagannath YS, et al. Opportunities to enhance patient and physician e-mail contact. Int J Med Inform 2003;70:1–9.
110. Kittler AF, Wald JS, Volk LA, et al. The role of primary care non-physician clinic staff in e-mail communication with patients. Int J Med Inform 2004;73:333–340.
111. Kawasaki S, Ito S, Satoh S, et al. Use of telemedicine in periodic screening of diabetic retinopathy. Telemed J E Health 2003;9:235–239.
112. Gaster B, Knight CL, DeWitt DE, et al. Physicians' use of and attitudes toward electronic mail for patient communication. J Gen Intern Med 2003;18:385–9.
113. Hirsch IB. The burden of diabetes (care). Diabetes Care 2003;26:1613–1614.
114. McKay HG, King D, Eakin EG, Seeley JR, Glasgow RE. The Diabetes Network Internet based physical activity intervention. A randomized study. Diabetes Care 2001;24:1328–1334.
115. Tate DF, Wing RR, Winett RA. Using Internet technology to deliver a behavioral weight loss program. JAMA 2001;285:1172–1177.
116. Gates GS, Coyle CG, Smith RD, Meutel JJ. Interactive diabetes education online: the development of MayoTrack and NovoTrack. International Diabetes Monitor 2003;15:1–6.
117. Bonomi AE, Wagner EH, Glasgow RE, VonKorff M. Assessment of Chronic Illness Care (ACIC): a practical tool to measure quality improvement. Health Serv Res 2002;37:791–821.
118. Loomis GA, Ries JS, Saywell RM Jr, Thakker NR. If electronic medical records are so great, why aren't family physicians using them? J Fam Pract 2002;51:636–641.
119. Chambliss ML, Rasco T, Clark RD, Gardner JP. The mini electronic medical record: a low-cost, low-risk partial solution. J Dam Pract 2001;50:1063–1065.
120. Nichols GA, Hillier TA, Erbey JR, Brown JB.Congestive heart failure in type 2 diabetes: prevalence, incidence, and risk factors. Diabetes Care 2001;24:1614–1619.
121. Selby J. Linking automated databases for research in managed care settings. Ann Intern Med 1997;127:719–724.
122. Zeng Q, Cimino JJ, Zou KH. Providing concept-oriented views for clinical data using a knowledge-based system: an evaluation. JAMA 2002;9:294–305.
123. Gorman CA. Electronic medical record—-promises, promises! Ulster Med J 1998;67:91–94.
124. Jorgensen B, Bjornsen S, Hanson P, et al. Integration an electronic medical record into a clinical office visit. Diabetes Nutr Metab 1998;11:22.
125. Bjornsen SS, Dinneen S, Drake J, et al. Diabetes education in the electronic era: old wine in new skins. Diabetes Nutr Metab 1998;11:48.
126. Bjornsen SS, Murphy M, Holm D, et al. A New Paradigm for Health Care Audits and Use of an Electronic Audit Tool. In: Health Service Research: Implications for Policy, Delivery, and Practice, Washington D.C., 1998, pp. 48.

8 Supporting Patients' Participation in Decision Making

Annette M. O'Connor, RN, MScN, PhD,
Dawn Stacey, BScN, MScN, PhD,
and France Légaré, MD, MSc, CCMF, FCMF

INTRODUCTION

Evidence-based medicine integrates clinical experience with patient's values using the best available evidence *(1)*. In the past, physicians acted as agents in the best interest of their patients *(2)*. These roles are now changing. Although physicians are still considered experts in diagnosing and identifying treatment options, patients are increasingly recognized as the best experts for judging values associated with options *(2–4)*. With the growing patient interest in participating in decision making about options, evidence-based decision aids have been developed to supplement physician counseling. These tools prepare patients for counseling by helping them (1) understand the probable consequences of options, (2) consider and clarify the value they place on the consequences, and (3) actively participating their physician when selecting the best option of treatment.

This chapter discusses practical and effective methods to help patients become involved in decision making. First, we explore the types of decisions in endocrine practice and the clinicians' roles in providing decision support. Next, we describe the

From: *Contemporary Endocrinology: Evidence-Based Endocrinology*
Edited by: V. M. Montori © Mayo Foundation for Medical Education and Research

---

Case Presentation Part I: Mrs. O.

Mrs. O., a 52-yr-old Asian woman, recently started on estrogen for hot flashes that disturbed her sleep and affected her ability to function at work and at home. She had a hysterectomy for fibroids 10 yr ago, but is otherwise healthy, with no risk factors for cardiovascular or thromboembolic disease, or breast cancer. A recent mammogram and breast exam were normal. Her mother was just hospitalized for osteoporotic fractures, which stimulated Mrs. O. to investigate her own risks.

Mrs. O.'s bone density test indicated osteoporosis (*T*-score = 2.5 standard deviations below normal). Her long-term treatment options were discussed. However, Mrs. O. was not sure of her preference and requested information and help with deliberation.

---

efficacy of practical tools, known as patient decision aids. Finally, we provide examples of how decision aids can be integrated into practice.

CLASSES OF DECISIONS IN ENDOCRINE PRACTICE

The ideal medical decision involves choosing an option that increases the *likelihood* of *valued* health outcomes and minimizes the chance of *undesired* consequences according to the best available scientific *evidence (1)*. In some cases, the best strategy is clear because the evidence of benefits and harms are known and the harms are minimal relative to the benefits. For these decisions, most clinicians would recommend an option and most informed patients, placing a greater value on benefits relative to harms, would see the value in taking it.

Unfortunately, many decisions in health care do not have clear answers because the benefit–harm ratios are unknown or the best choice depends on how patients value the benefits vs the harms of options. For these more difficult decisions, clinicians do not routinely recommend the option but provide access to information about benefits, harms, and scientific uncertainties so that patients can consider their associated values.

To guide practitioners and patients in understanding which decisions have clear answers and which ones do not, treatment options are being classified not only according to the strength of scientific evidence but also the magnitude of benefit–harm ratios *(5,6)*. When there is good evidence that benefits are large relative to harms, therapies are usually endorsed with stronger recommendations; in contrast, there is less endorsement when choices involve balancing benefits vs harms or when the evidence on outcomes is uncertain.

CLINICIANS' ROLES IN PROVIDING DECISION SUPPORT ACCORDING TO CLASS OF DECISIONS

There are both commonalities and differences in counseling according to the classifications for decisions. For both classes of decisions, the counselor's role is to facilitate the patient's participation in ways that respect the patient's values, personal resources, and capacity for self-determination. Patients feel welcome to participate in deliberation, planning, and implementing the negotiated option according to their needs. However, as described next, the directiveness, intensity, and focus of decision support are different.

Recommended Options

Counseling may be more directive when standards of care are involved. The rationale for the recommendation is provided as well as benefits and harms (*see* Case Presenta-

---

Case Presentation Part II:
Clinician Discusses Recommended Option (Calcium and Vitamin D)
With Mrs. O. Using a Motivational Counseling Style

Clarify Decision

Condition: "As you know, you have osteoporosis, which is . . ."

Evidence-based recommendation: "We routinely recommend taking calcium and vitamin D every day to because there is strong scientific evidence that the benefits are large compared to the [harms, side effects]."

Role: "But, **your opinion counts** in deciding whether to take it."

Benefits vs Harms

- On the benefit side.......Calcium and vitamin D prevents broken bones in the spine . . .
- On the harm side.........Most people (#) tolerate it well but a few (#) may have to stop it because of . . ."

Clarify Patient Values

- "What do you think?" "In your opinion, is lowering your chance of a broken spine more important to you than the side effects?"
- "Do you have other questions or concerns?"

Screen for Implementation Problems

- "How important is it for you to make this change?" (on a scale of 1 [low] to 10 [high])
- "How confident are you in making this change?" (on a scale of 1 to 10)

Refer for support if decisional or implementation difficulties detected.

---

tion Part II). Patients' beliefs and opinions are explored *(7)*. The majority of patients will acknowledge the greater value of the benefits compared to the harms.

Once agreement is reached on the best option, the focus of support can move from decision making to the more challenging task of implementing the decision, which frequently requires changing behavior and ensuring continuance of the chosen option. We know that greater than 50% of patients prescribed medications have difficulties with follow-though either because: (1) they are not convinced of the need or they have personal beliefs that do are not in accord with the benefits or risks associated with this medication; (2) someone important to them might not support this decision; or (3) there are too many barriers to making the changes necessary to take medications over the long term. As a consequence, from 15 to 25% do not fill their prescription and only 50% are taking treatment at 1 yr following a prescription *(8)*. Involving patients in their care can address these issues. Indeed, doing so improves control of their disease and continuance of therapy.

For implementation of the decision, a motivational interviewing strategy is effective in identifying patients' (1) beliefs, values, attitudes, priorities, motivations, and confidence in making the recommended change; and (2) personal barriers for uptake *(9)*. This counseling strategy reflects a change in emphasis from a passive "informed consent" process to a more active engagement, which has been called: "evidence-informed patient choice," "collaborative care," 'shared decision making," or "patient–physician concordance." The approach is of "patient-centered care" for which the patient is considered as a unique human being with the interaction aimed at seeing the situation through the individual patient's eyes (10–12). It includes sharing power and responsibility based on a therapeutic alliance in order to reach an agreement about the problem, the options and the role in decision making (13).

Close Call Decisions

Counseling for these types of decisions is usually nondirective, because the best choice for an individual depends on how the patient values the benefits, harms, and scientific uncertainties (see Table 1). There is no evidence-based "right" decision. Moreover, there is a need to describe options, benefits, harms, and scientific uncertainties in more detail in order to create realistic expectations, clarify values, and enable participation in decision making. To streamline the process, evidence-based decision aids have been developed to prepare patients for discussions with their practitioners. These improvements will lead to enhanced accountability, informed consent, and, in some situations, have the potential to reduce litigation (14).

Choices may or may not involve making a change in behavior (e.g., if status quo is an option or watchful waiting); in cases where it does, motivational and tailored interviewing described previously may be helpful to assist the individual with follow-through on their chosen option.

The criteria for judging success of counseling with these types of decisions can be challenging to identify because the outcomes are unknown or involve making value tradeoffs. For decisions requiring tradeoffs, we can expect that patients will experience both benefits and harms. The key is to determine the option whose potential harms patients find least objectionable, and whose benefits they value most. In other words, success is the extent to which the choice is informed and matches the patient's values. With this approach, it is assumed that patients may be more likely to stick with their choice and to express less regret over the negative consequences of the choice.

Patient Decision Aids

Patient decision aids (15) differ from conventional education materials by providing

---

Case Presentation Part III: Mrs. O.

Mrs. O.'s doctor told her that in the short term, because she was pleased with the relief of hot flashes, she could continue on estrogen for both menopausal symptoms and osteoporosis. However, the osteoporosis therapy needed to be taken long-term and she should consider other medication options (in addition to the calcium, vitamin D, and physical activity) to prevent further bone loss and subsequent fractures. The doctor arranged for her to review a decision aid outlining her options of staying on hormones for the year or switching to a bisphosphonate therapy now (see the appendix).

---

personalized information about the options, outcomes, probabilities, and uncertainties in sufficient detail for decision making, and by helping individuals clarify the personal desirability of the potential benefits relative to the potential harms (see Table 2). Many patient decision aids also include balanced examples of how others deliberate about options and guide people in the steps of collaborative decision making. They are deliv-

Table 1
Practitioners' Decision Support Process for Multiple Options
That Depend on Patient Values

Directiveness and Focus	No routine recommendation; usually no right or wrong choice. Nondirective counseling usually involving more detailed personalized information and values clarification. Focus on decision making is usually longer than for beneficial options. Choosing status quo (watchful waiting) is often a valid option; therefore focus on implementing change depends on choice.
Goals	*Decision Quality* **Informed** of available options, benefits, harms, probabilities, scientific uncertainties. **Choice matches patient values** for benefits, harms, scientific uncertainties.

Decision Support Process	**1. Clarify Decision and Decisional Support Needs**
	• Explain condition stimulating need for a decision.
	• Summarize options, benefits, harms, scientific uncertainties.
	• Assess preferred role in decision making.
	• Screen for decisional conflict regarding best option and deficits in knowledge, values clarity, and support.
	2. Address Decisional Support Needs
	• Provide or refer patient for decision support (with information, decision aids, and/or referral to other team members as needed).
	  – Guide patient in steps of decision making process.
	  – Provide information.
	  – Clarify values.
	  – Provide access to examples of others' decisions.
	  – Identify questions and leaning toward options.
	• Discuss understanding and questions, acknowledge values, and determine preferred option(s).
	3. Facilitate Progress in Stage of Decision Making
	• Obtain agreement regarding choice or commitment to take steps toward making a choice.
	4. Discuss Implementation of Choice (if choice involves change in status quo).
	• Assess patient's motivation and confidence to implement choice.
	• Discuss barriers to implementation and potential solutions.
	• Negotiate arrangements for implementation and follow-up.

ered as self-administered or practitioner-administered tools in one-to-one or group sessions. The media for delivery include decision boards, interactive computer programs, audio-guided workbooks, and pamphlets. Many developers now use more than one medium, several of whom are moving toward Internet-based delivery systems.

Effects of Decision Aids on Decision Quality

A systematic review of trials of patient decision aids *(15,16)* indicated that, when PtDAs are used as adjuncts to counseling, they have consistently superior effects relative to usual practices on the following indicators of decision quality:

• Increased knowledge scores, by 19 points out of 100 (95% confidence interval [CI]: 13,24);

Table 2
Patient Decision Aids: Key Elements

Minimal elements	Additional elements
• Information on options and their outcomes (benefits and harms)	• Information on the condition • Probabilities of benefits and harms • Methods for clarifying patient's values for (what matters most) benefits and harms • Balanced stories of others' experiences • Guidance/coaching in deliberating and communicating with their health practitioners

- Improvements in the proportion of patients with realistic perceptions of the chances of benefits and harms, by 40% (95% CI: 10, 90%);
- Lowered scores for decisional conflict (psychological uncertainty related to feeling uninformed), by 9 points out of 100 (95% CI: 6,12);
- Reduced proportions of patients who are passive in decision making, by 30% (95% CI: 10, 50%);
- Reduced proportions of people who remain undecided after counseling, by 57% (95% CI: 30, 70%); and
- Improved agreement between a patient's values and the option that is actually chosen.

In general, patient satisfaction with decision making has been high both for those who have had usual care or patient decision aids. A minority of studies (5 out of 15 trials; 33%) have shown an incremental benefit of patient decision aids on satisfaction. Patient decision aids have consistently shown no effect (beneficial or deleterious) on anxiety or depression.

More research is needed on which decision aids work best with which decisions and which types of patients. As well, evaluation is needed on their acceptability to diverse groups of practitioners and patients, their impact on patient–practitioner communication, and their effects on continuance with chosen options, preference-linked health outcomes, practice variations, and use of resources. There continue to be questions about the essential elements in decision aids and whether or not information is enough, as a minimum requirement.

There is a need to examine ways to integrate patient decision aids into clinical practice. In a recent qualitative study of practitioner's attitudes towards decision aids, response to open-ended questions suggested that there are four unique barriers/facilitators to implementing patient decision aids in general and specialty medical practices (17). The first barrier was awareness that the decision aid exists. Another barrier was accessibility to decision aids with recommendation from practitioners that this needs to be smooth, automatic, and timely. The third barrier was acceptability. Practitioners reported common logistical barriers (18); decision aids need to be compatible with their practice and personal beliefs, up-to-date, attractive, easy to use, and not require additional cost, time, or equipment. Finally, practitioners identified needing to feel motivated to use it by factors such as time saving, avoidance of repetition, not requiring extra calls from patients, potential to decrease liability, and improved rationing of health care with possibility of reducing wait-list pressures. For example, Internet-based decision aids have many advantages, including increased availability, decreased expenses, ease of updating, and access either within patients' homes, practitioners' offices, or public libraries *(19)*. However, Internet-based decision aids requiring Internet connection may impede access to patients who lack computer resources and skills.

Current strategies under evaluation to improve patient and practitioner access to decision aids include the use of nurse call centers and imbedding decision aids in the routine process of care in practice centers.

AN INVENTORY OF PATIENT DECISION AIDS

To improve access to decisions aids, the Cochrane Collaboration Systematic Review Team examining the effectiveness of decision aids established an Inventory of Patient Decision Aids *(15)*.

The inventory includes information on the topic, author, location, last update, delivery format, evaluation status, availability, and relevant publications. For decision aids that are available for use, there is a more detailed description of their contents and a quality rating; access to these aids is available at a patient-friendly A to Z library on the web. In the most recent update, more than 200 patient decision aids were identified. Several of these decision aids are available on the Internet. To obtain the most recent version of the inventory and access to the A to Z inventory of decision aids, visit the Ottawa Health Research Institute website www.ohri.ca/decisionaid and follow the links to the A to Z inventory.

Given the wide range of decision aids available and the diverse methodologies used in their development and evaluation, there is a need for standards. Currently, the International Patient Decision Aids Standards (IPDAS) Collaboration are developing criteria for their evaluation (*see* www.ohri.ca/decisionaid).

Example of a Decision Aid for Endocrine Practice

An example of a very simple decision aid is included in the appendix. The first page provides information about the condition, possible outcomes and consequences without treatment, evidence-based self-care recommendations, and options for treating the condition. The practitioner individualizes the options by highlighting those that are most suitable for the individual patient to consider. The second page guides patients to assess their decisional needs and to compare their options. The steps include:

1. Clarifying the decision: options, rationale, timing, and stage in decision making.
2. Clarifying the patient's preferred role in decision making.
3. Summarizing the options being considered with pros and cons for each option and ratings for personal values associated with the potential outcomes. A values clarification exercise is included for patients to begin to focus on which outcomes are most important to them. Patients are invited to add additional pros and cons before rating the importance they attach to each using a "1 to 5" star rating system. The final question asks patients for their overall leaning for or against the option.
4. Assessing current decision-making needs using the Decisional Conflict Scale.
5. Planning the next steps.

The completed Ottawa Personal Decision Guide can be shared with the patient's practitioner to communicate knowledge and values associated with a health-related decision "at a glance." Alternatively, the guide can be completed together with the practitioner to structure the process of decision making. In addition, it provides a generic process that can be applied to future health-related decisions. A similar guide is being used in nurse call centers and patient information services as part of the process of care. However, referrals to these types of services are intended to compliment and streamline the decision-making process rather than replace discussion with the patient's physician. Most patients have made it clear that individual consultation with their practitioner about options is extremely important *(3)*.

This Decisional Conflict Scale, used within this decision guide (*see* the appendix), was developed to determine whether a patient is experiencing uncertainty about the best course of action to identify the modifiable factors contributing to decisional conflict (e.g., feeling uninformed, unclear about values, unsupported in decision making) *(20)*. Decisional conflict is a state of uncertainty about the course of action to take and is frequently characterized by difficulty in making a decision, vacillation between choices, procrastination, being preoccupied with the decision, and having signs and symptoms of distress or tension.

The Decisional Conflict Scale has good reliability and validity in a variety of clinical settings *(20–26)*. Greater decisional conflict occurs in those who (1) delay decisions compared with those who implement and stick with decisions; (2) score lower on knowledge tests; (3) are in the early phases of decision making compared with later phases; or (4) have not yet received decision support compared with individuals who have. Those who have unresolved decisional conflict following counseling will be more likely to have downstream problems of failure to stick with chosen option, regret, and dissatisfaction; highlighting the need to resolve these issues at the time of decision making.

HOW DO CLINICIANS INTEGRATE DECISION AIDS INTO THEIR PRACTICE?

Practitioners are essential for clarifying the decision, identifying patients in decisional conflict or requiring decision support, referring patients to the appropriate resources including decision aids as part of the process of care, and following up on patients' responses in the decision aids to facilitate progress in decision making. Patients prefer face-to-face contact with a practitioner to individualize the information and guide them in decision making *(3)*. Patient decision aids are designed to enhance this interaction rather than replace it.

To use decision aids in practice, the following steps can be followed by your team:

1. *Clarify the decision.* Including specific options the patient needs to consider.
   a. *Refer patient to the decision aid.* Endorsement of patient information from one's personal practitioner is highly valued by patients *(3)*. Direct patients to the website (www.ohri.ca) to access a decision aid or provide them with photocopies.
2. *Explain how the decision aid is used in your practice.* Ask the patient to complete the decision aid in preparation for a follow-up discussion.
3. *Refer to the decision aid at follow-up discussion.* It is important that the practitioner acknowledge patient's responses to their decision aid. It can serve as a communication

tool to focus the patient–practitioner dialogue. At a glance, you can quickly learn how your patients see the decision. You can:

a. Clarify their understanding of the benefits and harms.

b. Acknowledge their values as revealed by the patient's rating of importance on the balance scale.

c. Answer their questions.

d. Facilitate decision making according to the patient's preference for decision participation and leaning toward options. This information helps you judge how quickly you can move from facilitating decision making to follow-up planning.

These steps can be completed by the individual practitioner or shared among team members. When shared within a clinical team, it is better to determine who on the team will be responsible for each part of the process. In the absence of staff to help with this process, referral to nurse call centers or patient information services may be an option to prepare patients for a dialogue.

This decision aid can also be used by patients when discussing their options and preferences with important others such as a spouse, family member, or friend.

Case Presentation Part IV: Mrs. O.

Mrs. O. completed the decision aid while the doctor saw other patients. The doctor then reviewed Mrs. O.'s responses to the decision aid (*see* the appendix), acknowledging the importance she placed on preventing fractures but her concerns about the long-term effects of continuing hormone therapy. Mrs. O.'s questions were answered about tapering her hormone therapy.

Together Mrs. O. and her doctor determined that alendronate was the "best" treatment option for her. Mrs. O. was motivated to take it and did not anticipate any barriers to taking it along with the calcium and vitamin D.

Evaluating the Patient's Responses to the Decision Aid

Practitioners can evaluate their usefulness in practice by noting whether (1) patients are better prepared to discuss options, (2) the need to repeat factual information is reduced, and (3) ascertainment of a patient's values is improved. Practitioners can also note whether, following counseling, patients resolve their decisional conflict (e.g., by repeating the Decisional Conflict Scale) and progress through the stages of decision making. If the practice is linked to a larger patient information system, the effects of introducing decision aids on renewal of prescriptions, satisfaction with counseling, health outcomes, and use of health services can also be monitored.

CONCLUSIONS

Patients with endocrine problems are likely to experience some difficulty in making health-related decisions. Decision aids improve the quality of patient decision making, facilitate the integration of patient values into evidence-based medical practice, and enhance the practitioner–patient interaction. The challenge is developing best practices for implementing decision aids as part of the process of care that will lead to better evidence-based decision making that matches patients' values.

APPENDIX: EVIDENCE-BASED OSTEOPOROSIS DECISION AID (27,28)

Mrs. O. Case Presentation

A. What is osteoporosis?

Osteoporosis is a condition of weak brittle bones that break easily, often without a fall, resulting in fractures of the wrist, spine, or hip. It is detected using a bone density test that measures the amount of bone loss. A result that is at least 2.5 "standard deviations" below normal confirms the diagnosis. This means people have lost at least 25% of their bone mass or density.

B. What are the possible problems from osteoporosis without treatment?

Hip fractures can cause severe disability or death.

- Among 100 women with normal bone density, about 15 may break a hip in their lifetime.

- Among 100 women with low bone density, approx 35–75 may break a hip in their lifetime. This number depends on amount of bone loss, age, and other bone or fall-related risk factors.

  Major bone related risks include
  —previous broken bones since age 50 (not from trauma)
  —family history of fracture (e.g., mother who broke a hip or wrist, spine)

  Major fall related risks
  —poor health
  —unable to rise from a chair without help
  —use of sedatives

- Spine fractures are more common and are disabling and painful. They can cause stooped posture and loss of height of up to 6 in.

- Talk to your practitioner about your personal risk of broken bones.

C. What are the recommended self-care options?

☑ Calcium   ☑ Vitamin D   ☑ Regular exercise

D. What are the treatment options?

Your doctor will advise you on the options for you to consider.

Bone-specific drugs
❑ Etidronate   ☑ Alendronate
❑ Risedronate   ❑ Calcitonin

Hormones that affect bones and other organs
☑ Hormone replacement therapy (estrogen alone or estrogen and progestin)
❑ Raloxifene
❑ Parathyroid hormone

Other
❑ Hip protector pads

E. Which option is best for you?

> ➤ Use the decision guide on the next pages to compare your options and identify your needs.
> ➤ Share your completed guide with your health professional at your doctor's office.

1. What decision do you face?   *alendronate or hormone therapy for osteoporosis*

What is your reason for making the decision?   *bone density low; need to prevent broken bones like my mother*

When does the decision have to be made?   *within 1 mo*

How far along are you with this decision? [*Check ✓ the box that applies to you*]

❏ not started thinking about the options   ❏ close to choosing one option

☑ is considering the options   ❏ already made a choice

2. What role do you prefer to take in decision making? [*Check ✓ the box that applies to you*]

❏ decide on my own after listening to the opinions of others

☑ share the decision with: *my doctor*

❏ someone else to decide for her, namely: _____

3. Details about how you see the options right now

1. What I know: List the options and their pros and cons. Underline the pros and cons that are most likely to happen.
2. What's important to me: show how important each pro and con is to you using one (★) star for a little important to five (★★★★★) stars for very important

	Reasons to choose option: "PROS"	Personal Importance	Reasons to avoid option: "CONS"	Personal Importance
Option #1 is: *Alendronate*	<u>Fewer broken hip and spine bones</u>	★★★★★	Side effects—heartburn	★★★★★
	Doing something	★★★★★	Personal costs	★★★★★
Option #2 is: *Hormone Therapy*	<u>Fewer broken hip and spine bones</u>	★★★★★	Risk of blood clot and stroke	★★★★★
	<u>Relieves menopause symptoms</u>	★★★★★	*My father died of stroke*	
	Doing something	★★★★★		

4. What are your current decision-making needs? [*Circle your answers to these questions.*]

What I know	Do you know which options you have?	(Yes)	No
	Do you know both the good **and** bad points of each option?	(Yes)	No
What's important	Are you clear about which good and bad points matter most to you?	(Yes)	No
How others help	Do you have enough support and advice to make a choice?	Yes	(No)
	Are you choosing without pressure from others?	(Yes)	No
How sure I feel	Do you feel sure about what to choose?	Yes	(No)

Decisional Conflict Scale © A. O'Connor 1993, Revised 2004.
Note: If you have many "no" answers, talk to your doctor.

5. What steps do you need to take to meet your needs? *Talk to my doctor and someone who has taken Alendronate; find out about tapering hormone therapy.*

APPENDIX: EVIDENCE-BASED OSTEOPOROSIS DECISION AID (27,28)

A. What is osteoporosis?

Osteoporosis is a condition of weak brittle bones that break easily, often without a fall, resulting in fractures of the wrist, spine, or hip. It is detected using a bone density test that measures the amount of bone loss. A result that is at least 2.5 "standard deviations" below normal confirms the diagnosis. This means people have lost at least 25% of their bone mass or density.

B. What are the possible problems from osteoporosis without treatment?

Hip fractures can cause severe disability or death.

- Among 100 women with normal bone density, about 15 may break a hip in their lifetime.

- Among 100 women with low bone density, approx 35–75 may break a hip in their lifetime. This number depends on amount of bone loss, age, and other bone or fall-related risk factors.

  Major bone related risks include
  —previous broken bones since age 50 (not from trauma)
  —family history of fracture (e.g., mother who broke a hip or wrist, spine)

  Major fall related risks
  —poor health
  —unable to rise from a chair without help
  —use of sedatives

- Spine fractures are more common and are disabling and painful. They can cause stooped posture and loss of height of up to 6 in.

- Talk to your practitioner about your personal risk of broken bones.

C. What are the recommended self-care options?

❏ Calcium   ❏ Vitamin D   ❏ Regular exercise

D. What are the treatment options?

Your doctor will advise you on the options for you to consider.

Bone-specific drugs
❏ Etidronate   ❏ Alendronate
❏ Risedronate   ❏ Calcitonin

Hormones that affect bones and other organs
❏ Hormone replacement therapy (estrogen alone or estrogen and progestin)
❏ Raloxifene
❏ Parathyroid hormone

Other
❏ Hip protector pads

E. Which option is best for you?

> ➢ Use the decision guide on the next page to compare your options and identify your needs.
> ➢ Share your completed guide with your health professional at your doctor's office.

1. What decision do you face? _____

What is your reason for making the decision? _____

When does the decision have to be made? _____

How far along are you with this decision? [*Check ✓ the box that applies to you*]

❏ not started thinking about the options   ❏ close to choosing one option

❏ is considering the options   ❏ already made a choice

2. What role do you prefer to take in decision making? [*Check ✓ the box that applies to you*]

❏ decide on my own after listening to the opinions of others

❏ share the decision with: _____

❏ someone else to decide for her, namely: _____

3. Details about how you see the options right now

1. What I know: List the options and their pros and cons. Underline the pros and cons that are most likely to happen.
2. What's important to me: show how important each pro and con is to you using one (★) star for a little important to five (★★★★★) stars for very important

	Reasons to choose option: "*PROS*"	*Personal Importance*	*Reasons to avoid option:* "*CONS*"	*Personal Importance*
Option #1 is:				
Option #2 is:				

4. What are your current decision-making needs? [*Circle your answers to these questions.*]

	What I Know	Do you know which options you have?	Yes	No
		Do you know both the good **and** bad points of each option?	Yes	No
	What's important	Are you clear about which good and bad points matter most to you?	Yes	No
	How others help	Do you have enough support and advice to make a choice?	Yes	No
		Are you choosing without pressure from others?	Yes	No
	How sure I feel	Do you feel sure about what to choose?	Yes	No

Decisional Conflict Scale © A. O'Connor 1993, Revised 2004.
Note: If you have many "no" answers, talk to your doctor.

5. What steps do you need to take to meet your needs?

REFERENCES

1. Sackett DL, Straus SE, Richardson WS, Rosenberg W, Haynes RB. Evidence-based medicine. How to practice and teach EBM, 2nd ed.Churchill Livingstone, Edinburgh, 2000.
2. Gafni A, Charles C, Whelan T. The physician-patient encounter: the physician as a perfect agent for the patient versus the informed treatment decision-making model. Soc Sci Med 1998;47:347–354.
3. O'Connor AM, Drake ER, Wells GA, Tugwell P, Laupacis A, Elmslie T. A survey of the decision-making needs of Canadians faced with complex health decisions. Health Expectations 2003;6: 97–109.
4. Martin S. "Shared responsibility" becoming the new medical buzz phrase. CMAJ 2002;167:295.
5. Chalmers, Clinical Evidence Volume 2, BMJ Publications, 1999. Available at [http://www.clinical evidence.com/ceweb/about/guide;sp] accessed Aug 23, 2005.
6. Harris RP, Helfand M, Woolf SH, et al. Current methods of the US preventive services Task Force: a review of the process. Am Prevent Med 2001;20:21–35.
7. Rutter D, Quine L. Social cognition models and changing health behaviours. In: Rutter D, Quine L, eds. Changing Health Behaviour. Intervention and Research with Social Cognition Models. 1st ed. Open University Press, Buckingham, 2002, pp. 1–27.
8. Vermeire E, Hearnshaw H, ValRoyen P, Denekens J. Patient adherence to treatment: three decades of research. A comprehensive review. J Clin Pharm Ther 2001;26:331–342.
9. Orbell S, Sheeran P. Changing health behaviours: The role of implementation intentions. In: Rutter D, Quine L, eds. Changing Health Behaviour. Intervention and Research with Social Cognition Models. 1st ed. Open University Press, Buckingham, 2002, pp. 123–137.
10. Mead N, Bower P. Patient-centredness: a conceptual framework and review of the empirical literature. Soc Sci Med 2000;51:1087–1110.
11. Stewart M. Towards a global definition of patient centred care. BMJ 2001;322:444–445.
12. Weston WW, Brown JB, Stewart MA. Patient-centred interviewing Part I: Understanding patients' experiences. Can Fam Physician 1989;35:147–151.
13. Brown JB, Weston WW, Stewart MA. Patient-centred interviewing Part II: Finding common ground. Can Fam Physician 1989;35:153–157.
14. Lester G, Smith S. Listening and talking to patients. A remedy for malpractice suits? West J Med 1993;158:268–272.
15. O'Connor AM, Stacey D, Entwistle V, et al. Decision aids for people facing health treatment or screening decisions [Cochrane Review]. In: The Cochrane Library, Issue 3. Update Software, Oxford, 2003.
16. O'Connor A. Using patient decision aids to promote evidence-based decision making. Am Coll Phys Evidence-Based Med 2001;6:101–102.
17. Graham ID, Logan J, O'Connor A, Weeks K. A qualitative study of physicians' perceptions of three decision aids. Patient Educ Counseling 2003;50:279–283.
18. Freeman AC, Sweeney K. Why general practitioners do not implement evidence: qualitative study. BMJ 2001;323:1100–1104.
19. Deyo RA. A key medical decision maker: the patient. BMJ 2001;323:466–467.
20. O'Connor AM, Jacobsen MJ, Stacey D. An evidence-based approach to managing women's decisional conflict. JOGNN 2003;31:570–581.
21. O'Connor AM. Validation of a decisional conflict scale. Med Decision Making 1995;15(1):25–30.
22. O'Connor AM, Tugwell P, Wells G, et al. Randomized trial of a portable, self-administered decision aid for post-menopausal women considering long-term preventive hormone therapy. Med Decis Making 1998;18:295–303.
23. Cranney A, Jacobsen MJ, O'Connor AM, Tugwell P, Adachi JD. A decision aid presenting multiple therapeutic options for women with osteoporosis: Development and evaluation. Med Decis Making 2001;21:547.
24. Grant FC, Laupacis A, O'Connor AM, Rubens F, Robblee J. Evaluation of a decision aid for autologous predonation for patients before open-heart surgery. CMAJ 2001;164:1139–1144.
25. Comeau, C. Evaluation of a decision aid for family members considering long-term care options for their relative with dementia. Unpublished master's thesis, University of Ottawa, Ottawa, Ontario, Canada, 2003.
26. Mitchell SL, Tetroe J, O'Connor AM. A decision aid for long-term tube feeding in cognitively impaired older persons. J Am Geriatr Soc 2001;49:1–4.
27. Cranney A, Simon LS, Tugwell P, Adachi R, Guyatt G. Postmenopausal osteoporosis. In: Tugwell P, Shea B, Boers M, et al. eds. Evidence-based Rheumatology. BMJ Books, 2004:183–243.
28. Brown JP, Josse RG. 2002 Clinical practice guidelines for the diagnosis and management of osteoporosis in Canada. CMAJ 2002;167:S1–S34.

9 Incorporating Evidence Into Health Policy Decisions

Eduardo Ortiz, MD, MPH
and Janelle Guirguis-Blake, MD

CONTENTS

INTRODUCTION

Evidence-based medicine (EBM) has been described as the integration of best research evidence with clinical expertise and patient values *(1)*. Other chapters in this book have provided an overview of EBM, especially as it relates to clinical practice; in this chapter, we will take a slightly different approach and look at the intersection between EBM and health policy.

INTERSECTION BETWEEN EVIDENCE-BASED MEDICINE AND HEALTH POLICY

The emergence of EBM as an explicit field in the 1990s has led to renewed interest in how health policy decisions are developed and implemented. Providing safe, effective, efficient, and high-quality care that results in the best possible outcomes is the optimal goal of any health care delivery system. Information obtained from well designed, well-conducted scientific studies has been shown to be the best source of

From: *Contemporary Endocrinology: Evidence-Based Endocrinology*
Edited by: V. M. Montori © Mayo Foundation for Medical Education and Research

evidence regarding what interventions or services result in the best outcomes in health care. Programs that implement these evidence-based practices should, therefore, produce the best outcomes for the overall population, but they may not necessarily result in the best outcomes for each individual nor do they apply in all situations and circumstances (2). Differences among individuals, co-morbidities, clinical expertise and skills, family and socioeconomic environments, and other factors can limit the generalizability of the findings, making them nonapplicable to many constituents served by policymakers. Local circumstances will, therefore, often dictate how evidence is translated into practice, or if at all. Policymakers must take into account a multitude of factors, including national character, local culture, resources, affordability of care, access to information, access to health care services, the legal environment, parochialism, and centralized vs decentralized policymaking processes, all of which can influence how scientific research is translated into practice (3). In a similar vein, even when good evidence about outcomes and effectiveness clearly exists and when the generalizability of the findings is considered applicable enough to drive health policy, successful implementation of such policies is often difficult.

Another issue that confronts policymakers is that evidence from high-quality scientific studies is often lacking, yet policymakers still have to contend with making health policy decisions. For example, in 1997 the minister for public health in England and Wales commissioned the former chief medical officer for England to "moderate a Department of Health review of the latest available information on inequalities in health . . . and in the light of evidence to conduct an independent review to identify priority areas in future policy development, which scientific and expert evidence indicates are likely to offer opportunities for Government to develop beneficial, cost-effective, and affordable interventions to reduce health inequalities" (4,5). At the time, a scientific advisory group was appointed to assist him with this task. The chairman of this advisory group asked another group of experts to examine the quality of the evidence underpinning the scientific advisory group's emerging recommendations and to identify any gaps. They were struck by the lack of empirical evidence available for the government to base policies or decide on priorities, even though a large amount of research in this area had been conducted and published in the United Kingdom. Although this is just one example where good evidence to guide policymakers is lacking, their experience reflects a commonly encountered problem faced by policymakers trying to incorporate evidence into their decision-making processes.

If clinicians are expected to base their decisions on research findings, should we not hold policymakers, whose decisions can have profound effects on millions of people, to the same standard? As in clinical care, the case for evidence-based policymaking is hard to refute (6,7). Proponents of EBM often assume that there is a direct linear relationship between research evidence and health policy—that scientific research should inform policymakers, which leads to the formulation of evidence-based policy (6). This view is based on a belief that evidence from scientific research forms the basis for what is factual and true as well as a belief that the knowledge and experience of health care professionals (e.g., physicians) allows their views and priorities to dominate health policies.

In reality, the relationship between good scientific evidence and health policy decisions is often weak or nonexistent. Black (6) talks about the relationship between research and policymaking and divides policymaking into three categories: (1) practice policies (use of resources by practitioners), (2) service policies (resource allocation and pattern of services), and (3) governance policies (organizational and financial structures) *(8)*. He posits that the linear relationship between evidence and health policy holds up fairly well for practice policy, although there are two areas that he views as problematic. First, differences can exist in the interpretation of the evidence. We will discuss this in more detail later in this chapter. Second, the generalizability of research findings can pose a problem. For example, practice policies governing surgical interventions are often difficult to devise because of individual variations among patients (e.g., anatomy, obesity, co-morbid conditions), surgeons (e.g., experience and skill), and external factors (e.g., availability of equipment) *(9)*. In the area of service policies (resource allocation and pattern of services), the relationship between scientific evidence and health policy is even weaker. Black *(6)* lists six reasons why scientific evidence may have little, if any, influence on service policies:

1. Policymakers have many competing interests with which they must contend; they, therefore, have goals and deliverables other than those related to clinical outcomes and effectiveness (e.g., social, financial, electoral, employment terms and conditions, unions, service agreements, resource allocation, and others).
2. Research evidence may be considered irrelevant or not applicable if it emanates from a different sector or specialty.
3. There is often a lack of consensus about scientific evidence because of its complexity or because of varying interpretations of the evidence.
4. Policymakers, who may not have a background in scientific research or EBM, may value other sources of information such as personal stories, personal experience, individual cases, colleague's opinions, expert opinions, and medical reports.
5. The social or political environment may not be conducive to policy changes (e.g., times of political unrest, budget deficits, involvement in war, government elections, and organizational changes).
6. Knowledge purveyors, those individuals whose task it is to bring the scientific evidence into the policymaking arena (e.g., civil servants working for the federal government), may not have the appropriate knowledge and skills to successfully inform policymakers on complex health issues.

Finally, in the area of governance policies (organizational and financial structures), scientific research has played a limited role in shaping health policy because governance policies are often driven by factors such as ideology, political expediency, financial constraints, and economic theory *(6)*.

Innvaer et al. *(10)* conducted a systematic review to summarize the evidence from interview studies with policymakers in order to identify facilitators of, and barriers to, the use of research evidence by health policy makers. They identified 24 studies involving 2041 interviews with health policymakers, with 11 of the studies involving US policymakers. The most commonly reported facilitators were as follows:

- Personal contact between researchers and policymakers (13 of 24 studies).
- Timeliness and relevance of the research (13 of 24 studies).
- Research that included a summary with clear recommendations (11 of 24 studies).
- Good quality research (6 of 24 studies).
- Research that confirmed current policy or endorsed self-interest (6 of 24 studies).
- Community interest or client demand for research (4 of 24 studies).
- Research that included effectiveness data (3 of 24 studies).

The most commonly reported barriers were as follows:

- Absence of personal contact between researchers and policymakers (11 of 24 studies).
- Lack of timeliness or relevance of research (9 of 24 studies).
- Mutual mistrust, including perceived political naivety of scientists and scientific naivety of policymakers (8 of 24 studies).
- Power and budget struggles (7 of 24 studies).
- Poor quality of research (6 of 24 studies).
- Political instability or high turnover of policymaking staff (5 of 24 studies).

Innvaer et al. *(10)* concluded that researchers who wish to see scientific evidence incorporated into health policy decision making should do the following:

- Have personal and close two-way communication with decision makers.
- Provide decision makers with a brief summary of their research with clear policy recommendations.
- Ensure that their research is perceived as timely, relevant, and of high quality.
- Include effectiveness data.
- Argue that their research results are relevant to current policy and demands from the community.
- Avoid getting involved in power and budget struggles.
- Be aware that policymakers and their staff can have high turnover rates.

FRAMEWORK FOR MAKING EVIDENCE-BASED DECISIONS

The process used to make decisions based on scientific evidence involves several steps. The first step is to define the issues, including the disease and/or condition, population of interest, interventions or services, and outcomes, and to arrange them in a conceptual framework that will guide the evidence review. It is extremely important to clarify the relevant outcomes of interest (for both benefits and harms) at the outset. Policy conflicts often occur not because of differences in the science but because of differences in the significance assigned to the outcomes. The next step is to systematically search for, obtain, and synthesize all of the relevant evidence, which includes specifying the criteria for including and excluding studies, systematically searching the databases to abstract the relevant studies, ensuring that the search is comprehensive, evaluating the quality and strength of the evidence, interpreting the data appropriately, and synthesizing the evidence. This process typically takes the efforts of a team that has experience and skills in information management and should include, at a minimum, a specialist in library sciences and information retrieval, an epidemiologist, a biostatistician, one or more clinicians—who may or may not be the content experts in that particular topic area—and one or more persons with content expertise. The synthesis of evidence clarifies the strength of the evidence, including gaps in evidence, and the magnitude of benefits and harms that can accrue as a result of intervening—or not intervening—in a defined population for a specific disease or condition. Because the available evidence rarely fits neatly into a pre-defined conceptual framework, there is often an element of generalization and extrapolation that must occur in order to decide the implications of applying the evidence to an intended population. The final step involves interpretation of the evidence and consideration of other important factors. Depending on the types of decisions being made, these may include things such as actual number of persons affected by the decision, individual preferences, cultural issues, religious beliefs, alternative possibilities, costs, and principles of self-determination to formulate policy decisions.

An example of a conceptual framework used to guide the evidence review is the analytic framework used by the US Preventive Services Task Force (USPSTF) for its recommendations on clinical preventive services (11). The USPSTF is an independent panel of experts in primary care and evidence-based medicine convened and supported by the Agency for Health Research and Quality (AHRQ) and charged by Congress to review the scientific evidence of clinical preventive services for the purpose of developing recommendations for the health care community (12). AHRQ supports 13 evidence-based practice centers (EPCs) for the sole purpose of conducting systematic reviews of the evidence surrounding various health-related topic areas (13). The USPSTF utilizes the EPCs to conduct reviews in clinical prevention topics, which then become the basis for formulating its recommendations. Consensus panels sponsored by the National Institutes of Health (NIH) have also begun using these EPC systematic reviews for their deliberations. Figure 1 depicts the analytic framework used by the USPSTF to review the evidence for breast cancer screening. This framework defines the population of interest (women 40 yr of age or older with no history or manifestation of breast cancer), screening tests (breast self-exam, clinical breast exam, mammography), intermediate outcomes (e.g., detection of earlier stage breast cancer), health outcomes (e.g., reduced breast cancer mortality or morbidity), and harms from screening and treatment (e.g., anxiety, labeling, over-diagnosis, procedures resulting from false-positive tests, increased mortality or morbidity, effects on quality of life).

RESOLVING CONFLICTS WHEN MAKING EVIDENCE-BASED DECISIONS

Making evidence-based decisions is complex. Clinical practice guidelines have developed as a means to overcome some of the problems inherent in making health care decisions including wide and inappropriate variations in practice patterns and health care utilization; high prevalence of suboptimal care, including the overutilization of ineffective services and the underutilization of effective services; and uncertainty about the health outcomes achieved by the use of various services. Guidelines can help clinicians make more informed decisions based on the best available evidence, serve as a means to educate providers and organizations, help to assess and ensure quality of care for individuals and populations, and guide decisions about resource allocation (14). Dr. David Eddy, an international leader in the field of EBM and health policy, talks about three places to look for sources of disagreements in guidelines, which are also potential sources of disagreement for other evidence-based policy decisions (15): (1) target of the decision (e.g., disease, patient, intervention, clinician-type); (2) objective of the decision (e.g., improve health outcomes for a population, reduce costs); and (3) rationale for the decision (e.g., methodology, intermediate vs patient oriented outcomes, perspective/values).

Synthesizing the Evidence

Disagreements in drawing conclusions and making recommendations based on the evidence can sometimes result from differences in deciding which studies to include when synthesizing the evidence. For example, the USPSTF uses explicit criteria to

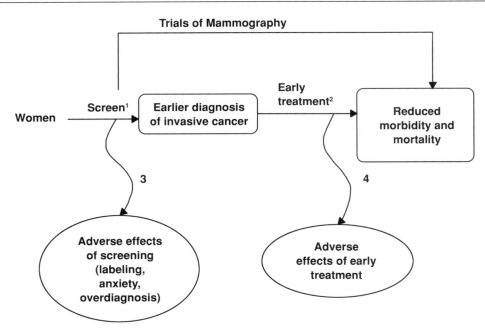

Fig. 1. US Preventive Services Task Force analytic framework used to review the evidence for breast cancer screening.

evaluate the methodological quality of a study in order to classify it into one of three quality categories: *good, fair,* or *poor*. A systematic evidence review on breast cancer screening with mammography and its effect on mortality was performed for the USPSTF *(16,17)*. The review identified eight randomized controlled trials (RCTs) and evaluated the quality of each study. Although all of these RCTs had methodological flaws, only one of them had flaws that were considered serious enough to warrant rejection of the study's results, thus meriting a *poor-quality* rating. The other seven studies were given a *fair-quality* rating because they had methodological flaws that could have led to potential biases; however, the biases were not considered severe enough to have accounted for the observed effects of mammography screening on mortality. The trials reported mortality reductions ranging from "no significant effect" to a "32% reduction" in breast cancer mortality. When the results of all seven trials were combined into a meta-analysis, the results demonstrated a statistically significant reduction in overall mortality of 16% (relative risk [RR] 0.84; 95% confidence interval [CI] 0.77–0.91).

In contrast to this finding, an earlier systematic review done for the Cochrane collaboration by Olsen and Gotzsche used a different grading scheme and came up with a different result *(18)*. This review identified a four-level scale to grade the evidence: *high-quality, medium-quality, poor-quality,* and *flawed*. This grading scheme is a bit unusual because most Cochrane reviews use a three-level scale to rate the validity of studies *(19)*. Having two different validity rating scales will almost inevitably lead to disagreements regarding which studies should be included in a scientific review. Whereas the Olsen and Gotsche review agreed with the USPSTF review that one RCT had serious flaws and that no RCT was of good quality, there were disagreements in the individual quality ratings of the other seven RCTs. Of these, three were assigned *medium-quality*, three were assigned *poor-quality*, and one was designated *flawed*. When a meta-analysis of the three *medium-quality* trials was performed, it led the authors to conclude that mammography screening had no significant effect on reducing breast cancer mortality (RR = 1.05, CI = 0.83–1.33).

Olsen and Gotsche further reported that a meta-analysis combining data from all 6 of the "nonflawed trials" showed a significant decrease in breast cancer mortality (RR = 0.80, CI = 0.71–0.89) as a result of mammography screening, which is similar to the result from the USPSTF review. Therefore, the methods used to determine the quality of the studies that are included in the evidence review and the way that results are combined across different studies can substantially influence the conclusions, even when they are based on the same evidence.

Assigning Values to Different Types of Outcomes: Health Outcomes vs Intermediate Outcomes

In incorporating evidence into clinical decision making, EBM focuses on the best available evidence that a service or intervention leads to improvements in important health outcomes. But what do we mean by *important outcomes*? By this we are referring to outcomes that patients actually experience and care about, both positive and negative. For example, patients tend to care about whether or not they die, so both disease-specific and overall mortality should be important health outcomes that are considered by policymakers. Patients also experience and care about things like having a heart attack or stroke, having an amputation, breaking a hip, developing bed sores, developing renal failure, losing their eyesight, having adverse reactions to a medication, and being able to perform activities of daily living. These can be thought of as *important patient oriented health outcomes,* which should be strongly considered when formulating health policy.

In contrast, many decisions in health care are based on information about intermediate outcomes, often resulting from the lack of adequate evidence that is available on important health outcomes. These intermediate outcomes, many of which are based on physiological, laboratory, biochemical, or pharmacological measures, are often used to determine the effects of a service or intervention. Some of these intermediate outcomes are appropriate as surrogate markers for important health outcomes because of adequate evidence that changes in the intermediate outcomes lead to changes in important health outcomes. For example, there is a large body of evidence that a reduction in blood pressure is associated with reductions in stroke, heart attack, renal failure, mortality, and other important health outcomes. Another important intermediate outcome is hemoglobin A1C, where improvements in hemoglobin A1C values are associated with decreases in important microvascular complications in patients with type 1 diabetes. In many other conditions, however, there is little or no evidence of a causal link between intermediate outcomes that are being measured and effects on important health outcomes. In order to determine whether or not an intermediate outcome can serve appropriately as a surrogate outcome, knowledge of the natural history of the disease and of the strength of association between changes in the intermediate outcome and important health outcomes is necessary.

For example, reduction in viral load is considered to be a valid surrogate measure for improved health outcomes in human immunodeficiency virus (HIV) infection but not in hepatitis C virus (HCV) infection. In HIV infection, more than 90% of untreated persons will progress to AIDS (with its attendant morbidity and mortality) within 8–10 yr, whereas only 10–20% of HCV-infected persons will develop cirrhosis over 20–30 yr *(20,21)*. Additionally, it is well established from scientific studies that anti-viral treatment of HIV, which results in a decrease in HIV viral load, will also decrease progression to AIDS. However it has not been established that anti-viral treatment of HCV infection will decrease progression to cirrhosis. Thus, in the case of HIV disease, a strong case can be made that a reduction in viral load (an intermediate outcome) is a meaningful end point because of its proven association with improved health outcomes. However, in HCV disease it would be difficult to make the same case based on existing evidence, even though a similar intermediate outcome (viral load) is being measured. In general, evidence-based expert panels should place a greater emphasis on patient oriented health outcomes (such as decreased morbidity or mortality) than on intermediate outcomes (such as laboratory and biochemical markers) whenever it is feasible.

Perspective of the Decision Makers and Stakeholders Who Will Be Affected by the Decision

It is important to consider the perspective of the decision makers, as well as the perspective and needs of the various stakeholders affected by health policy decisions. Stakeholders may include:

1. Patients or family members.
2. Individual clinical providers—e.g., primary-care clinicians, specialists, nurse practitioners, nurses, pharmacists, physical therapists.
3. Provider organizations—e.g., academic medical institutions, private sector fee-for-service hospitals, health maintenance organizations, Veterans Health Administration facilities, ambulatory care surgical facilities, rehabilitation facilities, nursing homes, home health care services.
4. Purchasing organizations—e.g., health insurance companies or employers.
5. Specialty societies—e.g., American Medical Association, American College of Physicians, American College of Surgeons.
6. Expert groups or panels—e.g., NIH consensus panels, USPSTF panel, guideline development panels.
7. Advocacy organizations—e.g., breast cancer advocacy groups, AARP.
8. Policymakers—legislative and executive branches of federal, state, and local governments.

The value attached to an outcome and the considerations influencing the decision depend upon the perspective of both decision makers and affected stakeholders. An individual may assign values different from that of an organization. A sick person may be more willing than a healthy person to tolerate medicines and surgical procedures associated with adverse effects. Policymakers must take into account the perspective of the person, group, or organization that will be affected by their decisions. One of the most common and important perspectives is that of the individual patient. However, other perspectives must also be considered; for example, that of the clinician. Even among clinicians, different types of clinicians may place different emphasis on different outcomes. A primary-care provider might focus more on outcomes related to the overall well-being of a patient—issues such as quality of life, balance of harms and benefits of an intervention, and ability to comply with treatment—whereas a subspecialist might tend to focus more on the direct benefits of a treatment on the targeted disease. In addition to evidence and perspective, clinical practice can be strongly influenced by local standards of care and concerns about medical liability.

Beyond the patient and clinician, other perspectives must also be taken into consideration, especially by policymakers who have to be responsive to a number of stakeholders. As one moves beyond the individual patient to a broader perspective, taking into account the needs, wants, and preferences of society, employers, or insurers, one can see that the outcomes emphasized can vary considerably.

Let's look at a concrete example: a study published in 2002 showed that prophylactic use of implantable cardiac defibrillators (ICDs) in patients with a previous myocardial infarction and reduced left ventricular ejection fraction reduced mortality after 20 mo from 19.8 to 14.2%, a 31% relative risk reduction and a 5.6% absolute risk reduction (number needed to treat of 18) (22). A patient who is a potential candidate for this therapy might logically want to receive such a defibrillator, because it has been demonstrated to reduce an important health outcome (i.e., death) by 31%, especially if the patient has insurance that will cover the cost of the device, the procedure, and the required follow-up care. An insurer or other payer may be concerned about the cost of this intervention, which has been conservatively estimated at $28,000 to $58,000 for the implantation (23) and which potentially could be used in 400,000 patients each year in the United States, costing payers an additional $12 billion annually (24). Payers could, thus, be justifiably concerned about the effects that this could have on their health care expenditures, despite the fact that it leads to reductions in mortality. An employer may be concerned that it will result in increased health care costs for its employees, which must then be covered by increases in the employer's health care expenditures. These increased expenditures must then be recouped by the employer through mechanisms such as increased productivity and sales, increased costs of goods and services to its customers, employee lay-offs, increased health care premiums for all employees, or decreases in other health care benefits for employees. Other employees may be concerned that they are not receiving the benefits of this intervention, yet their health care premiums and co-payments are increasing in order to pay for it, while other services are being scaled back or eliminated. From a societal perspective, concern arises because offering this service may lead to cuts in other health care services (e.g., preventive services), increases in health care costs for everyone, and increases in the number of uninsured Americans. Some clinicians are concerned because there are other simpler and less costly interventions that can reduce mortality as effectively but are not being optimally utilized. For example, the reduction in mortality that can be achieved with an ICD is comparable to that achieved by using β-blockers in patients with ischemic heart disease. Instead of spending this money on ICDs, why not spend a fraction of this money to do a better job of treating patients with ischemic heart disease with β-blockers, aspirin, and other medications that reduce mortality? In addition, a clinician might be concerned about the adverse effects of such an invasive intervention, which will undoubtedly result in complications that may increase certain morbidities and mortality.

A policymaker may consider one, several, all, or even none of these perspectives when making policy decisions. Policymakers will also bring their own perspectives to the table. Some of these perspectives will be influenced by their own individual experiences and beliefs that have been shaped over the years by their jobs, religion, race, education, families, and personal experiences with illness. Other perspectives will stem from their roles and responsibilities as policymakers. For example, in the case of ICDs, routine use could increase national health care expenditures by the billions. Given our current level of health care spending, with expenditures consuming approx 14% of the gross domestic product (GDP) and the growing number of uninsured Americans, even a policymaker who is convinced that using these devices will reduce mortality will need to consider the enormous cost of providing this service.

Factoring Costs Into the Equation

The practice of EBM involves using the best available evidence on important outcomes from systematic research as the foundation for clinical decisions (25). However, evidence must also be considered within the context of many other factors when making health-related decisions: clinical expertise and judgment; patient values, preferences, and circumstances; costs; and other important factors. Among these factors, cost is often ignored or de-emphasized, especially by patients and clinicians; yet it is also the proverbial "elephant in the room"—a very important consideration that is often at the forefront of many health policy decisions. For example, any decision to expand services or access in the Medicaid program can have an effect on a state's ability to provide other programs and presents a challenge when it is time to balance the state's budget. Likewise, when a health plan or insurer covers new and costly technologies, it often leads to increased costs for the health plan or insurer, increased out-of-pocket costs for the beneficiary, and/or decreases in coverage for other services.

Because we live in a world with limited resources, costs are an important consideration when making health policy decisions. The benefits of any intervention or service must be balanced by how much it costs to achieve that benefit. Some of this can be achieved through the use of economic studies, such as cost-effectiveness analyses, which incorporate the best available evidence into decision models that can inform policymakers on how resources can be used most effectively and efficiently. This is usually conducted from the societal perspective; that is, how to derive the most benefit per dollar for the population at large. Despite the potential utility of economic analyses, an economic analysis is only as good as the data used in the model (e.g., "garbage in, garbage out"). In addition, the data needed to conduct adequate economic analyses for the myriad of conditions facing decision makers are frequently not available or, if available, not robust enough to make good evidence-based decisions. Finally, health policy decisions are often made in contrast to the recommendations generated by economic analyses. This is because policymakers often weigh other factors more heavily when making policy decisions.

Despite the fact that the United States spends more money on health care (overall and as a percentage of its GDP) than any other country, measures of health outcomes are consistently worse than many developed countries that spend far less on health care (26). This frequently cited statistic argues against the assertion that higher spending equates to greater access or improved quality of care. In fact, data from the US health care system demonstrate that expenditures are not consistently directed toward services that are cost-effective. When one looks at the allocation of health care resources and what health care services are reimbursed, health policy decision makers, whether through conscious deliberation or other thought processes, prioritize certain types of health care services over others.

How do policymakers decide what services to cover and who has access to these services? One can make the case that policymakers should prioritize quality, access, and costs in making health policy decisions and that any politically viable legislation should contain all three elements (27). In addition, decisions should be based on evidence that each of these three elements will be significantly enhanced by policy that is enacted. But evidence is not the only driver of these decisions; in fact, in many cases, evidence is either not considered or ignored. Health policy decisions often occur without explicit consideration of the actual impact of the intervention or service on important patient-oriented health outcomes or on the benefit achieved per cost (e.g., using economic decision tools). Policymakers are influenced by many other considerations including advocacy groups, political action committees, lobbyists, constituents, individual stories, personal experiences and biases, and the current political or social climate (e.g., decisions made during an election year can vary from decisions made during non-election years, decisions made during wartime can vary from decisions made when the country is at peace, and so on).

For various reasons, health policymakers tend to favor acute care interventions over chronic care interventions. Likewise, they tend to prioritize interventions that utilize technology or involve invasive procedures over the delivery of preventive services. For example, Medicare will reimburse hospitals and providers for very costly services in an intensive care unit for a patient with a terminal illness at the end of life, yet it will not provide reimbursement for many routine preventive services. Another example can be seen in the fact that smoking cessation and weight reduction programs, which are cost-effective and can lead to decreases in cardiovascular morbidity and mortality, are usually not covered by payers; yet acute treatments for diseases that result from smoking or obesity, such as coronary artery disease or diabetes, are covered (28). If policymakers were to truly base policy decisions on the best available evidence of cost-effectiveness, reimbursement for smoking cessation initiatives and weight reduction programs in patients at risk for cardiac disease would be a priority over implantable cardiac defibrillators in patients with established cardiac disease.

Unfortunately, the scope of this chapter does not allow us to adequately address all the intricate issues involved in incorporating costs into health policy decisions. The bottom line is that if resources are limited, which is inevitably the case at some level for all health care delivery systems, then it is important to optimize the use of services that are cost-effective and improve important patient-oriented health outcomes while reducing the use of resources spent on ineffective or marginally effective services. The more that evidence is incorporated into these decisions, by using data from well-conducted randomized controlled trials, clinical practice guidelines, cost-effectiveness analyses, and other such decision aid tools, the easier it is to make effective and efficient health policy decisions that will lead to improved health outcomes.

Real-World Examples: Interpreting the Evidence

Another issue that is frequently encountered is that varying interpretations of the same evidence can often lead to different recommendations. For example, the USPSTF conducted a thorough review of the evidence for HCV infection in high-risk adults and concluded, "There is insufficient evidence to recommend for or against screening in this population" and gave it an "I" (insufficient evidence) recommendation. An NIH consensus panel and the Centers for Disease Control and Prevention (CDC) looked at similar data and came up with a different recommendation: "Groups at high risk for HCV infection should be screened." How can these groups of "experts" review the same data yet come up with different interpretations and recommendations?

There are several reasons for this discrepancy. One is the value placed on a reduction in viral load as a meaningful endpoint. The USPSTF viewed the reduction in viral load as an intermediate endpoint that has not been demonstrated to result in important patient-oriented health outcomes, whereas the NIH panel and the CDC viewed viral load reduction as an appropriate surrogate outcome. Another reason stems from a difference in perspective. The USPSTF frames issues from the perspective of the primary-care clinician, who is often taking care of many patients (e.g., primary-care physicians can have more than 2000 patients in their panels), dealing with multiple medical problems, and faced with limited time and resources with which to deliver comprehensive care, including preventive services; thus, the USPSTF must necessarily place a higher value on interventions with proven health benefits compared with those interventions with unknown or marginal health benefits. The NIH panel, on the other hand, may view HCV screening more from the perspective of the specialty physician, perhaps a gastroenterologist specializing in diseases of the liver or an infectious disease expert, both of whom may be more uniquely focused on hepatitis C and its possible health effects, or perhaps focused on research issues in patients with hepatitis C infection. Yet another perspective might come into play with the CDC (or the infectious disease specialist)—that of a public health official who wants to conduct disease surveillance and protect the public from a potential health risk. One can, thus, see that policy recommendations may be substantially influenced by how the evidence is interpreted, which may not necessarily result from problems with the science, but rather from differences in perspective and underlying biases that one brings to the table when evaluating the evidence. Thus, even though there is currently no good evidence that screening high-risk patients for HCV infection results in any important long-term health benefits, there may be other reasons for policymakers to conclude that screening is justified.

Another important but related factor that affects how evidence is interpreted and formulated into policy decisions, and which often leads to conflicting recommendations, involves the extrapolation of study results to various groups that could be affected by the recommendations. Recommendations on screening for subclinical hypo- and hyperthyroidism that have come out of different organizations illustrate this issue.

In 2000, the American Thyroid Association (ATA) recommended that adults be screened for thyroid dysfunction by measurement of the serum thyroid stimulating hormone (TSH) concentration, beginning at 35 yr of age and every 5 yr thereafter (29). The ATA further stated that the indication for screening is particularly compelling in women, but it may also be justified in men as a relatively cost-effective measure in the context of the periodic health examination. This recommendation was based on the following grounds: (1) high prevalence of the condition, (2) disease burden of overt hyperthyroidism and hypothyroidism, (3) existence of accurate screening tests, and (4) effective treatments in those in whom treatment is indicated.

In contrast, the USPSTF reviewed this topic area in 2003 and found insufficient evidence to recommend for or against routine screening for thyroid disease (30). In its rationale for this recommendation, the USPSTF stated:

"The USPSTF found fair evidence that the thyroid stimulating hormone (TSH) test can detect subclinical thyroid disease in people without symptoms of thyroid dysfunction, but poor evidence that treatment improves clinically important outcomes in adults with screen-detected thyroid disease. Although the yield of screening is greater in certain high-risk groups (e.g., postpartum women, people with Down syndrome, and the elderly), the USPSTF found poor evidence that screening these groups leads to clinically important benefits. There is the potential for harm caused by false positive screening tests; however, the magnitude of harm is not known. There is good evidence that over-treatment with levothyroxine occurs in a substantial proportion of patients, but the long-term harmful effects of over-treatment are not known. As a result, the USPSTF could not determine the balance of benefits and harms of screening asymptomatic adults for thyroid disease."

The key issue in the USPSTF rationale was its finding that there was "poor evidence that treatment can improve clinically important outcomes in *screen-detected persons.*" In other areas, they agreed with the ATA; for example, the USPSTF agreed regarding the four criteria used by the ATA to justify its recommendations. However, the USPSTF did not find adequate evidence that treatment of subclinical thyroid disease resulted in health benefits, and they did not feel it was appropriate to extrapolate the benefits of treating persons with clinically overt thyroid disease to similar benefits in asymptomatic persons (i.e., asymptomatic persons with subclinical thyroid disease whose thyroid function abnormalities were detected only because they were screened). This extrapolation, which was derived from the application of proven scientific study results from one group (symptomatic patients with clinically overt thyroid disease) to another group where benefits have not been proven (asymptomatic persons with subclinical thyroid disease) was made by the ATA on the basis of expert opinion, which led to the positive recommendation for screening. Additionally, the USPSTF took into account the harms of false-positive results and the harms of overtreatment, but it did not find adequate evidence to quantify these harms, which led to its current recommendation. Hence, even when the evidence base is the same, extrapolation and application of scientific results to other groups or individuals can lead to different conclusions and recommendations.

Let's talk about another example that relates to the screening of patients for subclinical thyroid disease to further illustrate the complexities of interpreting scientific data and turning it into policy recommendations. In 2001, representatives of the ATA, the American Association of Clinical Endocrinologists (AACE), and The Endocrine Society (TES) formed a planning committee for a Consensus Development Conference to address issues relating to the diagnosis and treatment of subclinical thyroid disease, including whether population-based or selective screening is supported by the evidence. An expert panel, which included national experts in the field of endocrinology and thyroidology (8 of the 13 panelists), clinical cardiology, cardiovascular epidemiology, biostatistics and epidemiology, EBM, health services research, general internal medicine, clinical decision making, women's health, and clinical nutrition, was convened to evaluate the evidence and make recommendations. The panel reviewed a comprehensive evidence report *(31)* developed by the Lewin Group, which contained 195 relevant articles, *Evidence Report: Subclinical Thyroid Disease.*

The panel also sat through 1 d of presentations by 12 speakers identified by the planning committee as experts in thyroid disease, clinical biochemistry, epidemiology, biostatistics, and clinical decision making, who presented reviews of selected areas considered important in the diagnosis and treatment of subclinical hypo- and hyperthyroidism, including epidemiology, laboratory testing, screening, symptoms, effects on bones, lipids, and the cardiovascular system, and effects of treatment. Using methods adapted from NIH consensus conferences and the USPSTF, the 13 panelists weighed the evidence from the evidence report, together with evidence presented at the conference, assessed the data for quality, scope, and relevance, and developed screening recommendations for subclinical hypo- and hyperthyroidism *(32)*.

The panel based its recommendation on many factors, but it was largely influenced by the belief that one of the most important criteria for recommending a screening test is that screening asymptomatic persons and treating them for the condition should result in measurable and improved health outcomes when compared to persons who are not screened and who would otherwise have presented with signs and symptoms of the disease. Similar to the USPSTF, the panel found insufficient evidence that screening results in important patient oriented health outcomes and that the benefits of screening outweigh the risks. Even though this panel viewed the evidence in a manner similar to the USPSTF, their final recommendations differed. Whereas the USPSTF recommended neither for nor against routine screening for thyroid disease in adults *(30)*, the expert panel recommended against routine screening in the asymptomatic general adult population. The panel did, however, encourage case-finding in certain high-risk groups.

This illustrates how different groups can look at the same evidence and come up with three separate conclusions. The ATA recommended screening; the USPSTF said that there was insufficient evidence to recommend for or against screening; and the expert panel convened by the Endocrinology and Thyroid Professional Organizations recommended against screening. In fact, when one looks at the various recommendations in this topic area, the differences in interpretation and extrapolation of the evidence are quite striking (Table 1).

BEYOND THE EVIDENCE: POLITICAL LOBBYING, ADVOCACY GROUPS, AND PERSONAL NARRATIVES

In an ideal world, policymakers would find, assess, and weigh all the evidence objectively; integrate this with important information on clinical circumstances, clinical expertise and judgment, patient preferences and values, and costs; obtain input from all of the different stakeholders; balance all of the various interests and concerns; and then make a determination that optimally benefits the majority of stakeholders. Unfortunately, this scenario rarely (if ever) occurs, and health policy is often influenced by factors other than the evidence. Let's discuss a few examples that illustrate this point.

During the 1980s and 1990s, there was a substantial amount of controversy over the management of low-back pain, especially the merits of surgical procedures in improving pain, function, and other important long-term outcomes. In December 1994, the Agency for Healthcare Policy and Research (AHCPR, which is now the Agency for Healthcare Research and Quality or AHRQ) released its guidelines on the assessment and treatment of acute low-back pain *(33)*. The guideline was the product of several years of work by a 23-member panel of experts that performed a systematic evaluation of all the available evidence on the various diagnostic and treatment modalities for managing acute low-back pain. Regarding surgical options, one of the panel's conclusions was:

Table 1
Current Thyroid Screening Guidelines of Various Organizations

Expert panel	Recommends against population-based screening for thyroid disease in adults based on the lack of evidence that screening improves important health outcomes and the potential for harm (2004).
USPSTF	Evidence is insufficient to recommend for or against routine screening for thyroid disease in adults (2004).
ATA	Recommends screening for thyroid dysfunction, beginning at age 35 (2000).
AACE	Recommends routine screening for subclinical thyroid dysfunction in adults (2004).
AAFP	Evidence is insufficient to recommend for or against routine screening for thyroid disease in adults (2004).
ACOG	Insufficient data to warrant routine screening of asymptomatic pregnant women. Testing may be indicated in women with a personal history of thyroid disease or symptoms of thyroid disease (2002).
IOM	Medicare should not cover screening for thyroid dysfunction as a preventive services benefit based on the lack of sufficient evidence of either net benefit or harm (2003).
ACP, AMA, AGS	No current guidelines or recommendations on screening for thyroid disease.

Abbr: USPSTF, United States Preventive Services Task Force; ATA, American Thyroid Association; AACE, American Association of Clinical Endocrinologists; AAFP, American Academy of Family Physicians; ACOG, American College of Obstetricians and Gynecologists; IOM, Institute of Medicine; ACP, American College of Physicians; AMA, American Medical Association; AGS, American Geriatric Society.

"Patients with acute low back pain alone, without findings of serious conditions or significant nerve root compression, rarely benefit from a surgical consultation. Within the first 3 months of acute low back symptoms, surgery should be considered only when serious spinal pathology or nerve root dysfunction obviously due to a herniated lumbar disc is detected. Many patients with strong clinical findings of nerve root dysfunction due to disc herniation recover activity tolerance within one month; no evidence indicates that delaying surgery for this period worsens outcomes. With or without an operation, more than 80% of patients with obvious surgical indications eventually recover."

In response to AHCPR's guideline, the North American Spine Society (NASS) created an *ad hoc* committee, which attacked the literature review and subsequent AHCPR practice guideline *(34)*. In a letter published in 1994 in the journal *Spine (34)*, the committee not only criticized the methods used in the literature review and expressed concern that the conclusions might be used by payers or regulators to limit the number and types of spinal fusion procedures, but it also charged that AHCPR had wasted taxpayer dollars on the study. At the same time, advocacy groups lobbied Congress and launched an aggressive letter-writing campaign that attacked the Agency and resulted in an effort by several congressional members to end the Agency's funding *(34)*. Clearly, the guidelines had challenged the interests of powerful stakeholders. Despite evidence that much of these surgeries were unnecessary and perhaps even harmful, a group of powerfully connected influential stakeholders was able to successfully lobby Congress and almost single-handedly bring about the demise of an entire agency whose mission was to improve the quality of health care in the United States. At the time, this guideline and other AHCPR-sponsored guidelines developed during the 1990s helped set the standard for how evidence-based guidelines should be developed. This example illustrates that even when guidelines are developed using stringent evidence-based methodology, other interests, including personal lobbying efforts and politics, may override the evidence.

Another example where policy decisions were influenced by advocates lobbying for a cause can be seen with the use of high-dose chemotherapy with autologous bone marrow transplantation (HDC-ABMT) in the 1990s for patients with advanced breast cancer *(36)*. This experimental therapy was designed to overcome some of the toxicity problems of chemotherapy, which destroys hematopoietic cells and is a major limiting factor in treating these patients. Small observational studies in the 1980s indicated a dramatic response to HDC-ABMT, which excited researchers and breast cancer advocates and led to a strong lobbying effort to cover the new treatment. However, insurers balked at covering this treatment, which could cost up to $140,000, in the absence of clear evidence of benefit. A review done by David Eddy in 1992 noted that the benefit seen in most phase II studies lasted only a few months and that there was a markedly increased risk of serious morbidity in patients treated with HDC-ABMT compared to conventional chemotherapy *(37)*. However, even in the absence of clear evidence of effectiveness, there was widespread enthusiasm for this therapy among patients with breast cancer and physicians, especially oncologists. A survey of oncologists revealed that nearly 80% believed it appropriate to offer HDC-ABMT to patients with locally advanced breast cancer *(38)*. As a result, the number of patients receiving HDC-ABMT in the United States increased from an estimated 680 persons in 1990 to an estimated 8200 persons in 1999, a 12-fold increase. Many breast cancer patients resorted to litigation to force insurers to cover this unproven and costly procedure, and many were successful in their efforts. The attention of providers, patients, payers, and policymakers thus became focused on covering HDC-ABMT rather than on evaluating its effectiveness.

An illustrative example is the story of Nelene Fox, a 38-yr-old mother of three from California *(39)*. Mrs. Fox was diagnosed with advanced breast cancer in 1993, failed treatment with conventional therapies, and advised by her doctors that her only chance for survival was HDC-ABMT. Her health maintenance organization (HMO) refused to pay for the procedure because the HMO believed there was insufficient scientific evidence of improved long-term survival or other improvements in important health outcomes. Her local community raised the money for to have the procedure, but she died soon after receiving treatment. Advocates and sympathizers believed that delays in getting treatment were responsible for her treatment failure and death. Her brother, a lawyer, sued the HMO and won damages of $89,000 for her family. Similar lawsuits and media publicity were successful in forcing insurance companies to cover the costs of this procedure. In addition, because patients with advanced breast cancer were told that HDC-ABMT showed promise, many patients refused to participate in randomized clinical trials of HDC-ABMT, thus causing significant delays in obtaining definitive study results about the true efficacy of treatment. Results of a major randomized controlled trial published in 2000 showed no survival advantage in HDC-ABMT patients compared to conventional chemotherapy *(40)*. The Executive Director of a breast cancer advocacy group (Breast Cancer Action) later had this to say about the use of HDC-ABMT:

"After putting thousands of women through the most aggressive cancer therapy ever devised, what we know today is that there is no proven advantage of this very punishing treatment. It seems ironic at best to continue to call this 'therapy.' It's time we stopped putting women at risk and spending hundreds of thousands of dollars on aggressive treatments that show little, if any benefit, and focused our research efforts instead on less toxic and more targeted therapies." (41)

Professional organizations and advocacy groups can also take positions counter to the evidence and attempt to influence policy decisions, especially if the evidence contradicts their preconceived beliefs or if the evidence supports policies or decisions that are viewed as potentially detrimental to the organization or the members it represents. When the expert panel convened by the ATA, AACE, and TES came out with their recommendation against routine screening for subclinical thyroid disease (32), there was an immediate backlash from the leadership of these specialty societies. Before the expert panel's paper was published, confidential copies were sent to the leadership of these societies for their review and comments. Even though all three organizations had originally sponsored and commissioned the panel, they now refused to endorse the report because it did not reach the conclusions that they had expected or desired. They initially asked the panel to engage in a dialogue with the leadership of the societies to discuss the panel's assessment of the evidence and to reconsider its conclusions—an attempt to influence the panel's deliberations and recommendations, after the fact. However, the panel felt that this would jeopardize its independence as well as the objectivity and validity of the report, so it declined; but the panel did agree to consider new studies or evidence that could be identified by the societies, which may not have been included in the earlier review. The refusal of the panel to amend its conclusions and recommendations resulted in veiled threats against several of the endocrinology leaders on the panel. Later, two leaders from each of the three specialty societies worked collaboratively to publish an opinion-based article in one of the specialty society's journals that rebutted the conclusions and recommendations of the panel (42). This article was not based on an independent review of the evidence; instead, the authors offered their own interpretations, conclusions, and recommendations based on their own clinical experience, their own personal opinions, and selective opinions from other "experts" in the field of endocrinology. In the article, they state,

"Our reasons for disagreement on these issues are centered on the consensus conference participants' heavy, if not exclusive, reliance on EBM methodology to substantiate these negative recommendations. Their negative recommendations are inappropriate, in our opinion, because they are based primarily on a lack of evidence for benefit rather than evidence for a lack of benefit."

Despite their acknowledgment throughout the article that there is no good evidence that demonstrates proven health benefits from screening asymptomatic persons for subclinical thyroid disorders, they repeatedly cite their "belief" that screening is indicated. It is interesting to note that the same societies that had originally convened the scientific panel and asked for the evidence review were now issuing their own set of guidelines and recommendations, not based on the best available evidence, but instead based on their own "expert opinion" because they did not like the findings and recommendations supported by the evidence.

From the previous examples, one can see that lobbying and other such efforts by advocates for a cause can often influence policy decisions in spite of the evidence. It is also important to understand that policymakers are often interested in the evidence to the extent that it supports their own predetermined beliefs or agendas. When the evidence differs from what they would like it to be, the complexity of formulating evidence-based decisions can even work in their favor, because data collection, analysis, interpretation, extrapolation, applicability, and other factors can vary considerably and often depend on the circumstances, which allows groups to manipulate different parts of the evidence process to support their own beliefs, needs, and wants.

BEYOND THE EVIDENCE: MEDICAL LIABILITY

Another factor that can override evidence and drive individual, organizational, or health policy decisions is the concern about medical liability. A recent article published in the *Journal of the American Medical Association* illustrates this issue *(43)*. In the article, Merenstein discusses a case where he (a resident-physician) participated with his patient in a shared decision-making process to discuss the benefits and harms of screening for prostate cancer with the prostate-specific antigen (PSA) test. During this encounter, the patient decided against screening. A few years later, when the patient visited a new physician, the new physician ordered a panel of lab tests without counseling the patient, which included a PSA test, and the patient was found to have metastatic prostate cancer. The patient sued Dr. Merenstein and his residency program. Although the clinician was found not to be liable, the jury found the residency program liable and awarded a $1 million settlement to the plaintiff. Since that award was made, most clinicians affiliated with the residency program now order PSAs routinely on their patients *(44)*.

POTENTIAL SOLUTIONS

In this chapter, we have described some of the challenges of incorporating evidence into health policy decisions, highlighting specific issues relating to the retrieval, synthesis, interpretation, and translation of evidence where divergent approaches and perspectives may result in conflicting conclusions and recommendations. Given the difficulties inherent in trying to accommodate all of these various stakeholders, methodologies, values, perspectives, and personal interests, what role can and should evidence play in making policy decisions about the health care of Americans?

One of the many solutions that could help facilitate this process is to standardize some of the methods used to make health care decisions. The GRADE working group is an informal collaboration of experts in the field of EBM that have worked together to formulate recommendations on grading the quality of evidence and strength of recommendations when developing guidelines. Standard use of such a process by guideline developers and health policymakers should lead to more transparent and consistent interpretation and conclusions from research findings. Their recommendations are summarized as follows:

First Steps
1. *Establish the process*—e.g., prioritize problems, select a panel, declare conflicts of interest, and agree on the group process.

Preparatory Steps
2. *Systematic review*—identify and critically appraise or prepare systematic reviews of the best available evidence for all important outcomes.

3. *Prepare evidence profile for important outcomes*—develop profiles for each sub-population or risk group; they should include a quality assessment and summary of findings.

Grading Quality of Evidence and Strength of Recommendations

4. *Quality of evidence for each outcome*—judged on information summarized in the evidence profile and based on specific criteria.

5. *Relative importance of outcomes*—only important outcomes should be included in the evidence profiles; they should be classified as critical or important to a decision.

6. *Overall quality of evidence*—should be judged across outcomes based on the lowest quality of evidence for any of the critical outcomes.

7. *Balance of benefits and harms*—should be classified as net benefits, trade-offs, uncertain trade-offs, or no net benefits based on the important benefits and harms.

8. *Balance of net benefits and costs*—are incremental health benefits worth the costs? Because resources are limited it is important to consider costs (resource utilization) when making a recommendation.

9. *Strength of recommendation*—recommendations should be formulated to reflect their strength; that is, the extent to which one can be confident that adherence will do more good than harm.

Subsequent steps

10. *Implementation and evaluation*—using effective implementation strategies that address barriers to change, evaluation of implementation, and keeping up to date.

Dr. David Eddy, who we spoke about earlier in the chapter, has also proposed a set of principles that can be used to guide health policy decisions *(46)*. He posits that there should be national agreement on a single set of principles, but he believes that, in the absence of national leadership, this is unlikely to occur. These 11 principles, which are outlined below, speak to many of the challenges that we have presented in this chapter and can serve as a useful guide to health policymakers:

1. The financial resources available to provide health care to a population are limited.
2. Because financial resources are limited, when deciding about the appropriate use of treatments, it is both valid and important to consider financial costs of the treatments.
3. Because financial resources are limited, it is necessary to set priorities.
4. A consequence of priority setting is that it will not be possible to cover (using shared resources) every treatment that might have some benefit.
5. The objective of health care is to maximize the health of the population served, subject to the available resources.
6. The priority a treatment should receive should not depend on whether the particular individuals who would receive treatment are our personal patients.
7. Determining the priority of a treatment will require estimating the magnitudes of its benefits, harms, and costs.
8. To the greatest extent possible, estimates of benefits, harms, and costs should be based on empirical evidence. A corollary is that when empirical evidence contradicts subjective judgments, empirical evidence should take priority.
9. Before it should be promoted for use, a treatment should satisfy three criteria:
   a. Compared with no treatment, there should be convincing evidence that the treatment improves health outcomes.
   b. Compared with no treatment, the beneficial effects on health outcomes should outweigh the harmful effects on health outcomes.
   c. Compared with the next best alternative treatment, the treatment should represent a good use of resources that maximizes the health of the population.

10. When making judgments about benefits, harms, and costs, to the greatest extent possible, the judgments should reflect the preferences of the individuals who will actually receive the treatments.

11. When determining whether a treatment satisfies the criteria of principle 9, the burden of proof should be on those who want to promote use of the treatment.

CONCLUSIONS

In this chapter, we attempted to shed light on some of the complex issues involved in trying to incorporate evidence into health policy decisions. Many factors must be taken into account when making these types of decisions. Accessing, synthesizing, evaluating, interpreting, and using evidence in day-to-day clinical decisions poses significant challenges in and of itself. Incorporating evidence into health policy decisions may be even more complex because these decisions can affect an entire population, and the needs, wants, interests, and perspectives of many more stakeholders with different agendas and variable amounts of influence must be taken into account. In addition, the decision-making process may be driven by politics, budgets, ideology, religion, culture, and many other factors beyond the scientific evidence.

Standardizing the methods used to access, synthesize, evaluate, and interpret scientific evidence can help ensure a more consistent and transparent decision-making process and provide policymakers with important information needed for making sound policy decisions. Other actions that can facilitate this process include establishing personal contact and maintaining good communication between researchers, clinicians, and policymakers; ensuring that the research is timely, relevant, and of high quality; providing policymakers with a brief summary that has clear policy recommendations; and including data on effectiveness and costs.

One must also understand that scientific evidence is but one piece of the entire puzzle that must be put together when making decisions or formulating health policy. Although EBM promotes the use of scientific evidence on important health outcomes as the foundation for the decision-making process, the entire puzzle cannot be completed without the other pieces in place (e.g., clinical judgment, individual patient and provider characteristics, clinical circumstances, patient preferences, available resources, and costs). Finally, as with most things, the use of evidence to guide health policy decisions can be used appropriately or misused. Policymakers can use evidence in an objective and judicious manner to try to accurately determine the magnitude of the benefits and harms of a service or intervention for a target population; they can use evidence selectively to support their preconceived beliefs; or they can ignore evidence entirely.

One could easily write an entire book on this subject and still not do it justice. We hope that this chapter will shed some light on this important topic and help you to better understand some of the issues surrounding how and why evidence is (and often is not) incorporated into health policy decisions.

ACKNOWLEDGMENT

The authors wish to thank Gurvaneet Randhawa, MD, MPH for his contributions to this chapter.

REFERENCES

1. Sackett DL, Straus SE, Richardson WS, Rosenberg W, Haynes RB. Evidence-Based Medicine. How to Practice and Teach EMB. Harcourt Publishers, London, 2000.
2. Goldman HH, Ganju V, Drake RE. Policy implications for implementing evidence-based practices. Psychiatr Serv 2001;52:1591–1597.
3. Eisenberg JM. Globalize the evidence, localize the decision: evidence-based medicine and international diversity. Health Aff 2002;21:166–168.
4. Macintyre S, Chalmers I, Horton R, Smith R. Using evidence to inform health policy: case study. BMJ 2001;322:222–225.
5. Acheson D. Independent inquiry into inequalities in health. London: Stationery Office, 1998.
6. Black N. Evidence based policy: proceed with care. BMJ 2001;323:275–279.
7. Ham C, Hunter DJ, Robinson R. Evidence based policymaking. BMJ 1995;310:71–72.
8. Webb A, Wistow G. Planning, Need and Scarcity. Allen and Unwin, London, 1986.
9. Pope C. Assessing evidence based medicine: an investigation of the practice of surgery. PhD thesis. University of London, London, 1999.
10. Innvaer S, Vist G, Trommald M, Oxman A. Health policy-makers' perceptions of their use of evidence: a systematic review. J Health Serv Res Policy 2002;7:239–244.
11. Available at: http://www.ahrq.gov/clinic/ajpmsuppl/harris1.htm. Accessed November 24, 2004.
12. Available at: http://thomas.loc.gov/cgi-bin/cpquery/?&db_id=cp106&r_n=hr305.106&sel=TOC_20879&. Accessed November 23, 2004.
13. Available at: http://www.ahrq.gov/clinic/epc/index.htm. Accessed November 23, 2004.
14. Field MJ, Lohr KN. Guidelines for Clinical Practice: From Development to Use. National Academy Press, Washington, DC, 1992.
15. Eddy DM. Clinical decision making: from theory to practice. Resolving conflicts in practice policies. JAMA 1990;264:389–391.
16. Available at: http://www.ahrq.gov/clinic/3rduspstf/breastcancer/brcanrr.pdf. Accessed October 25, 2004.
17. Humphrey LL, Helfand M, Chan BK, Woolf SH. Breast cancer screening: a summary of the evidence for the U.S. Preventive Services Task Force. Ann Intern Med 2002;137:347–360.
18. Olsen O, Gotzsche PC. Screening for breast cancer with mammography (Chochrane Review). In: The Cochrane Library, Issue 3. John Wiley and Sons, Chichester, UK, 2004.
19. Available at: http://www.cochrane.dk/cochrane/handbook/hbook.htm. Accessed October 24, 2004.
20. Centers for Disease Control and Prevention. 1993 revised classification system for HIV infection and expanded surveillance case definition for AIDS among adolescents and adults. MMWR Recomm Rep 1992;41:1–19.
21. Freeman AJ, Dore GJ, Law MG, et al. Estimating progression to cirrhosis in chronic hepatitis C virus infection. Hepatology 2001;34:809–816.
22. Moss AJ, Zareba W, Hall WJ, et al.; Multicenter Automatic Defibrillator Implantation Trial II Investigators. Prophylactic implantation of a defibrillator in patients with myocardial infarction and reduced ejection fraction. N Engl J Med 2002;346:877–883.
23. Owens DK, Sanders GD, Harris RA, et al. Cost-effectiveness of implantable cardioverter defibrillators relative to amiodarone for prevention of sudden cardiac death. Ann Intern Med 1997;126:1–12.
24. Stecker EC, Pollack HA. Implantable cardiac defibrillators. N Engl J Med 2002;347:365–367.
25. Sackett Dl, Straus SE, Richardson WS, Rosenberg W, Haynes RB. Evidence-Based Medicine: How to Practice and Teach EBM. Churchill Livingstone, London, 2000.
26. Starfield B, Shi L. Policy relevant determinants of health: an international perspective. Health Policy 2002;60:201–218.
27. Committing to Quality Facing Old Challenges, Setting New Standards. Presented by Mary Wakefield, May 28, 2004, San Diego, CA.
28. Coffield AB, Maciosek MV, McGinnis JM, et al. Priorities among recommended clinical preventive services. Am J Prev Med 2001Jul;21:1–9.
29. Available at: http://ngc.gov/summary/summary.aspx?doc_id=2361&nbr=1587#s24. Accessed October 25, 2004.
30. Available at: http://www.ahrq.gov/clinic/3rduspstf/thyroid/thyrs.htm. Accessed October 25, 2004.
31. Available at: http://www.endo-society.org/educationevents/print/upload/mgmt-subclinical-thyroid-disease.pdf. Accessed February 20, 2005.

32. Surks MI, Ortiz E, Daniels GH, et al. Subclinical thyroid disease: scientific review and guidelines for diagnosis and management. JAMA 2004;291:228–238.
33. Agency for Health Care Policy and Research (AHCPR). Acute Lower Back Problems in Adults. Clinical Practice Guideline 14. AHCPR Publication, Rockville, MD, 1994.
34. Gray BH, Gusmano MK, Collins SR. AHCPR and the changing politics of health services research. Health Aff 2003;Suppl Web Exclusives:283–307.
35. White A., et al. Letter to the editor. Spine 1994;19:109–110.
36. Mello MM, Brennan TA. The controversy over high-dose chemotherapy with autologous bone marrow transplant for breast cancer. Health Aff 2001;20:101–117.
37. Eddy DM. High-dose chemotherapy with autologous bone marrow transplantation for the treatment of metastatic breast cancer. J Clin Oncol. 1992;10:657–670.
38. Belanger D, Moore M, Tannock I. How American oncologists treat breast cancer: an assessment of the influence of clinical trials. J Clin Oncol 1991;9:7–16.
39. Sharf BF. Out of the closet and into the legislature: breast cancer stories. Health Aff 2001;20:213–218.
40. Stadtmauer EA, O'Neill A, Goldstein LJ, et al. Conventional-dose chemotherapy compared with high-dose chemotherapy plus autologous hematopoietic stem-cell transplantation for metastatic breast cancer. Philadelphia Bone Marrow Transplant Group. N Engl J Med 2000;342:1069–1076.
41. Available at: http://www.bcaction.org/Pages/SearchablePages/ConferenceCoverage/BCAConcernedPr.html. Accessed November 29, 2004.
42. Gharib H, Tuttle RM, Baskin HJ, Fish LH, Singer PA, McDermott MT. Subclinical thyroid dysfunction: a joint statement on management from the American Association of Clinical Endocrinologists, the American Thyroid Association, and the Endocrine Society. J Clin Endocrinol Metab 2005;90:581–585.
43. Merenstein D. Winners and Losers. JAMA 2004;291:15–16.
44. Krist A, Kuzel A, Woolf S, Johnson R. The impact of malpractice litigation on prostate cancer screening. North American Primary Care Research Group Annual Meeting. Orlando, FL, 2004.
45. GRADE Working Group. Grading the equality of evidence and strength of recommendations. BMJ 2004;328:1–8.
46. Eddy D. Clinical decision making: from theory to practice. Principles for making difficult decisions in difficult times. JAMA 1994;271:1792–1798.

III RESEARCH EVIDENCE FOR EVIDENCE-BASED ENDOCRINE PRACTICE

10 The Value of Observational Studies in Endocrinology

L. Joseph Melton III, MD, MPH

CONTENTS

INTRODUCTION
WHAT ARE OBSERVATIONAL STUDIES?
HOW DO OBSERVATIONAL STUDIES COMPLEMENT RANDOMIZED
    CONTROLLED TRIALS?
WHERE ARE THE OPPORTUNITIES FOR OBSERVATIONAL RESEARCH?
REFERENCES

INTRODUCTION

In the pantheon of information sources about what works in medicine and what does not, the place of honor goes to randomized controlled clinical trials (RCTs). A particularly important aspect is the ability to neutralize, by random assignment of the intervention, any unmeasured and unknown determinants of the disease outcome in the treated and untreated groups. Observational studies do not enjoy this advantage and, because of the resulting potential for bias, are often given less credence. However, observational designs may be the only ones possible for addressing important clinical questions. Thus, some disease determinants cannot be subjected to trial. It would obviously be unethical to randomize subjects to excessive weight gain or chronic elevations in blood glucose, although trials may be possible where interventions are directed at reducing blood glucose and weight. Similarly, it is generally infeasible to extend RCTs for a sufficient length of time to determine the effects of an intervention on long-term outcomes decades later. In addition, the fact that efficacy is demonstrated under the idealized conditions of a RCT does not necessarily mean that a specific treatment is as effective in routine clinical practice. Finally, and more importantly perhaps, many questions arise in medicine that RCTs were never designed to answer: what set of clinical characteristics best defines a disease entity? What is the magnitude of the disease burden on society? What risk factors are associated with the risk of developing a disease? And which ones influence prognosis? These issues can be addressed in observational studies, including descriptive, cross-sectional, cohort, and case–control

From: *Contemporary Endocrinology: Evidence-Based Endocrinology*
Edited by: V. M. Montori © Mayo Foundation for Medical Education and Research

studies. All of these applications of epidemiology are relevant to endocrinology, and the use of these designs will be reviewed in the material that follows.

WHAT ARE OBSERVATIONAL STUDIES?

Originally created to investigate epidemics of infectious disease, the field of epidemiology now encompasses studies of the distribution and determinants of disease generally in the population. To accomplish this, methodology has been developed that includes descriptive studies of the frequency and impact of disease, as well as analytic studies of risk factors for disease onset or progression. These observational studies differ critically from RCTs insofar as the "exposure" (e.g., risk factor, treatment) is not controlled by the investigators. Instead, study groups are identified who do and do not have the exposure of interest or, alternatively, have or have not already developed the disease outcome. Although exposures and outcomes may be assessed by sophisticated measurements, such research differs from clinical studies (*see* Chapter 11) in that the focus is on population health rather than on pathophysiological processes in individual subjects.

Certain classes of problems in endocrinology are best addressed using these observational approaches. In particular, it is necessary to know the impact of endocrine disorders, not only on the affected patients themselves, but on society in general, because this establishes national priorities for research support and for the instigation of control efforts. It is equally important to describe the frequency and natural history of endocrine conditions because this provides an opportunity to generate hypotheses about etiology that can be tested in more focused clinical investigations or in basic studies of underlying pathophysiological mechanisms. Natural history data also help quantify disease prognosis and facilitate the identification of high-risk populations for screening, prophylaxis, or therapy. These are very broad areas, and there are many gaps and discrepancies in currently available data. Opportunities abound, therefore, to apply these methods to help rationalize the care of patients with a range of endocrine disorders.

Descriptive Studies

As the name implies, descriptive studies aim to measure the impact of a disease on a population with respect to its frequency, morbidity, mortality, and/or cost. The frequency of disease occurrence must be expressed as a rate or ratio, in which the number of cases of the disease (numerator) is related to the underlying population at risk (denominator). There are two general approaches to collecting this information: longitudinal population surveillance studies and cross-sectional surveys. These methods are described in detail in a number of introductory textbooks on epidemiology (1–3). In a longitudinal study, all cases of a particular disease that arise in a defined population over a period of time (days, years) are identified; the primary purpose is to determine the incidence of the disease, i.e., the rate at which new events occur in the population over time.

The methodological issues involved here mainly relate to the accuracy of the numerator and denominator data. Specifically, the numerator depends on a precise definition of the disorder, as well as on complete ascertainment of all cases in the population of interest. Ascertainment, in turn, may depend on clinical, technical, or systems capabilities. Of particular interest are technological advances that enable the detection of previously

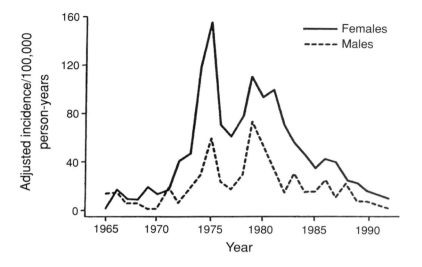

Fig. 1. Age-adjusted (to 1990 US caucasians) incidence of definite plus possible primary hyper-parathyroidism among Rochester, Minnesota, women (–) and men (---), 1965–1992, by year (5).

unrecognized cases of an endocrine disorder. For example, a dramatic increase in the apparent incidence of primary hyperparathyroidism (HPT) coincided with the addition of serum calcium determinations to routine chemistry panels *(4)*. In Rochester, Minnesota, the annual incidence of primary HPT increased from 7.8 cases per 100,000 between January 1, 1965 and June 31, 1974 to 51.1 per 100,000 in the following 12-mo period (*see* Fig. 1). The sharp rise and subsequent fall in apparent incidence is consistent with sweeping the population for previously undiagnosed HPT when serum calcium was added to the 12-test automatic screening panel at Mayo Clinic in July 1974. A similarly sharp increase and subsequent decline in the incidence of diabetes mellitus in Rochester was observed when blood glucose was added to the autoanalyzer panel in 1959 *(6)*.

The annual incidence of primary HPT fell subsequently to just 4.0 per 100,000 in 1992 (Fig. 1). These trends in incidence were associated with significant changes in the clinical spectrum of HPT at diagnosis (Table 1). For example, the proportion of patients who presented with possible complications of hyperparathyroidism declined dramatically from 22% in the era that predated opportunistic screening (1965–1974) to only 2% in 1983–1992 *(5)*. More generally, when some portion of the diseased population is systemically missed (e.g., the mild cases, and the elderly), as in studies of HPT prior to the mid-1970s, the resulting morbidity rates will be unduly low (ascertainment bias), and the clinical spectrum will be distorted to the extent that silent cases differ from those who present with symptoms. This almost always occurs in studies restricted to patients attended at major medical centers because patients are not referred randomly. Rather, there is appropriate but disproportionate referral of the small subset of patients who pose complex diagnostic or management problems (selection bias). The clinical spectrum of such patients may bear little resemblance to that of unselected community patients with the same diagnosis.

By contrast, a cross-sectional survey is done at a specific point in time to enumerate all existing cases in the population; one main purpose is to establish the prevalence of

Table 1
Clinical Characteristics of Rochester, Minnesota Residents Diagnosed
With Definite or Possible HPT From 1965 to 1992

Characteristic	Time period		
	1965–June 1974 (n = 63)	July 1974–1982 (n = 289)	1983–1992 (n = 123)
Mode of diagnosis, n (%)			
Histologic evidence	23 (36.5)	78 (27.0)	21 (17.1)
Inappropriately elevated immunoreactive parathyroid hormone level	25 (39.7)	135 (46.7)	49 (39.8)
By exclusion	13 (20.6)	60 (20.8)	31 (25.2)
Possible primary HPT	2 (3.2)	16 (5.5)	22 (17.9)
Presentation, n (%)			
Symptom or complication of primary HPT	14 (22.2)	23 (8.0)	2 (1.6)
Abnormal serum calcium level	47 (74.6)	264 (91.4)	119 (96.8)
Other biochemical abnormality	1 (1.6)	0 (0)	2 (1.6)
Autopsy finding	0 (0)	2 (0.7)	0 (0)
Uncertain	1 (1.6)	0 (0)	0 (0)
Maximum serum calcium level, mean mmol/L	2.72	2.72	2.67
Initial management, n (%)			
Surgery ≤ 6 mo after diagnosis	18 (28.6)	63 (21.8)	16 (13.0)
Surgery recommended but refused/ill	8 (12.7)	23 (8.0)	3 (2.4)
Decision to observe	35 (55.6)	203 (70.2)	104 (84.6)
Uncertain	2 (3.2)	0 (0)	0 (0)

Modified from ref. 5.

the disease (i.e., the proportion of the population affected at a given time). For example, the prevalence of self-reported diagnoses of diabetes mellitus has been estimated on numerous occasions by the National Health Interview Survey and there appears to have been a dramatic increase over the past half-century, especially in older age-groups (see Fig. 2). It is now anticipated that the estimated 10.9 million affected individuals (4.0% of the entire population) could rise to 29.1 million (7.2% of the US population) by 2050 (8). An increase in the prevalence of diabetes could certainly be owing to a rise in incidence associated with the ongoing epidemic of obesity. However, prevalence depends not only on the underlying incidence of a disease but on its duration as well, so any improvements in survival following the diagnosis of diabetes might also contribute to a rise in prevalence. Moreover, prevalence rates can also be affected by differential in- or out-migration of cases from the underlying population, although this is not as important a concern in a national sample as it could be in a local community survey. Because of these potential sources of error, prevalence rates are not as good as incidence rates for assessing trends in disease. Conversely, prevalence rates are preferred for evaluating the burden of disease in the population because the number of

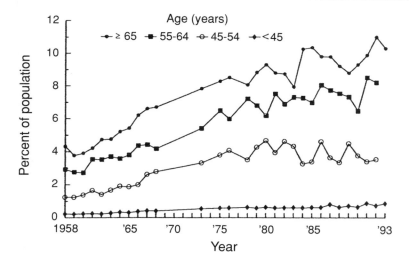

Fig. 2. Time trends in the percent of the population with diagnosed diabetes, by age, US, 1958–1993 *(7)*.

affected people in the community can be substantial, even when incidence rates are low, if their survival is good.

It is important to reemphasize that the prevalence cases are not necessarily representative of all cases that arose in the population. Those incidence cases of people who died early, those who were cured (if any) and those who moved away have been deleted, and the clinical spectrum of the remaining patients may differ. This is especially germane when assessing associations in cross-sectional studies, where an entire population is assessed simultaneously for the prevalence of a disease outcome and the prevalence of one or more risk factors. For example, in a representative sample of 84,572 US adults, only 2829 were thought to have diabetes. On questioning about numbness, pain or tingling, or decreased perception of hot or cold in the hands or feet over the previous 3 mo, 39.8% of women and 36.0% of men with type 2 diabetes reported symptoms of sensory neuropathy compared to 11.8 and 9.8%, respectively, among 20,129 of the nondiabetic women and men *(9)*. If neuropathy were associated with reduced survival, however, these figures would underestimate the association of neuropathy with diabetes. Note also that unaffected subjects in the original study population outnumbered those with diabetes by almost 30 to 1. Case–control studies (*see* Analytic Studies) can obtain similar information much more efficiently because smaller numbers of unaffected individuals need to be evaluated.

Analytic Studies

Enumerating those with a given endocrine disorder is not usually an end in itself. Instead, the emphasis more often is on discovering the causative agents or the factors that lead to disease progression and complications. In addition to cross-sectional studies as previously mentioned, associations between putative risk factors and disease can be formally tested using two main approaches: case–control and cohort studies (as described in detail elsewhere *[1–3]*). In a cohort study (*see* Fig. 3), a group of individuals with a particular factor thought to be related to disease etiology (exposed) and a comparable group without the characteristic (unexposed) we observed over time for

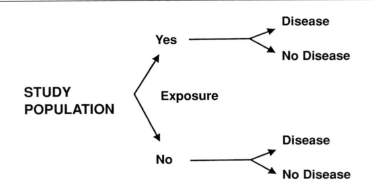

Fig. 3. Schematic of a cohort study.

the development of some disease outcome. To establish a positive association between the exposure and the occurrence of the outcome, it is necessary to show that the rate of developing disease is higher in the exposed than in the nonexposed group (relative risk). Such studies can be carried out prospectively (i.e., a concurrent cohort study where the exposure is assessed now and patients are followed into the future) or retrospectively (i.e., a historical cohort study where the exposure is assessed at some earlier time and disease outcomes are determined now).

The latter approach is especially valuable for evaluating late outcomes when a cohort can be identified whose past exposure status can be reliably assessed. Thus, Olmsted County, MN, women who had undergone bilateral oophorectomy 14 yr on average after a natural menopause in 1950–1987 were followed for up to 42 yr (median, 16 yr of follow-up per subject) for the occurrence of various fractures as of 2002. There was a significant increase in fractures of the hip, spine, and distal forearm (see Fig. 4), the fractures that are traditionally associated with osteoporosis (10). This is consistent with the hypothesis that androgens produced by the postmenopausal ovary are important for endogenous estrogen production, and therefore the preservation of bone mass, after menopause. However, it is important to keep in mind that the "intervention" (e.g., oophorectomy) in a cohort study is not randomly assigned as it is in a clinical trial. Rather, patients self-select into the exposed and unexposed categories and this may result in confounding (i.e., attribution of the outcome to the exposure itself when both the exposure and the outcome are related to some unmeasured third factor that is actually responsible). In the above example, it is conceivable that the elevated fracture risk was not a result of bilateral oophorectomy per se but rather the underlying indication for surgery because most oophorectomies are performed incidentally in the course of hysterectomy.

Case–control studies, on the other hand, are especially valuable for examining the etiology of relatively uncommon endocrine disorders. In a case–control study, one begins with a group of individuals who already have the disease being studied (cases) and a comparable group, matched on age and sex perhaps, without the disease (controls). Because the number of controls usually equals the number of cases (or some multiple thereof), this approach is more efficient than evaluating the entire population as in a cross-sectional study, where the great majority of subjects will not have the disease of interest. As shown in Fig. 5, the case and control groups are then compared for the prior

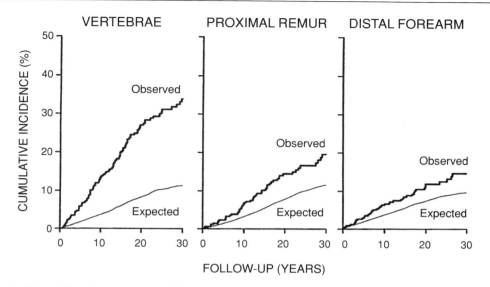

Fig. 4. Observed and expected cumulative incidence of subsequent fracture of the vertebrae ($p < 0.001$), proximal femur ($p < 0.001$) and distal forearm ($p = 0.012$) among Rochester, Minnesota, women who underwent bilateral (or second unilateral) oophorectomy following natural menopause in 1950–1987 *(10)*.

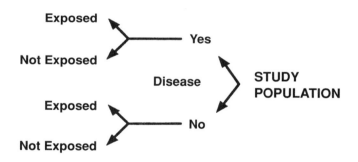

Fig. 5. Schematic of a case–control study.

presence or absence of factors thought to be related to disease occurrence (odds ratio). The odds ratio is a good estimator of the relative risk, which is the quantity actually desired, if: (1) the cases studied are representative of all cases in the underlying population in terms of the exposure of interest; (2) the controls are representative of all unaffected individuals in the population in terms of the exposure; and (3) the disease is rare. The latter condition is easily fulfilled in practice. If either the cases or the controls are unrepresentative of their respective groups, however, the odds ratio will not accurately reflect the true relative risk. Referral center cases and control subjects selected from these sources are rarely representative of the underlying general population in terms of potentially important risk factors. In addition, it is important that the exposure be assessed consistently in both cases and controls. Thus, all Olmsted County residents with diabetes mellitus (DM) by National Diabetes Data Group criteria were matched by age and sex to randomly sampled nondiabetic controls from the community, and both groups were then surveyed for gastrointestinal symptoms *(11)*. As shown in Table 2,

Table 2
Prevalence (%) of Gastrointestinal Tract and Neurological Symptoms
Among Olmsted County, Minnesota Residents With Diabetes Mellitus
Compared With Their Respective Community Controls

Symptoms/syndrome	Type 1 DM		Type 2 DM	
	Patients	Controls	Patients	Controls
Irritable bowel syndrome	10.9	7.6	5.1	8.3
Constipation symptoms and/or laxatives	27.0	19.0	17.0	15.0
Dyschezia	2.9	3.5	2.3	2.3
Fecal incontinence	0.7	1.2	4.6	1.8
Nausea and/or vomiting	11.6	10.6	6.0	5.5
Heartburn symptoms and/or antacids	18.8[a]	36.5	24.0	36.2
Autonomic neuropathy symptoms (overall)	9.4	5.9	7.8	7.3

[a]$p < 0.05$ (univariate association, subgroup with type 1 DM vs corresponding controls). Modified from ref. *11*. DM, diabetes mellitus.

only the lower prevalence of heartburn among those with type 1 diabetes was statistically significant. This indicates that physicians should not simply assume that all gastrointestinal tract symptoms in diabetic patients represent manifestations of autonomic neuropathy, as suggested by data from series of referral patients who may have been seen at a tertiary medical center precisely because they had developed such complications *(12)*.

Cohort studies are usually quite expensive and time-consuming because of the large number of subjects needed and the lengthy follow-up that is often required. Indeed, the disease outcome must be relatively frequent for such studies to be feasible in the first place. Therefore, these prospective studies are generally restricted to fairly common disorders, but they can be employed to examine smaller groups of people when they are at high risk of disease. Cohort studies are also needed if it is important to assess several different clinical outcomes resulting from a single risk factor. Retrospective case–control studies can generally be carried out much more quickly and inexpensively. This approach is required if multiple risk factors must be evaluated in conjunction with a single disease outcome. Because of their ability to evaluate many risk factors simultaneously, case–control studies are especially good for generating etiologic hypotheses.

HOW DO OBSERVATIONAL STUDIES COMPLEMENT RANDOMIZED CONTROLLED TRIALS?

Setting the Stage for Trials

Clinical trials generally depend on a large body of prior knowledge. In particular, observational studies often have a role in justifying an RCT by quantifying the magnitude of a disease problem (i.e., providing the motivation to develop a new therapy). Moreover, observational data are needed to define the natural history of the disease— data that may be necessary to design the trial. This is especially true for disorders like diabetes mellitus and osteoporosis, where there is a gradient of risk for adverse out-

Table 3
Projected Prevalence of Osteoporosis and/or Low Bone Mass (Osteopenia)
of the Hip in US Women and Men 50 yr of Age or Older in 2010 and 2020

	2002	*2010*	*2020*
Women			
Osteoporosis	7.8 million	9.1 million	10.5 million
Osteopenia	21.8 million	26.0 million	30.4 million
Men			
Osteoporosis	2.3 million	2.8 million	3.3 million
Osteopenia	11.8 million	14.4 million	17.1 million

Modified from ref. *13*.

comes (e.g., peripheral vascular disease, fractures) based on the perturbation of a clinical characteristic (e.g., high blood glucose, low bone mineral density) and the actual frequency of the disorder is somewhat equivocal. Thus, based on representative data from the National Health and Nutrition Examination Survey (NHANES III), it was possible to estimate that 7.8 million women and 2.3 million men in the US already have osteoporosis of the hip by World Health Organization criteria, but these figures could rise to 10.5 million and 3.3 million, respectively, by the year 2020 (Table 3). An additional 47.5 million Americans may develop low bone mass, or osteopenia (analogous to prediabetes), and would be at risk for osteoporosis *(13)*. Such numbers have spurred the development of new pharmacological agents (*see* Chapter 22), and stimulated the implementation of public health measures to control this growing problem *(14)*. In contrast, the number of US residents with hyperthyroidism, thyroiditis, or Addison's disease in 1996 was only 3.0 million, 1.5 million, and 13,335, respectively *(15)*. As a consequence, these conditions are the focus of much less commercial or public health interest.

Prospective clinical studies (*see* Chapter 11) are often needed to define the rate of change in disease markers. However, it is rarely feasible to study large enough groups for a sufficient length of time in order to quantify the hard clinical outcomes of greater interest to patients and their physicians. The same problem affects clinical trials, and intermediate or surrogate endpoints (e.g., bone mineral density and blood glucose control) are often employed to reduce costs. Much larger trials are needed to evaluate definitive outcomes (e.g., bone fractures and diabetic complications). Thus, large RCTs involving thousands of patients have provided unequivocal evidence that a number of antiresorptive agents (e.g., the aminobisphosphonates) can reduce fracture risk in postmenopausal women with established osteoporosis (*see* Chapter 22). However, the long-term effects of such treatments may remain unknown. Thus, in an observational study, Cauley et al. showed that elderly women who had taken hormone replacement therapy (HRT) for at least 10 yr after menopause, and who were still on it, experienced a substantial reduction in fracture risk *(16)*. However, postmenopausal women who had stopped therapy earlier had no reduction in fracture risk late in life, even though they had taken HRT for an average of 14.6 yr (Table 4). This is an important observation because lifetime compliance with any treatment regimen is likely to be modest. Moreover, it is difficult to provide complete assurance that a given treatment is safe because even the largest trials are unable to assess rare complications.

Table 4
Relative Risk of Fracture by Duration of HRT Compared to Non-HRT Users

Fracture site	HRT use ≤10 yr		HRT use ≥10 yr	
	Current	Past	Current	Past
Hip	0.81	0.97	0.27[a]	1.67
Wrist	0.75	0.79	0.25[a]	0.90
All nonspine	0.67[a]	0.92	0.60[a]	1.00

[a]$p < 0.05$.
Modified from ref. *16*.

Evaluating Treatment Effectiveness

Although randomized, controlled clinical trials represent the gold standard for assessing treatment efficacy, they may provide misleading information about the likelihood of success in the ordinary clinical practice environment (i.e., treatment effectiveness). In order to optimize internal validity, RCTs are usually restricted to homogenous samples of volunteers who meet rigorous inclusion and exclusion criteria. Those patients who have atypical disease manifestations or other comorbid conditions are likely to be excluded, along with those who cannot comply with the treatment regimen, have a poor prognosis, or are unable to provide informed consent. The results of most trials, therefore, apply to a highly selected subset of the potential target patient population. For example, participants were solicited by press release for a RCT of sodium fluoride therapy for the prevention of new vertebral fractures among women with established postmenopausal osteoporosis *(17)*. Subsequent enrollment depended upon screening by their own physician, where the presence of one or more vertebral fractures had to be verified and certain inclusion criteria met (*see* Fig. 6). Of 664 women who responded to the press release, only 44% had a radiographically confirmed vertebral fracture, and 50% were excluded (mostly for current use of estrogen or thiazide diuretics). The remaining 148 women were eligible for study, but 39% ultimately refused to participate. This left 91 women (14% overall) to be enrolled, only 44 of whom (7%) were randomized and actively continued in the trial. This experience is by no means unique among clinical trials, and it is often uncertain whether the positive effects seen in a given trial would be replicated in men, non-white women, elderly individuals, or those with particular characteristics (e.g., long-term corticosteroid users). The result is lack of evidence with respect to treatment effects in crucial subsets of the patient population.

By contrast, an observational cohort study could evaluate the effect of an intervention on the entire clinical spectrum of disease in the community. The results would be more generalizable than those from the trial cohort, and the data would reflect the ability to deliver the intervention effectively in the community, including actual treatment adherence rates among other factors. Such a study might show that societal costs were greater than anticipated, as therapeutic indications are expanded beyond the narrow RCT population, whereas benefits to society were less than expected. For example, among women in the Northern California Kaiser Foundation Health Plan who were newly diagnosed by bone densitometry with osteopenia or osteoporosis and started on pharmacologic therapy for osteoporosis, 22% had already stopped treatment after only

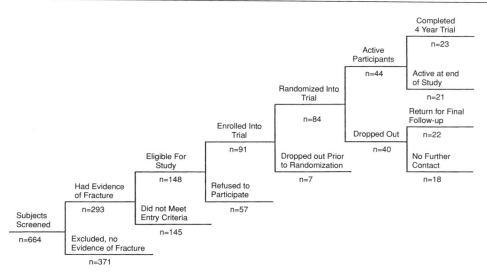

Fig. 6. Recruitment and participation in a clinical trial of sodium fluoride therapy *(17)*.

7 mo *(18)*. The predictors of treatment discontinuation (Table 5) suggest that, compared to trial participants, community women in general are less motivated by fear of osteoporosis and more bothered by potential treatment side effects. It is possible, of course, to resolve such concerns by carrying out RCTs to assess the effectiveness of preventive strategies within entire populations. This is rarely done because the logistic difficulties and costs involved in mounting such a trial are often perceived to be insurmountable. Under these circumstances, inferences about the effectiveness of a given treatment in the general population may be made from epidemiological observations. However, similar problems (i.e., selection bias and treatment adherence) can also plague observational studies if they are not carefully designed, as became evident in the controversy over HRT.

WHERE ARE THE OPPORTUNITIES
FOR OBSERVATIONAL RESEARCH?

There are practically unlimited opportunities to use observational studies to answer practical questions that arise in endocrine practice on a daily basis. This is an important consideration because shortcomings in the data currently available pose problems in implementing a rationale approach to the care of patients with most endocrine disorders. Thus, to ensure that substantial societal costs for treatment are rewarded with commensurate benefits, it is necessary to know (1) the likelihood of adverse outcomes among patients of different ages, genders, and races and with different risk factors; (2) the frequency and consequences (including cost and decreased quality of life) of these outcomes; (3) the effectiveness of treatment in reducing the risk; and (4) the tradeoff between the risks and costs of the adverse outcomes and the benefits, risks, and costs of treatment. Formal cost-effectiveness analyses are used to address these issues (*see* Chapter 14). However, such analyses are almost always flawed to some degree by the lack of empirical data on seemingly straightforward issues: the risk of disease in dif-

Table 5
Multivariable Analysis of Factors Associated With Early Treatment Discontinuation Among Postmenopausal Women Diagnosed With Osteopenia or Osteoporosis *(18)*

Variable	Odds ratio[a] (95% confidence interval)
Side-effect experience[b]	
Somewhat bothered	4.0 (2.5–6.5)
Very or extremely bothered	25 (16–39)
Self-reported exercise habits	
Exercise regularly (≥3 ×/wk)	0.7 (0.4–1.0)
Willingness to take prescribed medications	
Agree that they are willing	0.6 (0.4–0.9)
Perception of bone density test result	
Think test did not show osteoporosis or are uncertain	1.6 (1.0–2.5)

[a]Adjusted for age, bone density T-score, and the other factors shown in the table.
[b]Reference group comprised women who had no side effects or who were not at all bothered.

ferent subsets of the general population; the frequency of adverse outcomes in specific patient groups; the social and economic impact of these adverse outcomes; the actual long-term adherence to therapy; and the frequency or significance of treatment side effects. However, an important side benefit of such modeling exercises is the illumination of these critical gaps in knowledge, particularly with regard to practical problems in patient management *(19)*. This is information that often can be provided by observational studies, and the opportunity for such studies may be considerably enhanced in the future by ongoing improvements in electronic access to comprehensive patient data.

ACKNOWLEDGMENTS

The author would like to thank Mrs. Mary Roberts for assistance in preparing the manuscript. This work was supported in part by grant AG 04875 from the National Institutes of Health, US Public Health Service.

REFERENCES

1. Fletcher RH, Fletcher SW, Wagner EH. Clinical Epidemiology: The Essentials, 3rd ed. Williams and Wilkins, Baltimore, MD, 1996.
2. Greenberg RS, Daniels SR, Flanders WD, Eley JW, Boring JR. Medical Epidemiology, 2nd ed. Appleton and Lange, Norwalk, CT, 1996.
3. Gordis L. Epidemiology, 2nd ed. W. B. Saunders Company, Philadelphia, PA, 2000.
4. Heath H III, Hodgson SF, Kennedy MA. Primary hyperparathyroidism: Incidence, morbidity, and potential economic impact in a community. N Engl J Med 1980;302:189–193.
5. Wermers RA, Khosla S, Atkinson EJ, Hodgson SF, O'Fallon WM, Melton LJ III. The rise and fall of primary hyperparathyroidism: A population-based study in Rochester, Minnesota, 1965–1992. Ann Intern Med 1997;126:433–440.
6. Palumbo PJ, Elveback LR, Chu C-P, Connolly DC, Kurland LT. Diabetes mellitus: Incidence, prevalence, survivorship, and causes of death in Rochester, Minnesota, 1945–1970. Diabetes 1976;25: 566–573.
7. Kenny SJ, Aubert RE, Geiss LS. Prevalence and incidence of non-insulin-dependent diabetes. In: Diabetes in America, 2nd ed. National Diabetes Data Group, Bethesda, National Institutes of Health,

National Institute of Diabetes and Digestive and Kidney Diseases, NIH Publication No. 95–1468, 1995:47–67.

8. Boyle JP, Honeycutt AA, Narayan KMV, et al. Projection of diabetes burden through 2050: Impact of changing demography and disease prevalence in the U.S. Diabetes Care 2001;24:1936–1940.

9. Harris M, Eastman R, Cowie C. Symptoms of sensory neuropathy in adults with NIDDM in the U.S. population. Diabetes Care 1993;16:1446–1452.

10. Melton LJ III, Khosla S, Malkasian GD, Achenbach SJ, Oberg AL, Riggs BL. Fracture risk after bilateral oophorectomy in elderly women. J Bone Miner Res 2003;18:900–905.

11. Maleki D, Locke R III, Camilleri M, et al. Gastrointestinal tract symptoms among persons with diabetes mellitus in the community. Arch Intern Med 2000;160:2808–2816.

12. Melton LJ III, Ochi JW, Palumbo PJ, Chu CP. Referral bias in diabetes research. Diabetes Care 1984; 7:12–18.

13. National Osteoporosis Foundation. America's Bone Health: The State of Osteoporosis and Low Bone Mass in Our Nation. 1–55. National Osteoporosis Foundation, Washington, DC, 2002.

14. U.S. Department of Health and Human Services. Bone Health and Osteoporosis: A Report of the Surgeon General. U.S. Department of Health and Human Services, Office of the Surgeon General, Rockville, MD, 2004.

15. Jacobson DL, Gange SJ, Rose NR, Graham NMH. Short analytical review: Epidemiology and estimated population burden of selected autoimmune diseases in the United States. Clin Immunol Immunopathol 1997;84:223–243.

16. Cauley JA, Seeley DG, Ensrud K, Ettinger B, Black D, Cummings SR. Estrogen replacement therapy and fractures in older women. Study of Osteoporotic Fractures Research Group. Ann Intern Med 1995;122:9–16.

17. Tilley BC, Peterson EL, Kleerekoper M, Phillips E, Nelson DA, Shorck MA. Designing clinical trials of treatment for osteoporosis: Recruitment and follow-up. Calcif Tissue Int 1990;47:327–331.

18. Tosteson ANA, Grove MR, Hammond CS, et al. Early discontinuation of treatment for osteoporosis. Am J Med 2003;115:209–216.

19. Armstrong N. Research opportunities in diabetes. J Cardiovasc Nurs 2002;16:86–94.

11 Clinical Research Center-Based Investigations and Evidence-Based Medicine

William L. Isley, MD

Contents

INTRODUCTION

The last decade of the 20th century saw the emergence of a new paradigm in clinical decision making with the appearance of evidence-based medicine (EBM) *(1)*. The ultimate in the hierarchy of evidence in EBM is the randomized controlled clinical trial (RCT). Unfortunately, the *N*-of-1 RCT, ideal for evaluating the effectiveness of interventions in the individual patient, is rarely feasible or if feasible, is rarely conducted.

RCTs have become common place in the past 35 yr (beginning with the hypertension trials in the 1970s). Pragmatic drug RCTs enroll hundreds to thousands of participants in the community, outside the ivory towers of traditional medical academia. Their purpose is to assess the efficacy, and sometimes the safety and cost effectiveness, of experimental interventions in real patients cared for in real clinical settings.

The rise of the RCT in the hierarchy of evidence has meant the decline in priority of other forms of evidence to support clinical decision making, namely the clinical investigation.

Until the biomedical revolution inaugurated after World War II, unsystematic clinical observations and oligo-subject minimally systemized studies were the basis of much of clinical decision making, with the few observation masters passing on their conclusions in an authoritarian fashion as exemplified by the incomparable Sir William Osler. Some

From: *Contemporary Endocrinology: Evidence-Based Endocrinology*
Edited by: V. M. Montori © Mayo Foundation for Medical Education and Research

aspects of this paradigm still survive today, particularly in the surgical specialties and in the concept of "opinion leaders" used (and abused) by the pharmaceutical industry on a regular basis. The expansion of the National Institutes of Health (NIH) in the late 1940s saw the development of the modern biomedical research enterprise, with the clinical investigator being the hero of this paradigm of knowledge acquisition and application.

For those schooled in the 1970s, the burgeoning biomedical fields were to provide the basic knowledge of molecular biology, physiology, pathophysiology, and applied pharmacology in order to tackle disease in a far more sophisticated manner than the purported "ignorance" of our forebears. The triumph of Brown and Goldstein in the discovery of the low-density lipoprotein (LDL) receptor *(2)* and the subsequent modern assault on atherosclerosis from a metabolic standpoint exemplifies such exploits. The physician of the 1980s was to be an applied physiologist and pharmacologist *par excellence*.

To support this goal, highly trained researchers conducted standard metabolic studies of a highly selected and small group of research subjects. These studies involve tightly controlled experiments and intensively monitored observations conducted in a clinical research center (CRC). Whereas many CRC studies are done to marshal physiological and pathophysiological evidence for a therapeutic intervention's putative benefit while awaiting the outcome of RCTs, they cannot provide the ultimate "proof of the pudding" in most contexts. For example, in the field of endocrinology and metabolism, there are numerous CRC studies showing a positive benefit of insulin sensitizers (thiazolidinediones) on cardiovascular risk factors *(3)*, but there is a lack of RCTs showing that the effect of these agents on surrogate outcomes translate into improved cardiovascular health. Thus, those seeking to use evidence to support clinical decisions may deem clinical investigations peripheral or, sadly, irrelevant to their activity.

TYPES OF CLINICAL INVESTIGATORS

The "chemically pure" clinical investigator (CI) is often a full-time medical school faculty member who spends significant time in scientific pursuit. CIs generally have had substantial training in the art and science of detailed physiological studies in humans and practice their craft in the CRC or similar environment. CIs formulate hypotheses in their field of interest and secure funding, mostly from noncommercial sources, to perform the experiments to answer the questions of interest. CIs are solely responsible for reporting their findings to the scientific community.

The modern for-profit drug development enterprise has so changed the concepts of clinical investigation *(4)* that when asked to identify a clinical investigator today, physicians are likely to identify the local head of a "study center" (usually with an impressive sounding name) doing phase 2 and 3 drug development studies. This enterprise is often run by a clinician with little to no training in clinical investigations or lacking any particular expertise in the disease being studied, or a specialist far removed in time and training from traditional clinical investigation. Membership in learned societies such as the American Society for Clinical Investigation and the American Federation for Clinical Research are irrelevant to this undertaking.

Paramount concerns of drug development investigators are usually economic rather than scientific. The goal of research is to achieve Food and Drug Administration (FDA) approval of a drug or device, a new indication for an approved intervention, or to develop evidence of equivalence of the latest me-too drug. Funding of this investigator is based on the ability to recruit subjects and fill out case report forms, rather than on a track record of scientific achievement. Often these physicians take up drug development work because it is more lucrative that the delivery of clinical care. Their papers reporting results (if they are fortunate enough to be granted such status by the studies' sponsors) are often written or heavily censored by the pharmaceutical company or device maker sponsor. In light of this reality, and to differentiate these physicians from classical CIs, I have chosen to label such physicians "practice-based investigators" (PI).

Certainly there is a moderating position between the pure CI and the for-profit PI. This position is usually occupied by physicians who have clinical research training, with clinical appointments at medical schools, and who derive most or all of their income from the practice of medicine. These clinical researchers may conduct clinical care research, derive questions from their clinical practice, obtain funding from commercial interests as well as from nonprofit funding agencies (investigator-initiated studies), conduct studies or trials that are explanatory (highly selected subjects in tightly controlled environments) or pragmatic (usual patients in usual clinical practice), and publish the results without participation of the funding source in peer-reviewed journals.

Apart from the level of evidence they generate, the differentiation in the spectrum from CI to PI is appropriately made based on the flow of intellectual and financial capital. The CI formulates a scientific question and then obtains funding, often from noncommercial sources, to carry out clinical investigations necessary to answer that question in a CRC or similar environment. The flow of ideas is from the investigator to a funding organization. On the other extreme, the PI takes a question that is generated by industry and signs a contract to help answer that question in the context of the practice setting or nonacademic study center. The flow of ideas is from the sponsor to the investigator. The intermediate position, may have at times features that more closely resemble the CI (generation of ideas, independent conduct and report of findings, conduct of tightly controlled experiments) or the PI (management of large pragmatic trials, funded by for profit interests). All types of investigators are vital elements in the modern medical enterprise. In theory, the work of all is equally legitimate and should be of equal quality.

STRENGTHS AND WEAKNESSES OF CLASSICAL CLINICAL INVESTIGATION

With the change in the hierarchy of evidence for the practice of medicine, has the modern "classical" CI fallen on hard times? Has EBM devalued their trade to the point that it is largely irrelevant? The following discussion will seek to provide an answer to the latter question while assessing the strengths and weaknesses of the RCT and "classic" clinical investigation. However, prior to that exercise, we will briefly trace the sources of information that contribute to the greater body of medical knowledge.

In the perusal of the modern medical library, one will find works in epidemiology, biochemistry, cell biology, genetics, animal and human physiology, and pathophysiology, pharmacology, and standard medical texts and journals chronicling descriptions of diseases and their treatment (observations and RCTs). From the standpoint of the physician, the stream of knowledge pathway can be construed as in Fig. 1. Whereas basic science investigation (at the molecular and cellular level and animal studies) serves to inform ones basic body of knowledge, including the formulation of new

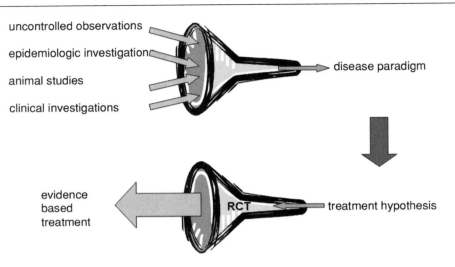

Fig. 1. The development of disease paradigms and the testing of potential therapies in the development of evidence-based medicine.

hypotheses and the refining of existing ones, it is only investigations in humans, the experimental animal of relevance, that should lead to actual changes in the practice of medicine. In a broad sense, the body of knowledge formulated by the many contributors previously mentioned and achieved through induction, allows one to reason deductively as to what interventions may be reasonable.

Epistemologically speaking, the nature of science, particularly in the fields of biology and medicine, is always changing and incomplete. Paradigms and hypotheses are continually being refined. Often the CI is forced to conclude that his or her investigations have resulted in a quantitative increase in the body of knowledge that is unknown as opposed to an absolute reduction in what is unknown. Unfortunately, the novice in science (which is often true in the PI environment) fails to appreciate this tension.

As previously described, the CI applies his trade in a carefully controlled environment (in-patient or out-patient CRC or similar facility); highly skilled personnel carry out classic clinical investigations that are unparalleled in their ability to define physiology and pathophysiology. The subjects are homogeneous and presumably healthy (for the study of normal physiology), or with a well-defined illness (for the study of pathophysiology), usually without concomitant significant disease or intake of medications that may potentially confound the findings of the studies. The knowledge acquired allows the investigator to formulate basic paradigms of bodily function and dysfunction. Thus the reasoning process is fundamentally inductive.

Furthermore, the investigator may alter the physiological system (with a hormone or drug) in a tightly controlled environment to precisely define the effects of the perturbation. Both common clinically monitored parameters (such as standard chemistry tests and commonly measured hormones) and analytes of pure research interest (such as the hormones leptin and ghrelin) can be assessed. Furthermore, highly invasive studies (catheterization of multiple vessels, muscle, or nerve biopsies) may be carried out in these willing and compensated subjects. What is deemed reasonable and acceptable to the watchful eyes of the institutional review board (IRB, usually local to the institution in the setting of the clinical investigation) can be accomplished. Similar studies might often be viewed extreme and unnecessary in the context of real world care and the study environment that approximates the real world, the pragmatic RCT.

Some shortcomings of the work of the CI as evidence for the practice of medicine are apparent. In experimental design, the CI may not use random allocation to the intervention or control conditions and blinding increasing the likelihood of bias. The relative short-term nature of the observations and interventions may be inadequate to extrapolate to years of disease and therapy. For a drug intervention where cumulative exposure may result in side effects, typical clinical investigation protocols are unlikely to realize the downside potential of the intervention in question. In a sense, CI knowledge thus acquired represents the ideal. Unfortunately, this ideal does not apply to most patients. Patients have one or more diseases, take one or multiple medications, do not consume a carefully controlled diet, and do not have highly regimented lifestyles. Deductions about physiological models are often isolated to healthy young men to the exclusion of older subjects and women in their reproductive years. Furthermore, the CRC environment often caters to the "professional subject" who may be unemployed or have unusual access to the study center (medical center employee or spouse of employee). These sources of selection bias may also limit the generalized conclusions reached from CRC data.

There are notable examples of findings in clinical investigation that did not confirm in clinical trials. Consider, for instance, the induction of idiosyncratic liver failure and death with the insulin sensitizer troglitazone in clinical trials and clinical practice occurring in the context of improvement of numerous physiological surrogates in short term studies. This example points out the inability of typical small-scale physiological studies to assess all aspects of potential drug toxicity (or efficacy). Thus, only weak inferences result from studies of physiological endpoints, surrogates for "hard" clinical outcomes (5). The clear superiority of the RCT to show real world evidence for benefit and/or harm is striking.

From these foundational paradigms, the scientist and clinician can reason deductively on how a patient's bodily function should behave in a particular situation (such as with the administration of a drug). The CRC environment allows testing of hypotheses developed with lesser levels of evidence (observational studies, animal studies, in vitro studies). Hypotheses generated from these lines of evidence can be further confirmed, modified, or rejected by the findings from CRC studies. Hypotheses confirmed or generated by the CI are then ultimately tested in an RCT. The CI develops and "fine tunes" the science; the investigators in RCTs (including PIs), test whether the application of the current understanding of the science has any real world value.

A now classic example of discrepancy between the results of clinical investigations refers to the disparity between the many physiological studies documenting beneficial effects of estrogen therapy on lipids and vasculature (and the accompanying compelling epidemiological studies showing improved cardiovascular health in postmenopausal women treated with estrogens) (6), and the recently completed HERS (7), and WHI (8) studies, showing no cardiovascular benefit, and perhaps cardiovascular harm. Given the large RCT findings, the informed clinician is left no choice but to conclude that the best evidence shows that for the average postmenopausal woman oral estrogen therapy is not cardioprotective. However, what should the practitioner conclude about the positive physiological studies? Assuming adequate clinical investigation rigor, we must conclude that the results of some of the surrogate physiological parameters were indeed in the direction of cardiovascular benefit. The disparity may be owing to a difference in effect between women without occult cardiovascular disease (protective or neutral) and women with occult cardiovascular disease (harmful). Or known potentially harmful effects (raising C-reactive protein or triglycerides) or unknown harmful effects may overwhelm known potentially beneficial effects (improved endothelial function, LDL cholesterol, and high-density lipoprotein [HDL] cholesterol).

Large RCTs must trump the knowledge from the CI environment because the RCT has addressed the question of relevance in real patients receiving health care (with their genetic and lifestyle diversity and varied concomitant disease and medications). Given the known findings of postmenopausal estrogen replacement therapy (ERT) and hormone replacement therapy (HRT), it may be reasonable for the clinician given the hierarchy of evidence to give ERT or HRT to women early after menopause for symptomatic relief, but not for long-term cardiovascular prevention, because the women studied in the large RCTs were older women, not women taking hormones soon after menopause. And this may be so until results from an ongoing large RCT of ERT on women shortly after menopause ultimately tests this hypothesis. Given the uncertainties surrounding this issue, risk attitudes—and other values and preferences of the patients—will have decisively important role in the decision (a reminder that according to EBM, the evidence alone never completely informs the decision and requires expert consideration of the circumstances and preferences of the patients).

STRENGTHS AND WEAKNESSES
OF RANDOMIZED CLINICAL TRIALS

The RCT is essentially a test based on deductions from scientific principles enunciated as the result of classic clinical investigation and other foundational work. The obvious strengths of the RCT relate to the ability to conceal the allocation of participants to the intervention or control and to produce two groups with the same prognosis (thanks to the random allocation of patients with equivalent distribution of known and unknown prognostic factors) such that differences in prognosis at the end of the trial can only be explained by differences in treatment effect. When researchers organize large pragmatic RCTs the large numbers of subjects enrolled allow for more precise findings with broader applicability. However, this strength of numbers and economy of scale may be its Achilles' heel as well. With heterogeneity of the study population comes confounding factors from concomitant diseases and medications. As a RCT becomes less like classic clinical investigation (from explanatory to pragmatic), it becomes more difficult to isolate the effect of the treatment from the other aspects of delivering the intervention. Thus, some mechanistic inferences become weaker while the applicability of the findings becomes more secure. As the population becomes less uniform, the ability to realistically isolate the effect of a single intervention in that population declines. Dropouts may be substantial with a real-world population rather than the more "professional" study population often enrolled in CI studies. Although the statistician may be able to preserve the protection from bias that randomization affords with an intention-to-treat analysis, this protection is inadequate in the face of large loss to follow-up.*

Montori and colleagues have recently reviewed common problems in RCT papers *(9)*. Such problems include faulty comparators (inflating treatment effect by comparing vs placebo or substandard treatment), composite endpoints (to inflate an effect or per-haps "find" an effect when there is not one), subgroup analyses, and small treatment effects. The latter is especially true for the modern "mega" RCT with thousands of subjects where a statistically significant effect may be seen, but the absolute effect of the benefit is very small. Analysis of the number needed to treat is often helpful for clinicians trying to discern the true size or importance of such statistical findings.†

Endpoints tend to be more clinically relevant, although perhaps less precise, in RCTs as compared with clinical investigations. Physiological parameters are measured with great precision in the CRC. Endpoints in RCT may be quite definite (death) or subject to regional practice patterns ("need" for and access to revascularization). Composite endpoints (a smorgasbord of events that may be possibly affected by the treatment in question) may further obscure what is actually happening in the RCT.

The RCT tends to average out effects across the study population. It fails to differ-entiate between subjects who are responders (and there may be heterogeneity of response among study subjects) and nonresponders. The assumption of uniformity is much less likely to be true in RCT. *Post hoc* analysis may identify subgroups with dif-ferent responses, though rarely are findings from such analyses clear cut or valid. There is generally too much heterogeneity in the population studied to differentiate distinct subgroups that benefit from those who do not. Fishing expeditions testing innumerable subgroups often lead to chance findings that cannot be confirmed in subsequent trials.

The RCT may also be plagued by the nature of the modern clinical investigator. The major endpoint trials are usually carried out by clinical trialists with both CI and PI backgrounds. Trials not funded by industry (where a new indication for a drug may not be at stake) are less tightly monitored during the actual performance of the trial, so the investigator is left more to his integrity to carry out the trial in a rigorous fashion. Studies carried out strictly under the auspices of industry have the advantage of more rigorous monitoring to meet FDA guidelines for potential new or expanded treatment indications, but a higher likelihood that much of the work is done in the PI environ-ment. As noted earlier, such physicians are often involved in the clinical investigation enterprise primarily for economic reasons and without adequate training in conducting studies or interest in the process other than financial remuneration. Many of the PI physicians can do an acceptable job. However, improper enrollment, protocol viola-tions, and failure to recognize or appropriately categorize adverse effects are some of the problems that plague the modern clinical investigation enterprise dominated by PIs. One may readily ask, if the quality of the investigator is suboptimal, can large numbers sufficiently obscure poor workmanship? The author has increasing doubts about large

---

*As in the recent statin acute coronary syndrome trials, PROVE-IT (N Engl J Med. 2004; 350:1495–504) and A to Z (JAMA. 2004;292:1307–1316) where >30% of subjects dropped out over 2 yr or less.

†As in the CAPRIE trial with clopidogrel where the results are statistically significant but the number needed to treat is approx 200 (Lancet. 1996; 348:1329–1339).

pharmaceutical company funded trials where a majority of the subjects are enrolled by the PI entrepreneur. Although rampant fraud has been documented (11), wholesale chicanery is probably rare. However, the fact that economics are now the paramount interest in most industry funded RCTs (by both the sponsor and most of the investigators) should raise concerns about potential compromises to the integrity of the data generated.

What is the physician to do with contradictory evidence from RCTs? For the clinical investigation situation, it is much more likely that one or more plausible explanations may be readily identifiable. The answers in the RCT environment are much less clear because of the many potential sources of influence on trial results, as well as the possibility that the prevailing hypothesis is actually incorrect. Publication bias (publishing only trials finding statistically significant treatment effects) is particularly problematic in industry-funded trials (12), in that they may provide the impression of false uniformity.

THE ROLE OF CLASSICAL CLINICAL INVESTIGATION IN THE 21ST CENTURY

Previously, we asked two questions: With the change in the hierarchy of evidence for the practice of medicine, has the modern "classic" CI fallen on hard times? Has EBM devalued his or her trade to the point that it is largely irrelevant? The author would answer these questions with a resounding, "No."

As already discussed, in the new paradigm of EBM, the CI will never provide the final answer about the efficacy or safety of treatments. However, without the CI, the entire superstructure of medical science is likely to collapse. Advances in the basic understanding of physiology and pathophysiology will come to a screeching halt. The inductive process of knowledge acquisition will be aborted. The science must advance well before the application of that science can proceed to testing in the RCT. Furthermore, from an economic standpoint, it is unjustifiable to contemplate carrying out a large multicenter RCT without encouragement from smaller more rigorous studies. Similarly, it is ethically unthinkable to subject large populations to interventions without having scrupulously evaluated the rationale for their use in a highly controlled environment such as the CRC. In short, the RCT cannot take place without the groundbreaking work of the CI.

Can classic clinical investigation become more like the pragmatic RCT? Definitely not, as its scientific rigor is vital to the integrity of its product, scientific understanding. Has the pragmatic RCT wandered too far from the moorings of the scientific method as performed most elegantly in humans in CRC? Possibly so, as has been mentioned in the earlier discussion. The RCT, although always likely to be an exercise in major monetary investment, may be too much governed by economic factors instead of scientific ones, particularly when its truth is linked to investors' returns. The recent fiasco with the coxibs and the selective publication of data (13) gives us ample pause to consider how pristine is the knowledge generated in the current environment. Furthermore, negative trials and trials that are not favorable to the industry sponsor's product (and thus industry's bottom line) are not likely to be become public.

Whereas the very recent trend for a registry of all trials will hopefully stop this practice (14), spinmeisters (opinion leaders) are likely to be given the new task of explaining the unexplainable. Only time will tell how this new approach to the dissemination of trial results will play out. The pure CIs are inclined to publish results contrary to their hypotheses, because their motivations come generally from science and knowledge rather than from economics. In fact, paradoxically finding contradictory findings may help the CI's funding because scientific bodies might conclude that we know even less about the field in question than we thought we did.

The CI is not dead. The rise of EBM has correctly placed the findings from clinical investigation as the shoulders over which patient important effects of promising treatments can be tested in RCTs. The displacement of classic clinical investigation from the hierarchy of evidence has not displaced it from its place as an invaluable discipline for the advancement of the science of medicine and patient care.

REFERENCES

1. Montori VM, Guyatt GH. What is evidence-based medicine? Endocrinol Metab Clin North Am 2002; 31:521–526
2. Brown MS, Goldstein JL. Receptor-mediated control of cholesterol metabolism. Science 1976;191: 150–154.
3. Parulkar AA, Pendergrass ML, Granda-Ayala R, Lee TR, Fonseca VA. Nonhypoglycemic effects of thiazolidinediones. Ann Intern Med 2001;134:61–71.
4. Angell M. The Truth About the Drug Companies: How They Deceive Us and What to Do About It. Random House, New York, NY, 2004.
5. Graham DJ, Drinkard CR, Shatin D. Incidence of idiopathic acute liver failure and hospitalized liver injury in patients treated with troglitazone. Am J Gastroenterol 2003; 8:175–179.
6. Fleming TR, DeMets DL. Surrogate end points in clinical trials: are we being misled? Ann Intern Med 1996; 125: 605–613.
7. Davison S, Davis SR. New markers for cardiovascular disease risk in women: impact of endogenous estrogen status and exogenous postmenopausal hormone therapy. J Clin Endocrinol Metab 2003; 88: 2470–2478.
8. Grady D, Herrington D, Bittner V, et al. For HERS Research Group. Cardiovascular disease outcomes during 6.8 years of hormone therapy: Heart and Estrogen/progestin Replacement. Study follow-up (HERS II). JAMA 2002;288:49–57.
9. Anderson GL, Limacher M, Assaf AR, et al. For the Women's Health Initiative Steering Committee effects of conjugated equine estrogen in postmenopausal women with hysterectomy: the Women's Health Initiative randomized controlled trial. JAMA 2004;291:1701–1712.
10. Montori VM, Jaeschke R, Schünemann HJ, et al. Users' guide to detecting misleading claims in clinical research reports. BMJ 2004;329:1093–1096.
11. Davis BR, Furberg CD, Wright JT Jr, Cutler JA, Whelton P; ALLHAT Collaborative Research Group. ALLHAT: setting the record straight. Ann Intern Med 2004;141:39–46
12. Eichenwald K, Kolata G. A doctor's drug trials turn into fraud. New York Times, May 17, 1999, Section A, pp.1.
13. Bhandari M, Busse JW, Jackowski D, et al. Association between industry funding and statistically significant pro-industry findings in medical and surgical randomized trials. CMAJ 2004;170:477–480.
14. Fitzgerald GA. Coxibs and cardiovascular disease. N Engl J Med 2004; 351:1709–1411.
15. DeAngelis CD, Drazen JM, Frizelle FA, et al. Clinical trial registration: a statement from the International Committee of Medical Journal Editors. JAMA 2004;292:1363–1364.

12

The Value of Systematic Reviews in Endocrinology

The Impact of the Cochrane Metabolic and Endocrine Disorders Review Group

Bernd Richter, MD, PhD

CONTENTS

INTRODUCTION

No one within endocrinology can keep up to date with the relevant evidence in their field of interest. The major bibliographic databases cover less than half the world's literature and are biased toward English-language publications. Of the evidence available in the major databases, only a fraction can be found by the average searcher. Textbooks, editorials, and narrative reviews that have not been prepared systematically may be unreliable. Much evidence is unpublished, but unpublished evidence may be important, particularly for adverse effects *(1,2)*. More easily accessible research reports tend to exaggerate the benefits of interventions.

The Cochrane Metabolic and Endocrine Disorders Review Group, through its input to the Cochrane Library (*see* The Cochrane Collaboration-The Cochrane Library), is trying to solve some of these problems. Published on a quarterly basis and made available both on CD-ROM and the Internet (*see* www.cochrane.org), the Cochrane Library

From: *Contemporary Endocrinology: Evidence-Based Endocrinology*
Edited by: V. M. Montori © Mayo Foundation for Medical Education and Research

is the best single source of reliable evidence about the effects of health care and should provide a sound basis for a genuine evidence-based endocrinology.

EVIDENCE-BASED MEDICINE: AN IMPORTANT ELEMENT OF "GOOD" MEDICINE

Contrary to the Cochrane Collaboration where consumers hold a key position from the very beginning, the evidence-based medicine (EBM) momentum surprisingly took some time to realize that the patient has a saying in the diagnosis and treatment of her condition.

The most cited EBM definition was created by David Sackett, one of the inaugurators of this innovative approach to medicine: "Evidence-based medicine is the conscientious and judicious use of current best evidence from clinical care research in the management of individual patients. The practice of evidence-based medicine means integrating individual clinical expertise with the best available external evidence from systematic research." *(3)* Three sentences later Sackett clarified, as one important element of individual clinical expertise, the "thoughtful identification and compassionate use of individual patients' predicaments, rights, and preferences in making clinical decisions about their care." This explanation was unfortunately overlooked by many and consequently led to a more concise description of EBM as "the integration of best research evidence with clinical expertise and patient values" *(4)*.

It should be noted that the term evidence is open to linguistic and philosophical interpretation (*see* Chapter 23). Probably, *evidence* should be seen in the context of falsification models to improve hypotheses which only approximate but never reach the *truth*. The neo-phenomenologist Hermann Schmitz illustrated this discourse as follows: "Admittedly the authority of reality which emerges in evidence is only a radiation of the primitive present and therefore not so unmistakable that confusing it with a mere apparent evidence could be ruled out in principle." Therefore, a somewhat cautious and humble approach to the complex nature of human disease seems advisable, indicating that different approaches to, and interpretations of, evidence are possible. A tyranny of evidence exclusively focusing on methodological high-level information like meta-analyses should be avoided because recognition of the whole body of knowledge is always necessary to individualize diagnostic and therapeutic procedures.

As a matter of course, *humane medicine* means much more than the integration of best research evidence with clinical expertise and patient values but also cannot exist without it. Some additional elements of better health care appear to be *clinical problem-solving* strategies to avoid typical errors in the diagnostic reasoning of physicians *(5)*, the empathic communication with patients utilizing *interpersonal skills* as well as the integration of core elements of *patient-centered medicine (6)* such as *narrative-based medicine (7)* to verge on a holistic medicine, which is treating sick people and not "diseases."

On the other hand, without a systematic way of searching for information, critical appraisal, and adequate summary of data, and transparent publication of results and procedures to continuously integrate updates and criticisms, medicine will never achieve good health care but keep talking about it forever.

Mike Clarke, the director of the UK Cochrane Centre, eloquently described the Cochrane Collaboration's systematic approach to nowadays information problems in medicine *(8)*:

". . . the results of a single trial will rarely be sufficient in many circumstances. Most trials are too small and their results are not sufficiently robust against the effects of chance. In addition, small trials might be too focused on a particular type of patient to provide a result that can be either easily or reliably generalised to future patients. Added to this, the amount of information about health care, including that coming from individual randomised trials, is now overwhelming.

. . . people making decisions about health care—including patients, health care professionals, policy makers and managers—need high quality information and, unfortunately, much of what is available is of poor quality. As a consequence, vast resources are wasted each year on health care that is not effective and may even be harmful, effective forms of care are often underutilised, and people sometimes suffer and die unnecessarily.

To help overcome these barriers to better health care, and to provide a key piece of the evidence needed for this, results from similar randomised trials need to be brought together. Trials need to be assessed and those that are good enough can be combined to produce both a more statistically reliable result and one that can be more easily applied in other settings. This combination of trials needs to be done in as reliable a way as possible. It needs to be systematic.

The traditional narrative review of health care is often not systematic. It may have been written by someone who is a recognised expert but who might simply not have the time to try to identify and bring together all relevant studies. Of more concern, they might actively seek to discuss and combine just those trials that confirm their opinions and prejudices. A systematic review aims to circumvent this by using a predefined, explicit methodology. The methods used will include steps to minimise bias in all parts of the process: identifying relevant studies, selecting them for inclusion, and collecting and combining their data. Studies should be sought regardless of their results.

A systematic review does not need to contain a statistical synthesis of the results from the included studies. This might be impossible if the designs of the studies are too different for an average of their results to be meaningful or if the outcomes measured are not sufficiently similar. If the results of the individual studies are combined to produce an overall statistic, this is usually called a meta-analysis. A meta-analysis can also be done without a systematic review, simply by combining the results from more than one trial. However, although such a meta-analysis will have greater mathematical precision than an analysis of any one of the component trials, it will be subject to any biases that arise from the study selection process, and may produce a mathematically precise, but clinically misleading, result."

THE COCHRANE COLLABORATION

The Cochrane Collaboration is a unique, worldwide nonprofit and independent organization, dedicated to making up-to-date, accurate information about the effects of health care readily available worldwide. It is now the largest organization in the world engaged in the production, dissemination, and maintenance of systematic reviews. The Cochrane Collaboration was founded in 1993 and named after the British epidemiologist, Archie Cochrane.

The collaboration aims to help people make well-informed decisions by preparing, maintaining, and promoting the accessibility of systematic reviews of the effects of interventions in all areas of health care. These reviews bring together the relevant research findings on a particular topic, synthesize this evidence, and then present it in a standard and structured way. Cochrane reviews have already contributed to many important improvements in health care. They are widely used in treatment guidelines and health policy documents.

There are currently around 10,000 people contributing to the work of the Cochrane Collaboration from more than 80 countries, and this involvement continues to grow.

There are currently 505 Cochrane Collaborative Review Groups, responsible for reviews within particular areas of health and collectively providing a home for reviews in all aspects of health care. These groups are spread around the world and are supported by regional Cochrane Centers. Those who prepare the reviews are mostly health-care professionals, researchers, and consumers who volunteer to work in one of the many Collaborative Review Groups, with Editorial Teams overseeing the preparation and maintenance of the reviews, as well as application of the rigorous quality standards for which Cochrane reviews have become known. Cochrane reviews' authors make a commitment to update their reviews as new evidence becomes available and as comments and criticisms from users of the Cochrane Library are received. The Collaboration promotes the involvement of consumers throughout the conduct of reviews, and reviews include consumer synopses written in lay language.

There are also Cochrane Methods Groups—with expertise in relevant areas of methodology, fields, or networks—with broad areas of interest and expertise spanning the scope of many review groups and a Consumer Network helping to promote the interests of users of health care. Each of these constituencies is represented on The Cochrane Collaboration Steering Group.

Most of the contributors do not receive any payment for the work they do within the collaboration. They are drawn to the collaboration through a wish to commit, either as a professional or as a consumer, to a movement that provides more sound evidence on which healthcare decisions can be made. Many members of the Cochrane Collaboration have pointed out that external perception is very important. Any perception that for-profit commercial organizations, notably but not exclusively, the pharmaceutical industry and medical device manufacturers, were influencing the conclusions of Cochrane reviews would damage a carefully nourished reputation for impartiality and scientific rigor. The debate about the conflict of interest issue within the Collaboration is going on but there is overwhelming consensus that there should be a clear barrier between the production of Cochrane reviews and any funding from commercial sources (any for-profit manufacturer or provider of health care, or any other for-profit source with a real or potential vested interest in the findings of a specific review). Although government departments, not-for-profit medical insurance companies, and health management organizations may find the conclusions of Cochrane reviews carry financial consequences for them, these are not included in this definition. Also not included are for-profit companies that do not have real or potential vested interests in the conclusions of Cochrane reviews. Thus, sponsorship of a Cochrane review by any commercial source or sources (as previously defined) is prohibited. To ensure the integrity (real and perceived) of the "firewall," it is also prohibited for a commercial source or sources (as previously defined) to sponsor Cochrane entities that produce Cochrane reviews, that is, Collaborative Review Groups.

The Cochrane Library

The major product of the Collaboration is the Cochrane Database of Systematic Reviews, which is published quarterly as part of the Cochrane Library. It currently contains the full text of more than 2400 Cochrane reviews, each of which will be kept up to date as new evidence accumulates. Moreover, there are also 1600 published protocols for reviews in progress. These outline how the reviews will be carried out and provide an explicit description of the methods to be used. Hundreds of newly completed reviews and protocols are added each year. In addition, a few hundred existing reviews are updated so substantively that they can be considered to be the equivalent of new reviews, and several hundred more are brought up to date by the addition of new information.

The Cochrane Database of Systematic Reviews is available on the Internet and on CD-ROM as part of the Cochrane Library. This is published by John Wiley and Sons Ltd. and is available on a subscription basis. The abstracts (i.e., summaries) of the reviews are available free of charge and provide a valuable source of health care information (9).

Additional coverage is provided worldwide through partnerships with information suppliers such as Ovid Technologies. The establishment of national contracts means that the Cochrane Library is available free of charge to users in Australia, Denmark, England, Finland, Ireland, Norway, Northern Ireland, South Africa, Spain, and Wales. For low- and middle-income countries the Cochrane Library is available through the Health InterNetwork Access to Research Initiative (HINARI). More countries are being added to this list each year.

The output of the Cochrane Collaboration also includes the Cochrane Central Register of Controlled Trials (CENTRAL), the Cochrane Database of Methodology Reviews, and the Cochrane Methodology Register with more than 7000 references to methodological publications, and three other databases of systematic reviews, health technology assessment reports, and economic evaluations.

Through extensive programs of the hand searching of journals (in which a journal is checked from cover to cover to look for relevant reports) and of electronic searching of bibliographic databases such as Medline and EMBASE, suitable records are added to CENTRAL, with coordination by the Cochrane Center in Rhode Island. At the moment, CENTRAL contains records for more than 400,000 reports of randomized controlled clinical trials, many of which are not included in any other electronic database.

Huge efforts are being made to continually improve the quality of Cochrane reviews. There are empirical studies demonstrating that, on average, Cochrane reviews are more likely to be valid than other reviews (10), although critical appraisal even of Cochrane reviews appears essential (11). Several major medical journals, including the *British Medical Journal*, *The Lancet*, and the *Journal of the American Medical Association* are now eager to publish versions of Cochrane reviews after they have appeared in the Cochrane Library, having recognized the importance of providing high-quality, up-to-date summaries of evidence to their readers.

To ensure the highest quality of Cochrane reviews, those who find gaps or faults in reviews are encouraged to submit comments. With the help of Criticism Editors, authors update their reviews according to this feedback. The most recent comments and criticisms are posted on the web (12).

THE COCHRANE METABOLIC AND ENDOCRINE DISORDERS REVIEW GROUP

In 1993, the Cochrane Collaboration was formally launched at the first Cochrane Colloquium in Oxford, United Kingdom. In 1994, a Cochrane Diabetes Group was registered, which had its Editorial Base in Leeds and was led by Professor Rhys Williams as coordinating editor. The group started with much enthusiasm but several years later, in 1998, they were unable to secure any further funding. Discussions started immediately on who might be willing to revive this Review Group. In the meantime, some of the diabetes reviews were redistributed among appropriate Review Groups to ensure their maintenance, and some of the gaps left by the Diabetes Group were filled by other Review Groups.

By mid-1999 it had been decided that Michael Berger and Bernd Richter from the Department of Metabolic Diseases and Nutrition at the Heinrich-Heine University in Duesseldorf, Germany, would take responsibility for taking over the work of the former Diabetes Group and expanding it into a Metabolic and Endocrine Disorders Group. The group was registered with the Cochrane Collaboration in early 2000.

The Editorial Base and the Editorial Team/Board

Cochrane Review Groups are composed of persons from around the world who share an interest in developing and maintaining systematic reviews relevant to a particular health area. Groups are coordinated by an Editorial Base which edits and assembles completed reviews into modules for inclusion in the Cochrane Library. The infrastructure of the Cochrane Metabolic and Endocrine Disorders Review Group (CMED) embodies the Editorial Base at Duesseldorf, Germany, a multi-disciplinary and international Editorial Team/Board, external referees and volunteers. CMED constantly tries to enlarge the Editorial Team, which should include people with a background in endocrinology, diabetology, metabolic disorders, as well as dietetics and nursing. Apart from clinical experts, consumers and methodologists/statisticians are involved.

The Editorial Base, which is responsible for the core functions of the group, amounts mainly to the following persons:

- The *coordinating editor* integrates the Editorial Team, establishes the infrastructure of the Editorial Base.
- The *review group coordinator* and an *assistant review group coordinator* is the primary contact for reviewers, administrative backbone of the group.
- The *trials search coordinator* helps reviewers with search strategies in electronic databases, overlooks hand search activities, establishes a specialized registrar.
- The *consumer coordinator* tries to increase consumer participation within CMED, increases CMED's output for consumers.
- The *comments and criticism editor* supervises incoming comments and criticisms of Cochrane reviews, negotiates directly with authors.

The Editorial Process

The editorial process of a Cochrane Review Group is quite complicated if compared to the peer-reviewed journals' one. In the first place, CMED tries hard to support authors from the very first contact. Therefore, nobody should feel rejected (which does not seem to happen too often with peer-reviewed journals). In the second place, the reviewer-CMED relationship is a long-term commitment from both sides, making it necessary to establish good communication in order to raise the quality of systematic reviews.

The editorial process spans a long time from title registration to protocol development to the finished review and updates of the review.

TITLES

Individuals who would like to do a review within the scope of the CMED should first contact the Review Group Coordinator (ebrahim@uni-duesseldorf.de). If not already done so, a copy of the Cochrane Reviewers' Handbook should be obtained, which is an excellent resource and gives guidance on all matters regarding systematic reviews and meta-analyses *(13)*. The Review Group Coordinator will check that the proposed subject has not already been reviewed within the Cochrane Collaboration. If it has not, the reviewer will be encouraged to develop a formal title in consultation with the Editorial Group. From the outset, reviewers should be aware of their responsibility to update and maintain their reviews after publication.

After negotiations on the proposed title, reviewers will submit a title registration form, which includes a detailed questionnaire on the proposed review. The proposed title will be circulated within the wider collaboration to identify common interests. The Trial Search Coordinator runs a quick search to provide authors with an approximate "confidence interval" ranging from a very-specific to a middle-sensitive search strategy. Should the specific search identify a great number of potential trials, authors might reflect upon their ability to cope with the foreseeable amount of work.

PROTOCOLS

Once the title has been accepted, the reviewer and their co-reviewers will be encouraged to attend a Cochrane workshop on protocol development, if they have not already done so. After attending the workshop, reviewers will prepare the final protocol.

The development of a high-quality protocol is a very important step in the production of a systematic review, at least demanding the same scientific rigor as to generate a good protocol for a multicenter randomized controlled clinical trial. Serious errors in the design of the protocol will unavoidably result in time-consuming and sometimes unsuccessful efforts to rectify problems. Hence, CMED provides templates and standard operating procedures to make life easier for systematic reviewers, but several drafts and revisions are often necessary before authors can proceed.

The reviewer will be required to submit a draft protocol within 6 mo of approval of the title (or as agreed with the Editorial Base), after careful proof-reading and completion of a checklist. The deadline aims to ensure that if someone submits a title but is unable to deliver the review, the topic can be made available to others.

The Trials Search Coordinator will set up a search strategy in cooperation with the authors to ensure quality of this very important step of the review production process. Many reviewers underestimate the difficulties to create and run good search strategies in various databases, and the help of an experienced information scientist or librarian is definitely recommended.

The protocol undergoes both a two-stage internal and an external refereeing process. The protocol is first checked by the core Editorial Base staff (coordinating editor, review group coordinator, trials search coordinator, and consumer coordinator) and suggestions for improvement are passed back directly to the reviewers, if necessary. The revised draft is checked again, regarding implementation of the recommendations, and then is passed on to the group's editors and external referees. External refereeing usually involves a clinical expert, a methodology expert, and a consumer. Additional authorities may be consulted if deemed appropriate. Every effort will be made to complete the refereeing process as quickly as possible, ideally within 4–6 wk. The review group coordinator will provide a summary of the comments received and ask the reviewer to make appropriate changes to the protocol. The final protocol will be proofread and edited by the review group coordinator (in consultation with the reviewer), approved by the coordinating editor, and submitted for publication in the Cochrane Library.

REVIEWS

Once the protocol has been accepted, the reviewer will proceed with preparing the final review. Advice on methodological issues and data extraction sheets, as well as translation of trials will be available from the Editorial Base. Sample letters are obtainable for identifying additional or unpublished information, for example from the pharmaceutical industry, and for contacting authors about missing or unclear data. There will be a deadline for the submission of the review of around 12 mo from the approval of the protocol (or as agreed with the Editorial Base). The finished review must be submitted to the Editorial Base in RevMan format (Cochrane software consisting of a word processor and a statistical package for meta-analyses), after careful proof-reading and completion of a checklist. Again, a template review should be used to help reviewers include all the relevant information in the right format.

The review will undergo a similar two-stage refereeing process as the protocol. Again, internal refereeing will be undertaken by the Editorial Base, and external refereeing by usually the same three referees who reviewed the protocol. Every effort will be made to complete the refereeing process as quickly as possible, again ideally within 4–6 wk. The final review will be proofread and edited by the review group coordinator (in consultation with the reviewer), approved by the coordinating editor, and submitted for inclusion in the Cochrane Library. Before publication, reviewers will have to sign a permission-to-publish form. Reviewers are encouraged to publish their reviews in print journals in addition to the Cochrane Library, but this should not delay publication in the Library.

UPDATING REVIEWS

Reviewers will be responsible for scanning the medical literature at least once a year to identify any newly published trial within the scope of their review and to update their review accordingly. This will be supplemented by searching activities of the group's trials search coordinator. Reviewers will also be responsible for replying to any comments or criticisms that have been received via the Cochrane Library's "Comments and Criticisms" facility. Any comments received will be summarized by the comments and criticism editor who will negotiate with the reviewers directly regarding required changes.

The reviewer will receive support from the Editorial Base for the task of updating the review, for example, by being notified of new trials published. Updated reviews will be passed to the Editorial Team and to external referees for comment in a similar manner as for the protocol and the review. If the Editorial Team recognizes that a review has become significantly out of date and the responsible reviewers do not take any action, the Editorial Team may either consider to transfer responsibility for the review to a third party or to withdraw the review from the Cochrane Library.

All contact reviewers receive a free subscription to the Cochrane Library after publication of their full review. This subscription may be withdrawn if the date of the latest search for new data lies back more than 1 yr.

The editorial process is illustrated in Fig. 1.

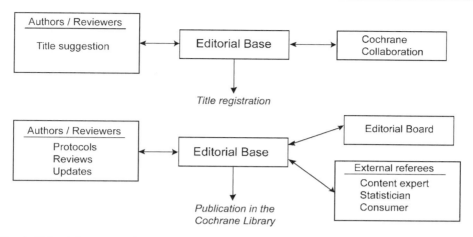

Fig. 1. Editorial process of the Cochrane Metabolic and Endocrine Disorders Review Group.

Scope of the Cochrane Metabolic and Endocrine Disorders Review Group

CMED is primarily but not exclusively concerned with the evaluation of randomized controlled trials and other controlled health care interventions relevant to the prevention, treatment or management, and rehabilitation of metabolic, nutritional, and endocrine disorders. The main disorders CMED is responsible for are diabetes mellitus and related disorders, additional metabolic and nutritional disorders (e.g., deficiency diseases), obesity, and other endocrine disorders.

The number of reviews required in the field of metabolic and endocrine disorders is very large. CMED seeks to encourage as many reviews as possible. However, CMED will also aim to maintain the quality of reviews. Therefore, a balance between quantity and quality has to be maintained, ensuring that all reviews meet a minimum standard, in order to preserve the high reputation of Cochrane reviews. Publication in the Cochrane Library must be seen as an indicator of quality. New reviewers may find the task daunting, but the Editorial Base will try to help new reviewers produce good reviews. Tools designed to help reviewers achieve a high-quality review can be found on the website of CMED (www.cc-endoc.info or www.cc-endoc.de).

Within 4 yr, the number of titles, protocols, and reviews CMED has to manage has risen exponentially and sum up to more than 100 projects at the moment. Approved protocols and review can be found in the Cochrane Library, registered titles and protocols in the editorial process may be inspected through the Cochrane Collaborations' Review Title Manager system *(14)*.

In June 2004, an Australian CMED Diabetes Satellite was launched by Professor Alan Pettigrew, chief executive officer of the National Health and Medical Research Council. The Australian satellite to CMED has been formed to support the work of this review group, particularly its work in diabetes. The role of the Australian Diabetes Satellite is to:

• Increase capacity within the Australian diabetes community to prepare and maintain Cochrane reviews.
• Support CMED in the production and updating of Cochrane reviews, specifically those related to the management of diabetes.

- Facilitate the dissemination of the results of relevant Cochrane reviews to clinicians, consumers, and policymakers in the Australian diabetes community.
- Identify and facilitate priority reviews relevant to diabetes that are needed to inform practice and policy in Australia.
- Promote the use of the Cochrane Library for informing practice and research in the Australian diabetes community.
- Collaborate with the Australasian Cochrane Centre and other Collaborative Review Groups based in Australia, satellites and entities to further the work of the Cochrane Collaboration in the Australasian region.

This initiative is very promising and could serve as a role model for other areas of the world. Perhaps, the next liaison could be a US Endocrinology Satellite?

Moreover, CMED is open to all kinds of help and collaboration, for example assistance in the form of editors, referees, consumer participation, hand searcher, methodological advice to name a few.

OUTCOMES

CMED focuses on outcomes that are important to patients and will encourage reviewers to use clinical events as outcomes, rather than, for example, biochemical proxy indicators. Outcomes considered important include patient-oriented endpoints like (health-related) quality-of-life, morbidity and mortality data, as well as specific indicators of health and well-being (including physical, emotional, and psycho-social dimensions), and costs. Evaluation of possible problems associated with interventions for metabolic and endocrine diseases, such as adverse effects of medication, have to be an integral part of every review. Some biochemical parameters, such as glycosylated haemoglobin as an indicator of metabolic control in diabetes mellitus, may be important in terms of explaining changes observed in patient-oriented parameters.

Consumer Participation

Consumer involvement and the investigation of patient-oriented outcome measures are a top priority for CMED. Contact has been made with a range of consumers and people representing consumer organizations, who are very keen to participate in the work of the group. Furthermore, the group makes its work accessible to the general public by collaborating with scientific journalists.

The integration of consumers is an integral part of CMED's philosophy. Various stages of participation are possible, ranging from advice on editorial issues to full integration into every element in the production of systematic reviews/meta-analyses. Because of the skewed distribution of Cochrane Review Groups, with headquarters mainly in Europe and other countries with advanced infrastructure, consumers from these areas have a better chance to influence Review Group's agendas. There is a danger that consumers' perspectives from other parts of the world are not perceived resulting in biased research. Therefore, a project to increase consumers' impact was launched: within CMED's scope, consumers' preferences and needs from as many countries as possible are going to be explored and evaluated. A structured questionnaire was developed and sent to various organizations. A network focusing on diabetes, obesity, and other endocrine diseases will be established. By the way of continuous publications in the Cochrane Library and on CMED's web site, consumers from various social and cultural backgrounds will have the opportunity to express their points of view. Thereby, CMED hopes to contribute to the dissemination of otherwise easily neglected sociocultural diversities of consumers' preferences, needs, and attitudes and to influence future research priorities and funding bodies to bridge the gap between easily identifiable and hidden health care topics.

SOME IMPORTANT ELEMENTS OF SYSTEMATIC REVIEWS/META-ANALYSES

This section cannot provide detailed advice of how to write a good systematic review/meta-analysis. For everybody being interested to embark on a Cochrane review adventure careful study of the Reviewer's Handbook is positively recommended *(15)*.

On the other hand, some hopefully useful hints from CMED are listed next in order to disclose some easily neglected or forgotten items in the review production and to counterbalance attitudes that denounce mega-analytic techniques as "mega-silliness *(16)*":

- *Sifting the literature:* from the very beginning on reviewers should name key words for identification of trials and continuously improve this by implementation of new items that are detected in the literature scan. After careful institution and run of a usually sensitive search strategy in various databases like Medline, EMBASE, the COCHRANE LIBRARY, and LILACS, authors are often confronted with thousands of titles and abstracts referring to the associated publications. At least two reviewers should check all the "hits" because there is a high possibility of missing important information if only one person it trying to deal with an enormous amount of abstracts. Information that is lost at this stage might never be found again. CMED recommends downloading search results to a Citation Manager (e.g., Reference Manager) in order to create a bibliography consisting of the title and abstract only. Time of publication, original language, authors' names, and key words may influence the reviewer's decision to include or exclude the publication for further scrutiny. In case of any doubt the original publication has to be investigated. The bibliography should be opened in a word-processor like Microsoft Word with the opportunity to transform the text (e.g., by the use of *macros*) into a composition which can easily be checked on a computer screen. Page breaks for every new title should be inserted so that the reviewer's eye always focuses on the same height of the screen avoiding constant eye movements diluting authors' concentration after a short time. Thereafter, if possible, the document could be transformed into PDF-format, because navigation in Acrobat (Reader) is very easy and the file might be comfortably shared among international collaborators via e-mail attachment. A logbook of the degree of agreement (positive hits, doubtful hits, otherwise interesting items) should be used, for example in spreadsheet format with automatically generated numbers covering the range of references that were detected in the literature search. Further on, CMED advocates calculation of inter-rater agreement on the literature scan and labeling of the studies where primary consensus was not reached. In case these studies should be included and subjected to a meta-analysis, a sensitivity analysis should be performed with inclusion and exclusion of these trials. There must be a reason why reviewers did not agree on this information at first and careful inspection of the publications might reveal subtle clinical ambiguities that would not have been discovered through the application of the usual quality criteria. Finally, reviewers should present an adapted flow diagram of the inclusion/exclusion procedure according to QUOROM standards *(17)* but should also make it clear in which database references were uniquely discovered.

- *Data extraction:* lengthy lists in spreadsheet format are discouraged because the reviewer has to constantly scroll up and down the document. A well-prepared Word document or even a specially designed database (e.g., in Access format) will be more helpful. Advice and templates are available from CMED. Authors should keep in mind that a thorough description of the included studies (e.g., mean age of participants, duration of disease) calls for *weighted* means and not for a simple calculation of the mean of means. For example, it would be wrong to compute a mean age of 50 yr from two trials reporting participants' mean age as 40 and 60 if trial 1 included 1000 and trial two 400 patients (54.3 yr is the correct result).

- *Study quality:* empirical evidence *(18)*, as well as theoretical considerations, suggest that although summary quality scores may in some circumstances provide a useful overall assessment, scales should not generally be used to assess the quality of trials in systematic reviews. The analysis of individual components of study quality overcomes many of the shortcomings of composite scores. The component approach takes into account that the importance of individual quality domains, and the direction of potential biases associated with these domains, will vary between the contexts in which trials are performed. In addition to the usual quality criteria such as concealment of allocation, blinding conditions, and drop-out rates, reviewers should consider *clinical* quality parameters when writing up the protocol. Furthermore, potential confounders, effect modifiers or covariates (e.g., dose of active treatment, choice of comparison treatment, length of follow-up, design of the study, compliance, age, and risk level) should be specified *a priori*. CMED encourages computation of inter-rater agreement of key domains of critically appraised study quality.

- *Heterogeneity:* inevitably, studies brought together in a systematic review will differ. Any kind of variability among studies in a systematic review may be termed heterogeneity. It can be helpful to distinguish between different types of heterogeneity. Variability in the participants, interventions, and outcomes studied may be characterized as clinical diversity (clinical heterogeneity), and variability in trial design and quality may be described as methodological diversity (methodological heterogeneity). Variability in the treatment effects being evaluated in the different trials is known as statistical heterogeneity, and is a consequence of clinical chance and/or methodological diversity among the studies. Meta-analysis should only be considered when a group of trials is sufficiently homogeneous in terms of participants, interventions and outcomes to provide a meaningful summary. The often used χ-squared test for homogeneity must be interpreted with care, because it has low power in the (common) situation of a meta-analysis when trials have a small sample size or are few in number. A recently developed statistic for quantifying heterogeneity is I^2 *(19,20)*. This describes the percentage of the variability in effect estimates that is caused by heterogeneity rather than chance. A value greater than 50% may be considered substantial heterogeneity. On the other hand, heterogeneity between study results should not be seen as purely a problem for systematic reviews, because it also provides a unique opportunity for examining why treatment effects differ in certain circumstances. The comprehensive consideration of heterogeneity will generally provide more insights than the mechanistic calculation of an overall measure of effect or the avoidance of pooling, which leaves the clinician without a single clear quantitative summary.

USE OF COCHRANE REVIEWS AND CONCLUSIONS

Cochrane reviews are being used to support health technology reports and the evidence-based practice guidelines development. Cochrane reviews provide, for example, the evidence base for the Reproductive Health Library, a World Health Organization-sponsored electronic publication containing Cochrane reviews, guidelines, and commentaries *(21)*. Moreover, Cochrane reviews are an important source of evidence for the regularly updated Clinical Evidence, which is distributed free to professionals within the UK National Health Service, to professionals in the United States (*BMJ Publishing*, courtesy of the Unit Health Foundation) and via the Internet to many low- and middle-income countries.

Hence, Cochrane reviews are essential tools for health care workers, researchers, consumers, and policymakers who want to keep up with the evidence that is accumulating in their field. Meta-analysis, if appropriate, will enhance the precision of estimates of treatment effects and possibly lead to a more timely introduction of effective treatments through reduction of the probability of false-negative results. In the near future, the Cochrane Collaboration will enlarge its scope to systematic reviews of diagnostic accuracy studies. Systematic reviews may also demonstrate the lack of adequate evidence and, thus, identify areas where further studies and funding are needed.

Above all, greater efforts are needed to reduce biases in the individual studies that will contribute to reviews *(22)* and to reduce publication bias. The latter could be achieved by registration of studies prior to their results being known, and by researchers recognizing that they have an ethical and scientific responsibility to report findings of well-designed studies, regardless of the results *(23)*.

Considerable challenges remain for the Cochrane Collaboration and CMED. Infrastructure funding prevails problematic. Efforts are needed to ensure international collaboration, especially from low- and middle-income countries. CMED realizes the necessity for higher quality systematic reviews, as well as the demand to maintain the enthusiasm of reviewers to update their reviews as the number of reviews increase. In an atmosphere of ever intensifying economic pressure CMED will keep its balance to guarantee as much objective appraisal of the evidence as possible *(24)*.

REFERENCES

1. Hemminski E. Study of information submitted by drug companies to licensing authorities. BMJ 1980;280:833–836.
2. Melander H, Ahlqvist J, Meijer G, Beermann B. Evidence b(i)ased medicine —selective reporting from studies sponsored by pharmaceutical industry: review of studies in new drug applications. BMJ 2003;326:1171–1175.
3. Sackett DL, Rosenberg WM, Gray JA, Haynes RB, Richardson WS. Evidence based medicine: what it is and what it isn't. BMJ 1996;312:71–72.
4. Sackett D, Straus SE, Richardson WS, Rosenberg W, Haynes RB. Evidence-Based Medicine. How to Practice and Teach EBM. Churchill Livingstone, London, 2000.
5. Barrows HS, Pickell GC. Developing Clinical Problem-Solving Skills. A Guide to More Effective Diagnosis and Treatment. Norton and Company, New York, NY, 1991.
6. Stewart M, Weston WW, McWilliam CL, Freeman TR. Patient-Centered Medicne. Transforming the Clinical Method. Sage Publications, Thousand Oaks, CA, 1995.
7. Greenhalgh T. Narrative based medicine: narrative based medicine in an evidence based world. BMJ 1999;318:323–325.
8. Cochrane Library. Accessed 8/18/05. Available at www.cochrane.org/docs/whycc.htm.
9. Cochrane Library. Accessed 8/18/05. Available at www.cochrane.org/reviews/index.htm.
10. Jadad AR, Cook DJ, Jones A, et al. Methodology and reports of systematic reviews and meta-analyses: a comparison of Cochrane reviews with articles published in paper-based journals. JAMA 1998;280:278–280.
11. Olsen O, Middleton P, Ezzo J, et al. Quality of Cochrane reviews: assessment of sample from 1998. BMJ 2001;323:829–832.

12. Update Software Ltd. Accessed 8/18/05. Available at www.update-software.com/comcritusers/.
13. The Cochrane Collaboration. Accessed 8/18/05. Available at www.cochrane.org/resources/handbook/index.htm.
14. The Cochrane Collaboration Review Titles Manager. Accessed 8/18/05. Available at www.cochrane.no/titles.
15. Higgins, JPT, Green, S, eds. Cochrane Handbook for Systematic Reviews of Interventions 4.2.5 [updated May 2005]. Accessed 5/31/05. Available at http://www.cochrane.org/resources/handbook/hbook/htm.
16. Eysenck HJ. An exercise in mega-silliness. Am Psychol 1978;33:517.
17. Moher D, Cook DJ, Eastwood S, Olkin I, Rennie D, Stroup DF. Improving the quality of reports of meta-analyses of randomised controlled trials: the QUOROM statement. Quality of reporting of meta-analyses. Lancet 199;354:1896–1900.
18. Jüni P, Witschi A, Bloch R, Egger M. The hazards of scoring the quality of clinical trials for meta-analysis. JAMA 1999;282:1054–1060.
19. Higgins JPT, Thompson SG. Quantifying heterogeneity in a meta-analysis. Stat Med 2002;21:1539–1558.
20. Higgins JPT, Thompson SG, Deeks JJ, Altman DG. Measuring inconsistency in meta-analyses. BMJ 2003;327: 557–560.
21. Reproductive Health Outlook. Accessed 8/18/05. Available at www.rho.org/html/who-rhlibrary.htm.
22. Chalmers I. Unbiased, relevant, and reliable assessments in health care. BMJ 1998:317:1167–1168.
23. Chalmers I, Altman DG. How can medical journals help prevent poor medical research? Some opportunities presented by electronic publishing. Lancet 1999;353:490–493.
24. Blumenthal D. Doctors and drug companies. N Engl J Med 2004;351:1885–1890.

13 Health-Related Quality-of-Life Assessment in Endocrinology

Elie A. Akl, MD, MPH
and Holger J. Schünemann, MD, PhD

CONTENTS

INTRODUCTION

One may judge the impact of drug interventions by examining a variety of outcomes. In some situations, the most compelling evidence of drug efficacy may be found in a reduction of mortality (e.g., tight blood pressure control in diabetes mellitus) *(1)*, rate of hospitalization (e.g., influenza vaccination of diabetic patients) *(2)*, rate of disease occurrence (e.g., intensive blood glucose control and incidence of microvascular complications) *(3)*, or rate of disease recurrence (insulin pump therapy and severe

From: *Contemporary Endocrinology: Evidence-Based Endocrinology*
Edited by: V. M. Montori © Mayo Foundation for Medical Education and Research

hypoglycemic episodes) *(4)*. Alternatively, clinicians frequently rely on direct physiological or biochemical measures of the severity of a disease process and the way drugs influence these measures—for example, left ventricular ejection fraction in congestive heart failure, thyroid stimulating hormone (TSH) levels in hypothyroidism, or glycosylated hemoglobin level in diabetes mellitus.

Clinicians and investigators have recognized that there are other important aspects that one can use to assess the usefulness of the interventions that these epidemiological, physiological, or biochemical outcomes do not address. These aspects include the ability to function normally; to be free of pain and physical, psychological, and social limitations or dysfunction; and to be free from iatrogenic problems associated with treatment. On occasion, the conclusions reached when evaluating different outcomes may differ: physiological measurements may change without people feeling better *(5,6)*, a drug may ameliorate symptoms without a measurable change in physiological function, or life prolongation may be achieved at the expense of unacceptable pain and suffering *(7)*. The recognition of these patient-important (vs disease-oriented) areas of well-being led to the introduction of a technical term: health-related quality of life (HRQL).

WHAT IS HEALTH-RELATED QUALITY OF LIFE?

The definition of quality of life has led to much debate. The term "quality of life" lacks focus and precision because it is an abstract concept. Because the patient's subjective well-being is influenced by many factors unrelated to the disease process or treatment (e.g., education, income, and the quality of the environment), investigators have adopted a narrower term, HRQL, that focuses on quality of life related to health. Arguably, other factors, such as income, that are not included in this narrower focus can influence health. Some definitions of HRQL stem from the recognition that HRQL is a multi-level concept: first, an overall assessment of well-being; second, several broad domains—physiological, functional, psychological, and social status; and, third, subcomponents of each domain—for example pain, sleep, activities of daily living, and sexual function within physical and functional domains.

It follows that HRQL is a multi-level and multi-factorial concept that represents the final common pathway of all the physiological, psychological, and social influences of the therapeutic process *(8)*. It follows also that when assessing the impact of an intervention on patients' HRQL, one may be interested in describing the patients' status (or changes in the patient status) as a whole, on a variety of domains or on a specific subdomain, and that different strategies and instruments are required for this exploration.

Definitions of HRQL, both theoretical and practical, remain controversial. Most HRQL measurement instruments focus largely on how patients are functioning (e.g., their ability to care for themselves and carry out their usual roles in life). Whereas this pragmatic view of HRQL has gained dominance, there remain those who argue that unless one is assessing individual patients' values of health states the outcome is health status and not HRQL *(9)*.

These issues can be clarified by thinking of a wheelchair-bound patient who, despite limitations, is happy and fulfilled and values life highly (more, for instance, than most people). On most domains of most HRQL instruments, this patient's assessment would suggest a poor HRQL, despite the high value placed on the health state. Investigators and those interpreting the results of HRQL measures should be aware of the varying emphasis put on individual patient values and preferences in the different types of instruments *(10)*.

HOW DO WE EVALUATE HEALTH-RELATED QUALITY OF LIFE?

Generic Instruments

Generic instruments are instruments that measure several different aspects of quality of life. These instruments usually provide a scoring system that allows aggregation of the results into a small number of scores and sometimes into a single score (in which case, it may be referred to as an index). Generic measures are designed for use in a wide variety of conditions. Numerous generic instruments are available: for example, the Medical Outcome Study Health Survey 36-Item Short Form (SF-36) *(11)*, the Euro-QoL (EQ-5D) *(12)*, the Nottingham Health Profile (NHP) *(13)*, the Duke-UNC Health Profile *(14)*, and the McMaster Health Index Questionnaire *(15)*.

Although generic instruments attempts to measure all the important aspects of HRQL, they may slice the HRQL pie quite differently. For example, the SF-36 profile consists of eight subscales that measure physical functioning, role-physical, bodily pain, general health, vitality, social functioning, role-emotional, and mental health. The EQ-5D includes five dimensions about mobility, self-care, usual activities, pain/discomfort, and anxiety/depression *(16)*.

Generic instruments offer a number of advantages to the clinical investigator. Their reliability and validity (*see* Key Measurement Properties of Health-Related Quality-of-Life Tools) have often been established in a variety of populations. When using them for discriminative purposes, that is for distinguishing between people with better and worse HRQL (*see* Key Measurement Properties of Health-Related Quality-of-Life Tools), one can examine and establish areas of dysfunction affecting a particular population. Identification of these areas of dysfunction may guide investigators who are constructing disease-specific instruments to target areas of potentially greatest impact on the quality of life. Generic instruments used as evaluative instruments, that is, to measure change in HRQL over time, allow determination of the effects of an intervention on different aspects of quality of life. The inclusion of several aspects of HRQL eliminates the necessity to use multiple instruments (thus saving time for both the investigator and the patient). Because they are designed for a wide variety of conditions, one can potentially compare the effects on HRQL of different interventions in different diseases. Instruments that provide a single score can be used in a cost-effectiveness analysis, in which the cost of an intervention in monetary values is related to its outcome in natural units.

The main limitation of generic instruments is that they may not focus adequately on the aspects of quality of life specifically influenced by a particular disease (e.g., diabetes mellitus). This may result in an inability of the instrument to detect a real effect in the area of importance (i.e., lack of responsiveness). In fact, disease-specific instruments offer greater responsiveness compared with generic instruments *(17,18)*.

Specific Instruments

Specific instruments focus on aspects of health status that are specific to the area of primary interest. The rationale for this approach lies in the increased responsiveness that may result from including only those aspects of HRQL that are relevant and important in a particular disease process or even in a particular patient situation.

The instrument may be specific to the disease (e.g., instruments for type 1 diabetes *[19]*, type 2 diabetes *[20]*, e.g., pituitary gland disease), specific to a population of patients (instruments designed to measure the HRQL of the frail elderly, for youth with diabetes *[21]*), specific to a certain function (e.g., emotional function or psychological stress in diabetic patients *[22]*), or specific to a given condition or problem which can be caused by a variety of underlying pathologies (e.g., peripheral neuropathy and foot ulcers *[23]*). Within a single condition, the instrument may differ according to the intervention administered. For example, while inhaled Insulin should result in improved HRQL by reducing the number of daily injections required *(24)*, diabetes self-management training may improve HRQL by providing self management and coping skills *(25)*. Appropriate disease-specific HRQL outcome measures should reflect this difference.

Disease-specific instruments may be used for discriminative purposes. They may aid, for example, in discriminating among patients with different levels of diabetes severity *(26)*. Disease-specific instruments can also be applied in clinical trial for evaluative purposes to establish the impact of an intervention on a metabolic control *(27)*. Guidelines provide structured approaches for constructing specific measures *(28)*. Whatever approaches one takes for the construction of disease-specific measures, a number of head-to-head comparisons between generic and diabetes-specific instruments suggest that the latter approach will fulfill its promise of enhancing responsiveness *(29–31)*. In addition to the improved responsiveness, specific measures have the advantage of relating closely to areas routinely explored by the physician. For example, Diabetes-39, a diabetes-specific measure of quality of life focuses on the patient's anxiety and worry, social and peer burden, sexual functioning, energy and mobility, and diabetes control *(32)*. Specific measures may therefore appear clinically sensible to the clinician.

The disadvantages of specific measures are that they are (deliberately) not comprehensive, and cannot be used to compare across conditions. When evaluating the results of highly specific instruments, one should be wary regarding the possibility that adverse effects of medications and other interventions could remain undetected. That is, a highly specific instrument is usually not designed to detect adverse outcomes of a treatment. The foregoing arguments and descriptions suggest that there is no one group of instruments that will achieve all the potential goals of HRQL measurement. Thus, investigators may choose to use multiple instruments *(33)*.

Preference Instruments

Economic and decision theory provides the underlying basis for utility or preference based measures. The key elements of a utility instrument are, first that it is preference-based, and second, that scores are tied to death as an outcome. Typically, HRQL can be measured as a utility using a single number along a continuum from "dead" (0.0) to full health (1.0). Specific measurement techniques allow the measure of preferences "for states" that some respondents consider worse than death. The use of these measures in clinical studies requires serial measurement of the preference respondents assign to specific health states throughout the study.

To measure utility, patients make a single rating that takes into account all aspects of their quality of life *(34)*. Respondents can make this rating in many ways. When completing the "standard gamble" (SG) patients choose between their own health state and a gamble in which they may die immediately or achieve full health for the remainder of their lives. Patients' utility or HRQL is determined by the choices they make, as the probabilities of immediate death or full health are varied. Strictly speaking only the SG yields utility scores because of theoretical assumptions that only the standard gamble fulfills. Other instruments provide what is widely known as preference-based scores; scores that are expressed on the same 0 to 1 scale as the SG. These preference-based scores may differ systematically; however, the tools used to obtain them are simpler to administer and conceptually less challenging for patients to complete. In this text, we will use the terms utility and preference scores interchangeably if they fulfill the same purpose of measurement. The "time tradeoff" (TTO), in which respondents consider the number of years in their present health state they would be willing to tradeoff for a shorter life span in full health represents one of the alternatives. A third technique is the use of a simple visual analog scale (VAS) presented as a thermometer, the feeling thermometer *(35)*. When comparing alternative interventions and the benefits or downsides they cause in utility scores it is important to consider the techniques used to measure these utilities.

A major advantage of utility measurement is its amenability to cost-utility analysis. In cost-utility analysis, the cost of an intervention is related to the number of quality adjusted life-years (QALYs) patients may gain through application of the intervention *(36)*. QALYs are the product of years lived multiplied by the utility score assigned to this time period. For example, 2 yr lived in a health status that corresponds to 0.5 on the 0 to 1.0 scale are equivalent to 1 yr at a utility of 1.0 or 10 yr at a utility of 0.1. The cost per QALY can be compared and provide a basis for allocation of resources among different health care programs.

However, utility or preference measurement has limitations. As previously described, utilities can vary depending on how they are obtained, raising questions of the validity of any single measurement *(37)*. In addition, utility measurement does not allow investigators to identify which aspects of HRQL are responsible for measured changes in utility. Finally, utilities share the disadvantage of health profiles, in that they may not be responsive to small but patient-important changes.

KEY MEASUREMENT PROPERTIES OF HEALTH-RELATED QUALITY-OF-LIFE TOOLS

Validity

Validity is the property of an instrument to measure what it intends to measure. Validity is best determined when a gold standard is available; however, in HRQL measurement a gold standard usually does not exist.

VALIDITY WHEN THERE IS A GOLD STANDARD

If a gold standard or criterion standard for some aspect of health exists, one determines validity of a new instrument using the concept of criterion validity. That is investigators determine whether the results of the measurements with the new instrument correspond to those of the criterion standard. The concept of a gold or criterion standard is most easily applied for physiological measures. For instance, experts may agree that blood glucose measured in samples obtained by venipuncture is a gold standard for measurement of glycemia, and fingerstick tests could be judged in relation to this criterion.

Although there is no gold standard for HRQL, there are instances in which there is a specific target for a HRQL instrument that can be treated as a criterion or gold standard. For instance, criterion validity is applicable when a shorter version of an instrument (the test) is used to predict the results of the full-length instrument (the gold standard). Another example is using a health-status instrument to predict mortality. In this instance, to the extent that variability in survival between patients (the gold standard) is explained by the questionnaire results, the instrument will be valid.

VALIDITY WHEN THERE IS NO GOLD STANDARD

If there is no gold or criterion standard, investigators employ validation strategies used by clinical and experimental psychologists; these strategies provide information about *face, content*, and *construct* validity.

Face validity refers to whether an instrument appears to be measuring what it is intended to measure. Content validity refers to the extent to which the domain of interest is comprehensively sampled by the items, or questions, in the instrument. Quantitative testing of face and content validity are rarely attempted.

The most rigorous approach to establishing validity is an approach that measures construct validity. A construct is a theoretically derived notion of the domain(s) that one wishes to measure. An understanding of the construct will lead to expectations and allows hypotheses about how an instrument should behave, related to other measures, if it is valid. The first step in constructing validation is to establish a "model" or theoretic framework, which characterizes the understanding of what investigators are trying to measure. Investigators then administer a number of instruments to a population of interest and examine the data. Validity is strengthened or weakened according to the extent to which the results confirm or refute the hypotheses. For example, a discriminative HRQL instrument may be validated by comparing two groups of diabetic patients; those who have diabetic foot ulcers and those who do not *(38)*. An HRQL instrument should distinguish between these two groups, and if it does not it is very likely that something has gone wrong. Another example is the validation of an instrument discriminating between people according to some aspect of emotional function. The correlation between the Diabetes Health Profile (DHP-1) and the Hospital Depression and Anxiety Scale supports the construct validity of this instrument in regards to measurement of depression *(20)*. We call construct validity that deals with measurements at one point in time *cross-sectional construct validity*. The principles of validation are identical for evaluative instruments, but their validity is demonstrated by showing that changes in the instrument being investigated correlate with changes in other related measures in the theoretically derived predicted direction and magnitude (*longitudinal construct validity*). For instance, the validity of the Diabetes Quality of Life Clinical Trial Questionnaire (DQLCTQ) was supported by two multinational clinical trials showing the association between the instrument and improved metabolic control *(27)*.

Validation is not an all-or-nothing process. We may have varying degrees of confidence that an instrument is really measuring what it is supposed to measure. *A priori* predictions of the strength of relationship with other measures that one would expect if a new instrument is really measuring what is intended strengthen the validation process. Without such predictions, it is generally easy to rationalize whatever correlations between measures are observed.

Validation does not end when the first validation study is published, but continues with repeated use of an instrument. Readers of studies that included HRQL outcomes should evaluate whether studies that support validity of an instrument exist and whether they support the use of an instrument for the given question.

Responsiveness

Responsiveness is the property of evaluative instruments (those designed to measure changes within individuals over time) to detect change. If a treatment results in an important difference in health status, investigators wish to be confident that they will detect that difference, even if it is small. Responsiveness will be directly related to the magnitude of the difference in score in patients who have improved or deteriorated (the signal) and the extent to which patients who have not changed obtain more or less the same scores (the noise). Readers of studies that evaluate change in HRQL should evaluate whether the instrument is able to differentiate the signal from the noise. If instruments are burdened with a low signal to noise ratio, then these instruments may fail to detect important changes in HRQL.

Reliability

Reliability is an important property of HRQL instruments. An instrument is reliable if the variability in scores between subjects (the signal) is much greater than the variability within subjects (the noise). Measures of reliability are Cronbach's coefficient, the item-total correlation and the test–retest correlation. Cronbach's coefficient measures how well the items within a scale measure a single underlying dimension or domain; coefficients between 0.7 and 0.9 are recommended, but we refer readers to other texts for a description of the exact methodology (39). The item-total correlation coefficient measures the correlation of each of the items to the total scale; each item should correlate at least 0.2 with the remainder of the scale. Test–retest correlation reflects the reproducibility (test–retest reliability) of measures in the same patients (39).

INTERPRETATION OF HEALTH-RELATED QUALITY-OF-LIFE SCORES

A final key property of a HRQL instrument is interpretability. For a discriminative instrument, we could ask whether a particular score signifies that a patient with diabetes is functioning normally, or has mild, moderate, or severe impairment of HRQL. For an evaluative instrument we might ask whether a particular change in score represents a trivial, small but important, moderate, or large improvement or deterioration, respectively. Considerable research has focused on establishing what constitutes the minimal important difference (MID) in HRQL. One can define the MID as "the smallest difference in score in the outcome of interest that informed patients or informed proxies perceive as important, either beneficial or harmful, and which would lead the patient or clinician to consider a change in the management" (40). However, any change in management will depend on the downsides, including cost, associated with that outcome and the values and preferences patients place on these outcomes.

A number of strategies are available for trying to make HRQL scores interpretable and describe the MID (35), but the methodology is complex. Knowing the change or difference in score that is meaningful enables the estimation of the number of patients who need to be treated for one individual to have an additional clinically meaningful improvement (41).

HEALTH-RELATED QUALITY OF LIFE IN ENDOCRINOLOGY

Instruments Used to Evaluate Health-Related Quality of Life

GENERIC INSTRUMENTS AND THEIR MEASUREMENT PROPERTIES

We review here three instruments, the SF-36, the EQ-5D, and the WHOQOL-100 as examples of generic instruments that investigators evaluated and used in endocrinology. We will focus on diabetes because among the endocrinological disorders HRQL is most extensively studied in diabetic patients.

SF-36

The SF-36, developed by Ware et al., is one of the most popular and most widely used generic measurements of HRQL *(42)*. It has been translated into more than 40 languages and normal values for the general population in many countries are available. It provides a profile with eight subscales that measure physical functioning, role-limitations/physical, bodily pain, general health, vitality, social functioning, role-limitations/emotional, and mental health. The SF-36 has been used widely in patients with endocrinological disorders. In one study, the SF-36 had poor predictive validity regarding glycemic control but correlated with the number of complications in patients with diabetes *(33,43)*. Two other studies showed that the SF-36 and diabetes-specific instruments examine somewhat different and complementary aspects of HRQL. In one study, the Diabetes Quality of Life (DQOL) Questionnaire, a diabetes-specific instrument, correlated more with lifestyle issues, particularly in younger patients, whereas the SF-36 provided more information about functional health status *(33)*. In another study the Diabetes Care Profile (DCP), another diabetes-specific instrument, was superior to the SF-36 in assessing the impact of acute complications and/or interventions on HRQL. Conversely, the SF-36 was superior in examining relationships between the patient's experience of living with diabetes and other chronic diseases with HRQL *(44)*. The estimates of internal consistency (Cronbach's α) for SF-36 subscales in measuring HRQL in patients with type 1 and 2 diabetes range from 0.78 to 0.91 *(33)*.

EuroQoL EQ-5D

The EQ-5D is a generic instrument designed for self-completion and postal surveys *(12)*. The EQ-5D includes five questions about mobility, self-care, usual activities, pain/discomfort, and anxiety/depression *(16)*. One further question elicits whether the present health state is better, much the same, or worse than the general level of health over the past 12 mo. The EQ-5D also contains a VAS on which patients rate their present health on a scale like a thermometer from 0 to 100. It has been tested for validity, reliability, and for use in different health states and diseases, as well as in the general populations of several countries *(12)*.

For example, in a study assessing HRQL in patients with type 2 diabetes, the EQ-5D average scores were lower than that of the similarly aged healthy population. The EQ-5D scores were associated with gender, diabetes complications, treatment type, age, obesity, and hyperglycemia *(45,46)*. In the United Kingdom Prospective Diabetes Study (UKPDS) investigators used the EQ-5D to estimate the impact of diabetes-related complications on HRQL *(47)*. The test–retest analysis indicated relatively high intra-patient variability, but the 4-mo interval between surveys was longer than the usually recommended 2-wk periods to assess test–retest reliability in stable patients. In that study, the EQ-5D also showed weak responsiveness *(47,48)*.

WHOQOL-100

The WHOQOL-100 is a generic HRQL instrument developed through an international collaboration of 15 field centers. The aim of the project was to develop a cross-culturally applicable instrument that covers the respondent's overall quality of life and general health, as well as quality of life domains referring to physical health, psychological state, social relationships, and environment *(49)*. Each domain contains several facets, each of them consisting of four questions.

In a Croatian study exploring its psychometric properties in patients with type 2 diabetes, the WHOQOL-100 had discriminated groups of patients who have different disease characteristics *(49)*. In terms of reliability, it had a Cronbach's coefficient of 0.76–0.95 and a test–retest correlation coefficient of 0.75–0.91 *(49)* Over the 2-mo follow-up period of the study, the scores of an intervention group started on insulin therapy improved compared with a control group providing information about the responsiveness of the instrument.

Specific Instruments and Their Measurement Properties

We review and compare here 10 of the mostly used diabetes-specific HRQL instruments: the Appraisal of Diabetes Scale (ADS), the Audit of Diabetes-Dependent Quality of Life (ADDQL), the DHP, the Diabetes Impact Measurement Scales (DIMS), the DQOL, the Diabetes-39 (D-39), the Diabetes Specific Quality of Life Scale (DSQOLS), the Questionnaire on Stress in Patients with Diabetes-Revised (QSD-R), the Well-Being Enquiry for Diabetics (WED), and the Diabetes Quality of Life Clinical Trial Questionnaire-Revised (DQLCTQ-R).

GENERAL DESCRIPTION OF INSTRUMENTS

Table 1 lists information related to diabetes-specific HRQL instruments. Investigators developed and validated most of these instruments in the last 10 yr *(50)*. The DIMS and the DQLCTQ-R measure HRQL in clinical trials *(27,51)*, and the DQOL was specifically designed to assess the impact of intensive diabetes management on HRQL for the Diabetes Control and Complications Trial *(52)*. The WED, on the other hand, is intended for use in clinical settings *(53)*. Some of the diabetes-specific HRQL instruments were developed for either type 1 (e.g., DQOL, DSQOLS) or type 2 diabetes patients (e.g., DHP), but all, except for the DSQOLS, have been evaluated in both type 1 and type 2 diabetes *(50)*.

These HRQL instruments can be self-administered and are available in English, either as the original language or as a translation. The DQLCTQ-R is a composite of generic and specific instruments including the SF-36 and Diabetes DQOL *(27)*. Whereas items within the ADS and ADDQL produce a single index, items within the remaining instruments are partitioned into three to eight dimensions. All instruments include items or domains of psychological and social well-being *(50)*.

VALIDITY OF INSTRUMENTS

Criterion validity of disease-specific instruments in diabetes has not been investigated extensively *(50)*. To explore content and face validity, the developers of D-39,

QSD-R and WED involved patients in the development process, whereas the developers of ADDQL, DHP-1, DQOL, and DSQOLS involved both patients and experts.

Instrument developers tested construct validity through correlation with other instruments and global judgments of health, and comparisons with clinical and sociodemographic variables. However, most studies did neither construct theoretic frameworks nor did they provide hypotheses Table 1 summarizes results of these studies and shows that the ADDQoL, DHP-1, DSQOLS, D-39, and QSD-R have better evidence for construct validity than the other instruments.

RELIABILITY OF INSTRUMENTS

Table 1 also summarizes the results of reliability studies. The D-39, ADDQL, ADS, and DHP have item-total correlations greater than the 0.2 value (*see* Reliability) *(20,31, 54,55)*. The D-39, ADDQL, ADS, DHP, DSQOLS, and WED have Cronbach's levels greater than 0.7, the criterion recommended for studies involving groups of patients. ADS and DQOL have good test–retest reliability for group evaluation *(52,55)*.

RESPONSIVENESS OF INSTRUMENTS

Few of the reviewed instruments have been formally assessed for responsiveness *(50)*. Four domains of the DQLCTQ-R (treatment satisfaction, health/distress, mental health, and satisfaction) were responsive to clinical changes in metabolic control in diabetes *(27)*.

The responsiveness of DQOL was assessed in two studies. In the first study, the DQOL showed significant improvements in the total scores and all subscales in patients with end-stage renal disease receiving a combined pancreas and kidney transplant compared with those receiving a kidney transplant alone *(56)*. In the second study, only the DQOL scale of satisfaction showed an improvement in patients receiving an implantable pump compared with patients on standard insulin treatment *(57)*.

The authors of the DSQOLS assessed its responsiveness to a teaching program for Type 1 diabetics *(19)*. The program produced statistically significant improvements in the dimensions of social relations, physical complaints, worries about the future, diet restrictions, and treatment satisfaction.

Preference Based Instruments

A study assessing the value of the VAS, the SG, and SF-36 in measuring HRQL of hospitalized diabetic patients showed that VAS values were related to some of the SF-36 subscale scores but the SG values had no relation to any SF-36 subscale scores *(43)*.

Researchers have also assessed the properties of the TTO technique in assessing HRQL in patients with diabetic retinopathy. Both the SG and TTO methods demonstrated strong validity for utility assessment in patients with retinal disease (32.5% were diabetics) when evaluated against visual acuity in the higher sight eye and the VF-14 score *(58)*. The mean utility value for the diabetic retinopathy in 95 patients was 0.77 (0.73 to 0.81) with the TTO method and 0.88 (0.84 to 0.92) with the SG method. The length of time of visual loss and amount of formal education did not appear to affect the utility value *(59)*.

EXAMPLES OF STUDIES ASSESSING HEALTH-RELATED QUALITY OF LIFE IN DIABETES

Key Epidemiological Studies

There are a large number of epidemiological studies assessing the relationship between HRQL and diabetes, its duration, its type, the presence of complications, the treatment regimen, and metabolic control.

A systematic review *(60)* showed that people with diabetes have worse HRQL than people with no chronic illness, but better HRQL than people with most other serious chronic diseases. The review also showed that although duration and type of diabetes are not consistently associated with HRQL, the complications of diabetes are the most important disease-specific determinants of HRQL.

There is conflicting evidence about the relationship between the duration of diabetes and HRQL. Several studies found that increased duration of diabetes was associated with decreased HRQL in both type 1 and type 2 diabetes *(61–63)*, whereas other studies have found no significant association *(64–66)*.

The type and therapy of diabetes may also affect HRQL. Jacobson and colleagues showed that type 2 diabetic patients not on insulin reported higher HRQL than type 2 diabetic patients on insulin. Type 2 diabetic patients on insulin reported better HRQL than type 1 patients on insulin *(33)*. Whereas some investigators believe that these patterns of HRQL may be a function of diabetes type, others suggest that they are the result of other factors, such as treatment regimen or age *(60)*. Although a number of studies showed that increasing treatment intensity in patients with type 2 diabetes from diet and exercise alone, to oral medications, to insulin, is associated with worsening HRQL *(33,67,68)*, two others did not *(66,69)*.

Findings about the relationship between glycemic control and HRQL in diabetic patients depend on the type of HRQL instrument used. Although studies using generic measures have found no relationship *(44,70,71)*, most studies using diabetes-specific instruments have found that higher levels of HbA1c are associated with greater impairment of HRQL *(72,73)*. Thus, the benefits of good metabolic control may outweigh the increased burden of diabetes management.

As to the effect of diabetes-related complications on HRQL, there is strong and consistent evidence suggesting that the presence of complications is associated with worsened HRQL *(33,66,74)*. Both the severity and number of complications predict the effect on HRQL *(33,74)*.

Key Trials

We review here the findings of key trials in diabetes research: primarily the Diabetes Control and Complications Trial (DCCT) and the UK Prospective Diabetes Study Group (UKDPS). We also review the effect of interventions such as self-management, training, continuous subcutaneous insulin infusion, diabetes screening, home-based management, and inhaled insulin on HRQL.

In the DCCT, the investigators evaluated the effect of intensive diabetes treatment on HRQL of patients with type 1 diabetes. They measured HRQL using the DQOL, the Symptom Checklist-90R, and SF-36 *(75)*. All analyses of HRQL, psychiatric symptom indexes, and psychosocial event data showed no differences between intensive

Table 1
Summary Table of Ten Diabetes-Specific HRQL

Instrument	Author, year	Development process	Setting and translations
Appraisal of Diabetes Scale (ADS)	Michael P. Carey, 1991	Theory and previous research	US outpatients (55)
Audit of Diabetes-Dependent Quality of Life (ADDQL)	Clare Bradley, 1999	Existing instruments, discussions with health professionals and patients	UK outpatients (31) Translated to more than 15 languages including French, Italian, Polish, and Portuguese for Brazil and Spanish for Mexico.
Diabetes Health Profile (DHP)	Keith A. Meadows, 1996	Literature review, review of instruments, interviews with type 2 patients and health care professionals	UK outpatients (20,95) Netherlands outpatients (96) Denmark outpatients (95) Translated to Danish, Dutch, English for Australia, English for South-Africa, Flemish, French, German, German for Switzerland, Hebrew, Italian, Polish, Russian, Spanish, Urdu
Diabetes Impact Measurement Scales (DIMS)	Thomas T. Aoki and G. Steven Hammond, 1992	Literature review, review of instruments, and discussions with clinicians	US outpatients (51) Translated to French, Italian
Diabetes Quality of Life Measure (DQOL)	Alan M. Jacobson, 1988	Literature reviews, discussion with clinicians and type 1 diabetics	US outpatients (33,64) Translated to Chinese, French, Spanish
Diabetes (D) 39	J. G. Boyer, 1997	Literature review, existing instruments, and interviews with diabetics and health professionals	US outpatients (54) Translated to multiple languages including UK English, Danish, Dutch, Finnish, French, German, Italian, Norwegian and Swedish

Dimensions/domains [items]	Scale	Reliability[1]	Validity

One domain (7)	5-point scale	α = 0.73
		ITC = 0.28–0.59
		TRC = 0.85–0.89
			Diabetic Daily Hassles
			  Scale r = 0.59
			Diabetes Regimen Adherence
			  Questionnaire-R r = 0.17
			Diabetes Health Belief
			  Questionnaire
			  r = 0.31–0.42
			Perceived Stress Scale
			  r = 0.49
			Psychiatric Symptom
			  Index r = 0.39–0.55

One domain (13)	Each item is scored
	  for on a 7-point
	  scale and
	  for importance
	  on a 3-point
	  scale.
		α = 0.84
		ITC=0.37–0.67
			Global judgment (QOL)
			  r = 0.31
			Global judgment (QOL
			  without diabetes)
			  r = 0.47

Psychological
  distress (14)
Barriers to activity (13)
Disinhibited eating (5)
	4-point scale	ITC = 0.47–0.75
		αa = 0.70–0.88
		  (20)
			Hospital Anxiety
			  and Depression Scale
			  r = 0.28–0.62 (20)
			SF-36 r = 0.17–0.68 (20)
			SF-36 r = 0.07–0.65 (96)

Well-being (11)
Social-role fulfillment (5)
  fulfillment (5)
Diabetes-related
  morale (11)
Non-specific symptoms (11)
Specific symptoms (6)
	4- to 6-point
	  scale
		α = 0.60–0.85	Global judgment patient
			  (general health)
			  r = 0.27–0.47
			Global judgment clinician
			  (general health)
			  r = 0.29–0.45

Worries about future
  effects of diabetes (4)
Worries about social/
  vocational issues (7)
Impact of treatment (20)
Satisfaction with
  treatment (15)
	5-point Likert
	  scale
		α = 0.67–0.92 (52)
		α = 0.52–0.88 (64)
		α = 0.47–0.87 (33)
		TRC = 0.78–0.92
		  (52)
			Symptom Checklist
			  90 r = 0.40–0.60
			  (52,97)
			Bradburn Affect Balance
			  Scale
			  r = 0.27–0.57 (52,97)
			Psychological adjustment
			  to illness
			  r = 0.06–0.63 (52,97)
			SF-36 r = 0.00–0.60 (33)
			Duke Health Profile (64)
			General Health Perceptions
			  Profile (64)

Anxiety and worry (4)
Social and peer burden (5)
Sexual functioning (3)
Energy and mobility (15)
Diabetes control (12)
	7-point scale	α = 0.81–0.92
		ITC = 0.50–0.84
			SF-36 r = 0.15–0.71
			Global judgment of quality
			  of life r = 0.21–0.44
			Global judgment of diabetes
			  severity r = 0.15–0.56

(continued)

Table 1 *(continued)*

Instrument	Author, year	Development process	Setting and translations
Diabetes Specific Quality of Life Scale (DSQOLS)	Uwe Bott, 1998	Existing instruments and discussions with type 1 diabetics.	German general practice *(19)* Translated to UK English
Questionnaire on Stress in Patients with Diabetes-Revised (QSD-R)	G. Duran and P. Herschbach, 1997	Literature review and interviews with clinicians and diabetics, self-administered	Germany in-patients and outpatients *(22)* Translated to English
Well-Being Enquiry for Diabetics (WED)	E. Mannucci, 1996	Diabetologists, psychiatrists, nurses and diabetics	Italy outpatients *(53)* Italian, English
Diabetes Quality of Life Clinical Trial Questionnaire-Revised (DQLCTQ-R)	W. Shen, 1999	Composite of generic and specific instruments including SF-36 and DQOL, content based on patient focus groups and expert clinician panels	Canada, France, Germany, US, outpatients *(27)* Original in English, Translated to French and German

*a*ITC = item-total correlation; α = Cronbach's α; TRC = test–retest correlation

Dimensions/domains [items]	Scale	Reliability[a]	Validity

Worries about future (5)
Social relations (11)
Leisure time
  flexibility (6)
Daily hassles (4)
Diet restrictions (5)
Physical complaints (8)
Treatment satisfaction (10)
	6-point scale	α = 0.70–0.88	Positive Well-Being Scale
			  r = 0.35–0.53
			Treatment satisfaction
			  (r = 0.28–0.43)

Depression/fear of future (6) Leisure time (4) Partner (6) Work (6) Treatment regimen/diet (9) Physical complaints (6) Hypoglycemia (4) Doctor–patient relationship (4)	5-point scale	α = 0.69–0.81 TRC = 0.45–0.73	Complications ($p < 0.05$) State-Trait Anxiety Inventory r = 0.33–0.71

Serenity (10)
Discomfort (10)
Impact (20)
Symptoms (20)
	5-point scale	α = 0.81–0.84
		TRC=0.68–0.89
			Diabetes Quality of Life
			  Measure r = 0.05–0.68
			State-Trait Anxiety Inventory
			  r = 0.13–0.63
			Hamilton Depression Rating
			  Scale r = 0.29–0.49
			Bulimic Investigation Test
			  Edinburgh r = 0.26–0.35

Physical Function; Energy/
Fatigue; Health Distress;
Mental Health; Satisfaction;
Treatment Satisfaction;
Treatment Flexibility;
  and Frequency
  of Symptoms.
57 items in total
	Varies	α = 0.77–0.90.	Scale discriminates between
			  type of diabetes, metabolic
			  control, gender, and
			  self-perceived control
			  of diabetes.

and conventional diabetes treatment. Authors concluded that "under careful treatment conditions, such as those followed in the DCCT, patients undergoing intensive diabetes treatment do not face deterioration in the quality of their lives, even while the rigor of their diabetes care is increased."

In the UKDPS, the investigators evaluated the impact of therapeutic policies shown to reduce the risk of complications in patients with type 2 diabetes on HRQL (46). They used the EQ-5D and a disease-specific questionnaire (measuring mood disturbance, cognitive mistakes, symptoms, and work satisfaction) to measure HRQL. The results of both questionnaires showed that the therapy had no effect on HRQL; effects on other clinical endpoints were also similar in the three intensive agents (chlorpropamide, glibenclamide, or insulin).

A systematic review confirmed that intensive treatment does not impair HRQL and that having better glycemic control and perceived ability to control their disease result in improved HRQL (60). Another systematic review about the effectiveness of self-management training in type 2 diabetes found that HRQL was examined in three studies (25). Kaplan et al. noted an increase in HRQL at 18 mo for an intervention subgroup that received intensive counseling on both diet and physical activity (76). Two studies of brief interventions (education program for insulin-treated diabetic patients and a brief office-based intervention) failed to demonstrate improved HRQL (77,78).

A systematic review about the effects of continuous subcutaneous insulin infusion (CSII) therapy in diabetic patients found five studies that included HRQL as an outcome. Two of the five studies found improvements on CSII (79,80), whereas the other three studies found no difference (81–83). Weintrob et al. recently conducted a randomized controlled trial in children with type 1 diabetes (84) assessing HRQL with the Diabetes Treatment Satisfaction Questionnaire (DTSQ) (85) and the Diabetes Quality of Life Questionnaire for Youth (DQOLY) (21). By the end of the study, the DTSQ total score was significantly higher in the CSII group.

To assess the impact of diabetes screening on HRQL, investigators used the SF-36 at baseline and 1 yr after screening for diabetes (86). HRQL scores were similar in patients with and without a new diagnosis of diabetes discovered through systematic screening and remained stable over the year after screening.

Siminerio et al. conducted a systematic review to compare the effects of routine hospital admission to outpatient or home-based management in children newly diagnosed with type 1 diabetes who are not acutely ill (87). One study assessed parental quality of life and reported no differences in any of the subscales of the Parental Diabetes Quality of Life Scale (satisfaction, diabetes impact, diabetes worry) between the two groups at either of the time points assessed (87). On the whole, the data suggested that outpatient or home management treatment does not lead to any disadvantages in terms of metabolic control, acute diabetic complications and hospitalizations, psychosocial variables and behavior, or total costs.

Royle et al. (24) conducted a systematic review to compare the efficacy, adverse effects and patient acceptability of inhaled vs injected insulin. Inhaled insulin maintained a glycemic control comparable to that of patients taking multiple daily injections. The key benefit appeared to be a significant improvement in HRQL, presumably owing to the reduced number of daily injections required.

BEST INSTRUMENTS

As previously discussed, there is no one group of instruments that will achieve all the potential goals of HRQL measurement. Thus, investigators may choose to use multiple instruments including both generic and disease-specific ones. The SF-36 remains the most popular and widely used generic instrument and has the best measurement properties among generic instruments used in diabetes research. It also allows comparisons with other diseases and a large general research effort about its interpretability exists. As for diabetes-specific instruments, the ADDQL, DHP, DSQOLS, D-39, and QSD-R all show good evidence for validity and reliability. Among these the DSQOLS has the strongest evidence for responsiveness. Although the DQOL is reported as most widely used diabetics-specific instruments, the evidence for its reliability and validity is weaker. The choice among these instruments will depend on the study type and population.

EXAMPLES OF INSTRUMENTS USED IN OTHER ENDOCRINOLOGICAL DISORDERS

Researchers have used both generic and disease-specific instruments to measure HRQL in a number of endocrinological disorders. Examples include the SF-36, the Grave's Ophthalmopathy Quality of Life (GO-QOL) questionnaire, and the Quality-of Life-Assessment of Growth Hormone (GH) Deficiency in Adults questionnaire (QoL-AGHDA).

Bianchi et al. *(88)* used the SF-36 to measure and compare the HRQL of patients with thyroid disease to that of the Italian general population. All domains, except bodily pain, indicated impaired HRQL in thyroid disease. HRQL was impaired also in the absence of altered hormone levels. Mood and behavior disturbances were prevalent among a large proportion of patients and were significantly associated with poor HRQL *(88)*.

The GO-QOL questionnaire is a validated questionnaire for use in Grave's ophthalmopathy *(89)* Park et al. *(90)* showed that the majority of patients with Grave's ophthalmopathy reported impaired HRQL on the instrument's dimensions of daily activities and self confidence.

The QoL-AGHDA is a validated and commonly used instrument in growth hormone deficiency HRQL research *(91)*. In one study, patients with hypopituitarism and GH deficiency undergoing GH replacement therapy in an RCT showed a progressive score improvement compared to control patients *(92)*.

USERS' GUIDE TO HEALTH-RELATED QUALITY OF LIFE IN DIABETES

Standard Users Guide Questions

For clinicians looking at a study assessing HRQL as an outcome and asking the question "will this treatment make the patient feel better?" Guyatt et al. *(93)* proposed a guide for assessing the validity of the study methods, interpreting the results and applying the results to patients.

This users' guide includes the following assessments:

Are the results valid?
Primary Guides
- Have the investigators measured aspects of patients' lives that patients consider important?
- Did the HRQL instruments work in the intended way?

Secondary Guides
- Are there important aspects of HRQL that have been omitted?
- If there are tradeoffs between quality and quantity of life, or if an economic evaluation has been performed, have the most appropriate measures been used?

What are the results?
- How can we interpret the magnitude of the effect on HRQL?

How can I apply the results to patient care?
- Will the information from the study help patients make informed decisions about treatment?
- Did the study design simulate clinical practice?

EXAMPLE

Clinicians frequently face the situation when a study reports the absence of a statistically significant effect of an intervention on HRQL. We will follow the users' guide questions to evaluate such a study.

Are the Results Valid?

First, in assessing whether the investigators measured aspects of patients' lives that diabetic patients consider important, one should look at whether the instrument developers involved diabetic patients in the development process (e.g., D-39). If not, the instrument developers should at least cite prior work showing that the aspects they measured are important for patients with diabetes.

Second, whether the HRQL instrument worked in the intended way depends on the psychometric properties of the instrument, responsiveness being the most important property in clinical trials assessing the effectiveness of an intervention. Whereas the "no effect" result could be a true one, it could also be a false "no effect" result related to the nonresponsiveness of the instrument. The latter becomes less likely with a diabetes-specific instrument and with stronger published evidence of the instrument responsiveness in populations similar to that of the trial (e.g., DSQOLS). Another possibility is that the "no effect" result might be a mixed response by different subgroups included in the study averaging to a null effect. In that case a subgroup analysis, if provided by the authors, can help assess the impact in the subgroup that the individual patient matches the most. However, the more subgroup analyses the authors undertake, the greater is the risk of a spurious conclusion. Clinicians should be cautious and apply criteria to distinguish subgroup analyses that are credible from those that are not *(94)*.

Are there important aspects of HRQL that have been omitted? This is less likely if the instrument is diabetes-specific. In fact, disease-specific instruments aim to cover most aspects of HRQL that are specific to the disease. The caveat is that sometimes these instruments do not cover symptoms related to the side effects of treatments. Generic instruments might better cover them as part of their comprehensive coverage all relevant areas of HRQL. Clinicians should assess whether the diabetes-specific instrument under consideration covers such symptoms.

Finally, is the HRQL instrument appropriate to assess tradeoffs between quality and quantity of life and conduct economic evaluations? Preference instruments are the appropriate ones for such purposes as they allow standardized comparisons across treatment modalities and different conditions. Researchers use these instruments to generate QALYs. This measure accounts for both quality and quantity of life and is used to conduct economic analyses of clinical practices.

What Are the Results?

After having assessed the validity of the study, one should interpret the importance of the magnitude of the intervention effect on HRQL. In our example, the results suggest the lack of statistically significant results (Fig. 1). Do these results also exclude a patient important effect? The first step is to decide what is the MID for the change in HRQL score for both harm and benefit (*see* Interpretation of Health-Related Quality-of-Life Scores). If the lower limit of the confidence interval is smaller (more negative) than the MID for harm (negative value), then one cannot exclude a harmful effect of the intervention (Fig. 1, case 1). If the upper limit of the confidence interval is higher than the MID for benefit (positive value), then one cannot exclude a patient important beneficial effect of the intervention (Fig. 1, case 2). If the limits of the confidence interval are larger than the MID for harm and small than the MID for benefit, one can conclude with confidence that, in addition to a lack of statistically significant effect, the results suggest the lack of patient important effects (Fig. 1, case 3). Cases 4 and 5 show results that clearly demonstrate patient-important benefit and harm, respectively.

How Can I Apply the Results to Patient Care?

Assuming the results suggest the absence of any clinically or statistically significant effect, how can they help our patient make an informed decision about the intervention under consideration? Let us consider two cases. In the first one, the intervention (e.g., a more intensive Insulin regimen) is aimed at improving glycemic control and long-term microvascular outcomes. In this case the patient's interest with quality-of-life outcome stems from a concern of negative effect of the intensive regimen on HRQL. Thus, the absence of any effect of intervention on HRQL will encourage the patient to accept the intervention. In the second case, the intervention (e.g., behavioral program of coping skills training) is aimed primarily at improving quality of life in adolescent diabetic patients. The absence of any effect of the intervention on HRQL will make this intervention useless to our patient.

Finally, did the study design simulate clinical practice? Unlike clinicians, clinical investigators try to maintain patients on drug medication as long as possible, sometimes in spite of side effects. Because of these side effects such trials risk providing inaccurate estimates of the impact of the medication on HRQL. The more the study design simulate clinical practice the less the risk.

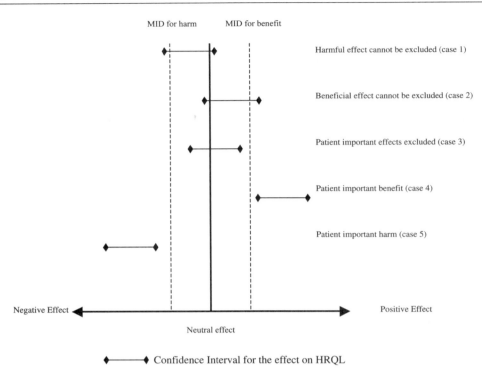

MID for harm   MID for benefit

Harmful effect cannot be excluded (case 1)

Beneficial effect cannot be excluded (case 2)

Patient important effects excluded (case 3)

Patient important benefit (case 4)

Patient important harm (case 5)

Negative Effect   Positive Effect

Neutral effect

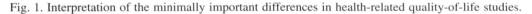 Confidence Interval for the effect on HRQL

Fig. 1. Interpretation of the minimally important differences in health-related quality-of-life studies.

RESOURCES FOR EVALUATION OF HEALTH-RELATED QUALITY OF LIFE IN ENDOCRINOLOGY

Databases

- The Quality of Life Instruments Database (QOLID) was initiated in 2002 by the Mapi Research Institute (http://www.qolid.org). The database provides a list of diabetes-specific instruments. A basic level of QOLID providing brief and descriptive information for each instrument is accessible to all users free of charge. A paid membership is required to access QOLID's advanced level. The advanced level provides a greater degree of practical information on the instruments and, when available, includes the review copy of the questionnaire, its translations, and the user manual.
- METRIC (http://www.measurementexperts.org).

Journals

- *Quality of Life Research*
- *Diabetes Care*
- *British Medical Journal*
- *Health and Quality of Life Outcomes*
- *Journal of American Medical Association*
- *Journal of Clinical Epidemiology*
- *Medical Care, Social Science and Medicine*

Instrument	Author, year	Development process	Setting and translations	Dimensions/domains [items]	Scale	Reliability[a]	Validity
SF-36 (33)	J.E. Ware, 1990	The 149-item Functioning and Well-Being Profile (FWBP) was based on review of previous instruments. The FWBP was the source for questionnaire items and instructions adapted for use in the SF-36.	Original English, translated to more than 40 languages	Physical functioning (10) Role limitations/physical (4) Pain (2) General health perceptions (5) Emotional well-being (5) Role limitations/emotional (3) Energy/fatigue (5) Social functioning (2)	Varies (yes/no, 3-, 5-, 6-point scales)	α = 0.78 to 0.91 (33) α = 0.67 (GH) and 0.88 (43)	DQOL r = −0.003 to 0.60 (33)
EQ-5D	The EuroQol Group, 1987		Initially developed simultaneously in Dutch, English, Finnish, Norwegian, and Swedish Translated to more than 40 languages	Five items: Mobility, Self-care, Usual activities, Pain/Discomfort, Anxiety/Depression. score between −0.59 and 1, where 1 represents perfect health, 0 represents death and scores less than 0 represent health states perceived by the patient to be worse than death	Three ordinal response levels. Tariff score is calculated using differences between values rather than using the values themselves	ITC = 0.41–0.72 (tariff scores) ITC = 0.64–0.82 (VAS score) (47)	Lower scores in patients with some DM2-related complication, deficient glycemic control and on insulin control and treatment (98) The inability to record relatively small changes in quality of life associated with less serious complications (47)

(continued)

199

Table 2 *(continued)*

Instrument	Author; year	Development process	Setting and translations	Dimensions/domains [items]	Scale	Reliability[a]	Validity
							EQ-5D values for diabetic patients reporting excellent, very good, good, fair and poor states of health on a self-rating health status item (0.95, 0.92, 0.83, 0.64, 0.27 respectively) (45) The EQ5D utility and Euroqol VAS scores correlated well (Pearson coefficient 0.633 [99])
WHOQOL-100	WHOQOL Group (100)	Focus groups, expert panels. international collaboration of 15 simultaneously involved field centers, aimed to develop a QoL assessment that would be applicable cross-culturally	Available in more than 40 languages	Overall QoL and general health plus six domains: physical domain, psychological domain, level of independence, relationships, environment and spirituality/religion/ personal beliefs domain. Each domain contains several facets, each consisting of four items. Total of 100 items.	5-point scale	α = 0.76–0.95 TRC = 0.75–0.91 (49)	Discriminant validity in differentiating groups of patients who have different disease characteristics (49)

[a]ITC = Item-total correlation; α = Cronbach's α; TRC = Test-retest correlation

SUMMARY

In summary, numerous HRQL instruments exist for the assessment of HRQL in patients with endocrinological disease. Several instruments have shown good measurement properties and generic instruments allow assessment of HRQL across diseases and populations. Disease-specific instruments have the advantage of greater responsiveness to changes in treatment but they may not capture important side effects of interventions. We provide a comprehensive list of instruments investigators and clinicians can use. More research exploring the application of HRQL instruments in clinical practice and the interpretability of HRQL scores and changes in HRQL scores is needed. Until now the evidence suggests that HRQL improves with few interventions in diabetes, but more research is needed to explore strategies that consistently show improvement in HRQL.

REFERENCES

1. Grossman E, Messerli HF, Goldbourt, U. High blood pressure and diabetes mellitus: are all antihypertensive drugs created equal? 2000;160:2447–2452.
2. Heymann AD, Shapiro Y, Chodick G, et al. Reduced hospitalizations and death associated with influenza vaccination among patients with and without diabetes. Diabetes Care 2004;27:2581–2584.
3. UK Prospective Diabetes Study (UKPDS) Group. Intensive blood-glucose control with sulphonylureas or insulin compared with conventional treatment and risk of complications in patients with type 2 diabetes (UKPDS 33). Lancet 1998;352:837–853.
4. Weissberg-Benchell J, Antisdel-Lomaglio J, Seshadri R. Insulin pump therapy: a meta-analysis. Diabetes Care 2003;26:1079–1087.
5. Packer M. How should we judge the efficacy of drug therapy in patients with chronic congestive heart failure? The insight of the six blind men. J Am Coll Cardiol 1987;9:433–438.
6. Franciosa J, Jordan R, Wilen M. Minoxidil in patients with chronic left heart failure: contrasting hemodynamic and clinical effects in a controlled trial. Circulation 1984;70:63–68.
7. Danis M, Gerrity MS, Southerland LI, Patrick DL, et al. A comparison of patient, family, and physician assessment of the value of medical intensive care. Crit Care Med 1988;16:594–600.
8. Schipper H, Clinch J, Powell, V. Definitions and conceptual issues. In: Spilker B, ed. Quality of Life Assessments in Clinical Trials. Raven Press, New York, 1990, pp. 11–24.
9. Gill T, Feinstein A. A critical appraisal of the quality of quality-of-life measurements. JAMA 1994; 272:619–626.
10. Guyatt G, Cook D. Health status, quality of life, and the individual patient. A commentary on: Gill TM, Feinstein AR. A critical appraisal of quality of life measurements. JAMA 1994;272:630–631.
11. Ware J, Sherbourne CD. The MOS 36-item short-form health survey (SF-36). Med Care 1992;30: 473–483.
12. Kind P. The EuroQol instrument: an index of health related quality of life. In: Spilker B, ed. Quality of Life and Pharmacoeconomics in Clinical Trials, 2nd ed. Lippincott—Raven Publishers, Philadelphia, PA, 1996, pp. 191–201.
13. Hunt SM, McKenna SP, McEwen J, Backett EM, Williams J, Papp E. A quantitative approach to perceived health status: a validation study. J Epidemiol Community Health1980;34:281–286.
14. Parkerson GR Jr, Gehlbach SH, Wagner EH, James SA, Clapp NE, Muhlbaier LH. The Duke-UNC Health Profile: an adult health status instrument for primary care. Med Care 1981;19:806–828.
15. Sackett DL, Chambers LW, MacPherson AS, Goldsmith CH, Mcauley RG. The development and application of indices of health: general methods and a summary of results. Am J Public Health 1977; 67:423–428.
16. Dolan P, Gudex C, Kind P, Williams A. A social tariff for EuroQol: results from a UK general population survey. Discussion paper 138. York: Centre for Health Economics, The University of York, 1995.
17. Wiebe S, Guyatt G, Weaver B, Matijevic S, Sidwell C. Comparative responsiveness of generic and specific quality-of-life instruments. J Clin Epidemiol 2003;56:52–60.

18. Guyatt GH, King DR, Feeny DH, Stubbing D, Goldstein RS. Generic and specific measurement of health-related quality of life in a clinical trial of respiratory rehabilitation. J Clin Epedemiol 1999;52:187–192.

19. Bott U, Muhlhauser I, Overmann H, Berger M. Validation of a diabetes-specific quality-of-life scale for patients with type 1 diabetes. Diabetes Care 1998;21:757–769.

20. Meadows K, Steen N, McColl E, et al. The Diabetes Health Profile (DHP): a new instrument for assessing the psychosocial profile of insulin requiring patientsdevelopment and psychometric evaluation. Qual Life Res 1996;5:242–254.

21. Ingersoll GM, Marrero DG. A modified quality-of-life measure for youths: psychometric properties. Diabetes Educator 1991;17:114–118.

22. Herschbach P, Duran G, Waadt S, Zettler A, Amm C, Marten-Mittag B. Psychometric properties of the questionnaire on stress in patients with diabetes-revised (QSD-R). Health Psychol 1997;16:171–174.

23. Vileikyte L, Peyrot M, Bundy C, et al. The development and validation of a neuropathy- and foot ulcer-specific quality of life instrument. Diabetes Care 2003;26:2549–2555.

24. Royle P, Waugh N, McAuley L, McIntyre L, Thomas S. Inhaled insulin in diabetes mellitus. Cochrane Database Syst Rev 2004;3:3.

25. Norris SL, Engelgau MM, Narayan KM. Effectiveness of self-management training in type 2 diabetes: a systematic review of randomized controlled trials. Diabetes Care 2001;24:561–587.

26. Fitzgerald JT, Davis WK, Connell CM, Hess GE, Funnell MM, Hiss RG. Development and validation of the diabetes care profile. Eval Health Prof 1996;19:208–230.

27. Shen W, Kotsanos JG, Huster WJ, et al. Development and validation of the Diabetes Quality of Life Clinical Trial Questionnaire. Med Care 1999;37:AS45–AS66.

28. Guyatt G, Bombardier C, Tugwell P. Measuring disease-specific quality-of-life in clinical trials. CMAJ 1986;134:889–895.

29. Bech P, Moses R, Gomis R. The effect of prandial glucose regulation with repaglinide on treatment satisfaction, wellbeing and health status in patients with pharmacotherapy naive Type 2 diabetes: a placebo-controlled, multicentre study. Qual Life Res 2003;12:413–425.

30. Abetz L, Sutton M, Brady L, McNulty P, Gagnon DD. The Diabetic Foot Ulcer Scale (DFS): a quality of life instrument for use in clinical trials. Pract Diabet Int 2002;19:167–175.

31. Bradley C, Todd C, Gorton T, Symonds E, Martin A, Plowright R. The development of an individualized questionnaire measure of perceived impact of diabetes on quality of life: the ADDQoL. Qual Life Res 1999;8:79–91.

32. Guyatt G, Walter S, Norman G. Measuring change over time: assessing the usefulness of evaluative instruments. J Chronic Dis 1987;40:171–178.

33. Jacobson AM, de Groot M, Samson JA. The evaluation of two measures of quality-of-life in patients with type I and type II diabetes. Diabetes Care 1994;17:267–274.

34. Torrance G. Measurement of health state utilities for economic appraisal: a review. J Health Econ 1986;5:1–30.

35. Schünemann HJ, Juniper E, Guyatt G. Measurement of health status. In Armitage P, Colton T, eds: Encyclopedia of Biostatistics. John Wiley and Sons, Chichester, 2005, pp 2393–2399.

36. Mehrez A, Gafni A. Quality-adjusted life years, utility theory, and healthy-years equivalents. Med Decis Making 1989;13:142–149.

37. Sutherland H, Dunn V, Boyd N. Measurement of values for states of health with linear analog scales. Med Decis Making 1983;3:477–487.

38. Ragnarson Tennvall G, Apelqvist J. Health-related quality of life in patients with diabetes mellitus and foot ulcers. J Diabetes Complications 2000;14:235–241.

39. Fitzpatrick R, Davey C, Buxton MJ, Jones DR. Evaluating patient-based outcome measures for use in clinical trials. Health Technol Asses 1998;2:1–74.

40. Schünemann H, Puhan M, Goldstein R, Jaeschke R, Guyatt GH. Measurement properties and interpretability of the Chronic Respiratory Disease Questionnaire (CRQ). J COPD 2005;2:81–89.

41. Guyatt GH, Juniper EF, Walter SD, Griffith LE, Goldstein RS. Interpreting treatment effects in randomised trials. BMJ 1998;316:690–693.

42. Ware JE, Snow KK, Kosinski M, Gandek B. SF-36 Health Survey: Manual and Interpretation Guide. The Health Institute, New England Medical Center, Boston, MA, 1993.

43. Ohsawa I, Ishida T, Oshida Y, Yamanouchi K, Sato Y. Subjective health values of individuals with diabetes in Japan: comparison of utility values with the SF-36 scores. Diabetes Res Clin Pract 2003;62:9–16.

44. Anderson RM, Fitzgerald JT, Wisdom K, Davis WK, Hiss RG. A comparison of global versus disease-specific quality-of-life measures in patients with NIDDM. Diabetes Care 1997;20:299–305.
45. Koopmanschap M, Board CA. Coping with type II diabetes: the patient's perspective. Diabetologia 2002;45:S18–S22.
46. UK Prospective Diabetes Study Group. Quality of life in type 2 diabetic patients is affected by complications but not by intensive policies to improve blood glucose or blood pressure control (UKPDS 37). Diabetes Care 1999;22:1125–1136.
47. Clarke P, Gray A, Holman, R.Estimating utility values for health states of type 2 diabetic patients using the EQ-5D (UKPDS 62). Med Decis Making 2002;22:340–349.
48. Jenkinson C, Gray A, Doll H, Lawrence K, Keoghane S, Layte R. Evaluation of index and profile measures of health status in a randomized controlled trial: comparison of the Medical Outcomes Study 36-Item Short Form Health Survey, EuroQol, and disease specific measures. Med Care 1997;35:1109–1118.
49. Pibernik-Okanovic M. World Health Organisation quality of life questionnaire (WHOQOL-100) in diabetic patients in Croatia. Diabetes Res Clin Pract 2001;51:133–143.
50. Garratt AM, Schmidt L, Fitzpatrick R. Patient-assessed health outcome measures for diabetes: a structured review. Diabet Med 2002;19:1–11.
51. Hammond GS, Aoki TT. Measurement of health status in diabetic patients: diabetes impact measurement scales. Diabetes Care 1992;15:469–477.
52. The DCCT Research Group. Reliability and validity of a diabetes quality-of-life measure for the Diabetes Control and Complications Trial (DCCT). Diabetes Care 1988;11:725–732.
53. Mannucci E, Ricca V, Bardini G, Rotella CM. Well-being enquiry for diabetics: a new measure of diabetes-related quality of life. Diabetes Nutr Metab 1996;9:89–102.
54. Boyer JG, Earp JA. The development of an instrument for assessing the quality of life of people with diabetes. Diabetes-39. Med Care 1997;35:440–453.
55. Carey MP, Jorgensen RS, Weinstock RS, et al. Reliability and validity of the appraisal of diabetes scale. J Behav Med 1991;14: 43–51.
56. Nathan DM, Fogel H, Norman D, et al. Long-term metabolic and quality-of-life results with pancreatic/renal transplantation transplantation in insulin-dependent diabetes mellitus. Transplantation 1991;55:85–91.
57. Selam JL, Micossi P, Dunn FL, Nathan DM. Clinical trial of programmable implantable insulin pump for type I diabetes. Diabetes Care 1992;15:877–885.
58. Sharma S, Brown GC, Brown MM, Hollands H, Robins R, Shah GK. Validity of the time trade-off and standard gamble methods of utility assessment in retinal patients. Br J Ophthalmol 2002;86: 493–496.
59. Brown MM, Brown GC, Sharma S, Shah G. Utility values and diabetic retinopathy. Am J Opthamol 1999;128:324–330.
60. Rubin RR, Peyrot M. Quality of life and diabetes. Diabetes/Metabol Res Rev 1999;15:205–218.
61. Aalto AM, Uutela A,Aro AR. Health related quality of life among insulin-dependent diabetics: disease-related and psychosocial correlates. Patient Educ Counsel 1997;30:215–225.
62. Glasgow RE, Ruggiero L, Eakin EG, Dryfoos J, Chobanian L. Quality of life and associated characteristics in a large national sample of adults with diabetes. Diabetes Care 1997;20:562–567.
63. Klein B, Klein R, Moss SE. Self-rated health and diabetes of long duration. The Wisconsin Epidemiologic Study of Diabetic Retinopathy. Diabetes Care 1998;21:236–240.
64. Parkerson GR Jr, Connis RT, Broadhead WE, Patrick DL, Taylor TR, Tse CK. Disease-specific versus generic measurement of health-related quality of life in insulin-dependent diabetic patients. Med Care 1993;31:629–639.
65. Wredling R, Stalhammar J, Adamson U, Berne C, Larsson Y, Ostman J. Well-being and treatment satisfaction in adults with diabetes: a Swedish population-based study. Qual Life Res 1995;4:515–522.
66. Peyrot M, Rubin RR. Levels and risks of depression and anxiety symptomatology among diabetic adults. Diabetes Care 1997;20:585–590.
67. Petterson T, Lee P, Hollis S, Young B, Newton P, Dornan T. Well-being and treatment satisfaction in older people with diabetes. Diabetes Care 1998;21:930–935.
68. Keinanen-Kiukaanniemi S, Ohinmaa A, Pajunpaa H, Koivukangas P. Health related quality of life in diabetic patients measured by the Nottingham Health Profile. Diabet Med 1996;13:382–388.
69. Mayou R, Bryant B, Turner R. Quality of life in non-insulin dependent diabetes and a comparison with insulin-dependent diabetes. J Psychosom Res 1990;34:1–11.
70. Weinberger M, Kirkman MS, Samsa GP, et al. The relationship between glycemic control and health-related quality of life in patients with non-insulin-dependent diabetes mellitus. Med Care 1994;32: 1173–1181.

71. Bagne CA, Luscombe FA, Damiano A. Relationships between glycemic control, diabetes-related symptoms and SF-36 scales scores in patients with non-insulin dependent diabetes mellitus. Qual Life Res 1995;4:392–393.

72. Naess S, Eriksen J, Midthjell K, Tambs K. Diabetes mellitus and psychological well-being. Results of the Nord-Trondelag health survey. J Diabetes Complications 1995;23:179–188.

73. Trief PM, Grant W, Elbert K, Weinstock RS. Family environment, glycemic control and the psychosocial adaptation of adults with diabetes. Diabetes Care 1998;21:241–245.

74. Peyrot M, Rubin RR. A new quality of life instrument for patients and families. Paper presented at the Psychosocial Aspects of Diabetes Study Group Third Scientific Meeting. Madrid, 1998.

75. Diabetes Control and Complications Trial (DCCT) Research Group. Influence of Intensive Diabetes Treatment on Quality-of-Life Outcomes in the Diabetes Control and Complications Trial. Diabetes Care 1996;19:195–203.

76. Kaplan RM, Hartwell SL, Wilson DK, Wallace JP. Effects of diet and exercise interventions on control and quality of life in non-insulin-dependent diabetes mellitus. J Gen Intern Med 1987;2:220–227.

77. de Weerdt I, Visser AP, Kok GJ, de Weerdt O, van der Veen EA. Randomized controlled multicentre evaluation of an education programme for insulin-treated diabetic patients: effects on metabolic control, quality of life, and costs of therapy. Diabetic Med 1991;8:338–345.

78. Glasgow R, Toobert D, Hampson S. Effects of a brief office-based intervention to facilitate diabetes dietary self-management. Diabetes Care 1996;19:835–842.

79. Chantelau E, Schiffers T, Schutze J, Hansen B. Effect of patient-selected intensive insulin therapy on quality of life. Patient Educ Couns 1997;30:167–173.

80. Beck-Nielsen H, Richelsen B, Schwartz Sorensen N, Hother Nielsen O. Insulin pump treatment: effect on glucose homeostasis, metabolites, hormones, insulin antibodies and quality of life. Diabetes Res 1985;2:37–43.

81. Boland EA, Grey M, Oesterle A, Fredrickson L, Tamborlane WV. Continuous subcutaneous insulin infusion. A new way to lower risk of severe hypoglycemia, improve metabolic control, and enhance coping in adolescents with type 1 diabetes. Diabetes Care 1999;22:1779–1784.

82. Tsui E, Barnie A, Ross S, Parkes R, Zinman B. Intensive insulin therapy with insulin Lispro: a randomized trial of continuous subcutaneous insulin infusion versus multiple daily insulin injection. Diabetes Care 2001;24:1722–1727.

83. Connis RT, Taylor TR, Gordon MJ, et al. Changes in cognitive and social functioning of diabetic patients following initiation of insulin infusion therapy. Exp Aging Res 1989;15:51–60.

84. Weintrob N, Benzaquen H, Galatzer A, et al. Comparison of continuous subcutaneous insulin infusion and multiple daily injection regimens in children with Type 1 diabetes: a randomized open crossover trial. Pediatrics 2003;112:559–564.

85. Bradley C. Diabetes Treatment Satisfaction Questionnaire. In: Bradley C, ed. Handbook of Psychology and Diabetes: A Guide to Psychological Measurement in Diabetes Research and Practice. Harwood Academic, London, 1994, pp. 111–152.

86. Edelman D, Olsen MK, Dudley TK, Harris AC, Oddone EZ. Impact of diabetes screening on quality of life. Diabetes Care 2002;25:1022–1026.

87. Siminerio LM, Charron-Prochownik D, Banion C, Schreiner B. Comparing outpatient and inpatient diabetes education for newly diagnosed pediatric patients. Diabetes Educ 1999;25:895–906.

88. Bianchi GP, Zaccheroni V, Solaroli E, et al. Health-related quality of life in patients with thyroid disorders. Qual Life Res 2004;13:45–54.

89. Terwee CB, Gerding MN, Dekker FW, Prummel MF, Wiersinga WM. Development of a disease specific quality of life questionnaire for patients with Graves' ophthalmopathy: the GO-QOL. Br J Opthamol 1998;82:773–779.

90. Park JJ, Sullivan TJ, Mortimer RH, Wagenaar M, Perry-Keene DA. Assessing quality of life in Australian patients with Graves' ophthalmopathy. Br J Opthamol 2004;88:75–78.

91. McKenna SP, Doward LC, Alonso J, et al. The QoL-AGHDA: an instrument for the assessment of quality of life in adults with growth hormone deficiency. Qual Life Res 1999;8:373–383.

92. Mesa J, Gomez JM, Hernandez C, Pico A, Ulied A; Grupo Colaborador Espanol. Growth hormone deficiency in adults: effects of replacement therapy on body composition and health-related quality of life. Med Clin (Barc) 2003;120:41–46.

93. Guyatt GH, Naylor CD, Juniper E, Heyland D, Jaeschke R, Cook D. Therapy and understanding the results. Quality of Life. In: Guyatt GH, Rennie D, eds. Users' Guides to the Medical Literature: A

Manual for Evidence-Based Clinical Practice. JAMA and Archives Journals, Chicago, IL, 2002, pp 309–327.

94. Meadows KA, Abrams S, Sandbaek, A. Adaptation of the Diabetes Health Profile (DHP-1) for use with patients with Type 2 diabetes mellitus: psychometric evaluation and cross-cultural comparison. Diabetic Med 2000;17:572–580.

95. Goddijn P, Bilo H, Meadows K, Groenier K, Feskens E, Meyboom-de Jong B. The validity of the Diabetes Health Profile in NIDDM patients referred for insulin therapy. Qual Life Res 1996;5:433–442.

96. Jacobson A. The diabetes quality-of-life measure. In: Bradley C, ed. Handbook of Psychology and Diabetes: A Guide to Psychological Measurement in Diabetes Research and Practice. Harwood Academic. London, 1994, pp. 65–87.

97. Mata Cases M, Roset Gamisans M, Badia Llach X, Antonanzas Villar F, Ragel Alcazar J. Effect of type-2 diabetes mellitus on the quality of life of patients treated at primary care consultations in Spain. Aten Primaria 2003;31:493–499.

98. Redekop WK, Koopmanschap MA, Stolk RP, Rutten GE, Wolffenbuttel BH, Niessen LW. Health-related quality of life and treatment satisfaction in Dutch patients with type 2 diabetes. Diabetes Care 2002;25:458–463.

99. Szabo S, On behalf of the WHOQOL Group S. The World Health quality of life WHOQOL assessment. In: Spilker D, ed. Quality of Life and Pharmacoeconomics in Clinical Trials. Raven Press, Philadelphia, PA, 1996, pp. 355–362.

14 Decision Analysis in Endocrinology

Evelyn Mentari, MD
and David Aron, MD, MS

CONTENTS

INTRODUCTION

Decision making under conditions of uncertainty characterizes medical practice. Clinicians are constantly faced with decisions that have implications on potential benefits, risks, gains, and losses not only for the patients, but also for several different stakeholders. These stakeholders include patients, providers, hospitals, payors, and society. The challenge of clinical medicine is to account for many different possibilities under conditions of considerable uncertainty. Medical literature often provides focused evidence regarding particular clinical problems, but this constitutes only a portion of the information required to fully evaluate a decision *(1–3)*. Decision analysis is a mathematical tool designed to facilitate complex clinical decisions in which many variables must be considered simultaneously. This analytical procedure selects among available diagnostic or therapeutic options based on the probability and predetermined value (utility) of all possible outcomes of those options. Decision analysis provides a systematic framework for organizing all data relevant to the decision, clearly defines the relationship between possible courses of action and their associated outcomes, and assigns a numerical value to various courses of action, simplifying comparisons between them. The role of decision analysis is to provide a systematic, nonbiased data review, which results in a suggested management strategy *(4)*. Decision analysis provides an organized method in which all possible outcomes are considered, so that relevant uncertainties are less likely to be overlooked *(5)*. By making the assumptions explicit decision analysis clarifies the management strategies. Not every decision is worth all the effort of a formal decision analysis. Decisions vary in the degree of complexity, time dependence, and uncertainty. Decision analysis is most helpful for important, unique, complex, nonurgent, and high-stakes decisions that

From: *Contemporary Endocrinology: Evidence-Based Endocrinology*
Edited by: V. M. Montori © Mayo Foundation for Medical Education and Research

Table 1
The Six General Steps in Decision Analysis

1. Construct a decision tree.
2. Determine and assign probabilities.
3. Assign utilities to each potential outcome.
4. Determine the expected utility.
5. Choose the course of action with the highest expected utility.
6. Evaluate the resistance of the chosen course of action to changes in probabilities and utilities.

involve uncertainty. This chapter provides a primer on the principles of decision analysis. In addition, a recent cost-effectiveness analysis of the diagnosis and treatment of adrenal incidentaloma is discussed in detail to illustrate the application of decision analysis.

PRINCIPLES OF DECISION ANALYSIS

Most biological events occur randomly and cannot be precisely predicted (6). There is substantial variation in duration and severity of disease between individuals. Choosing a treatment option in the setting of unpredictable effects is a difficult problem, and *expected value decision making* is a useful tool. When individual outcomes are uncertain, *expected value* is the result that is expected on the average. In preparing to perform a decision, one first must define the problem with a clear statement of the strategies to be examined. Two or more strategies may be included. There are many types of problems that may be analyzed. For example, established vs novel, conservative vs aggressive, or medical vs surgical strategies may be compared. In addition, decision analysis can look at patient care on a variety of levels. Analyses can be made for a specific, individual patient (7). Strategies for classes of patients with specific characteristics and situations can be formed. Estimates of clinical and economic outcomes can be used in health policy development. Clinical decisions have effects over different time frames. An important step in defining a decision problem is to decide the time horizon for outcomes to be evaluated. For example, if strategies for diabetes treatment are to be compared, a period of weeks to months may be appropriate for evaluating the risk of hypoglycemic episode. However, this relatively short time horizon would not be appropriate when the study outcome is diabetic retinopathy. In this case, a time horizon of years would be a better choice. The same time horizon must be applied to all strategies and outcomes in a single model. After choosing a problem and a time horizon, one can proceed to carry out a formal analysis following six general steps (Table 1). In the interests of full disclosure, it is worth pointing out that important insights can be gained from the careful construction of the decision tree itself, even in the absence of actual mathematical computation to "solve" the problem. This phenomenon has been referred to as "decision therapy."

The Decision Tree

In a decision tree, the term *decision alternative* refers to one of the potential strategies to be analyzed. Each alternative should be listed. Figure 1 shows a sample decision

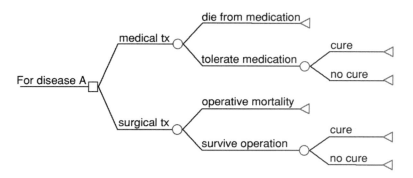

Fig. 1. Decision tree for medical vs surgical treatment.

tree that outlines strategies of medical vs surgical treatment for disease The decision itself is represented by a box called a *decision node*. All of the possible outcomes for each decision alternative are listed. An event that has outcomes under the control of chance is denoted by a *chance node*. The symbol for a chance node is a circle. The series of events leading to the clinical outcomes is represented by a series of chance nodes and decision nodes. The decision tree is usually written from left to right, with the initial decision node on the far left and the final outcomes on the far right. A final outcome is represented by a *terminal node*. There may be any number of outcomes at a chance node. The listed outcomes need to include all possible outcomes and must not overlap in definition. In addition to this assumption of mutual exclusivity, structuring a tree in this fashion assumes that the probability of occurrence of one event does not influence the probability of occurrence of other event(s). The decision tree structure should be as similar as possible for all strategies, because differences may lead to a structural bias in the analysis.

The Markov Model

A static decision tree is sometimes limited in its ability to represent complex and dynamic clinical situations. More elaborate models may be necessary to represent factors such as the passage through multiple health states, the results of prolonged treatment and monitoring, and costs and savings from initially aggressive strategies. One useful model is the Markov model *(8,9)*. In Fig. 2, a Markov model is used for decision analysis of screening for mild thyroid failure. Each oval represents a health state. The arrows represent the possibility of transition from one health state to another. From published literature the *transition probability*, or probability that a patient will move from one health state to another in a specified time period, may be obtained. The specified time period is termed a *cycle of the model*. Like each terminal node in a static decision tree, each health state in the Markov model is associated with a specific clinical measure, utility, or cost. The model more easily represents recurring events because it includes the possibility of cycling through health states. However, it is important to be aware of an assumption fundamental to the model. The *Markovian* assumption is that the future is determined only by the individual's present health state—events prior to that health state or how long it took to arrive there do not affect the individual's future, an assumption that may not hold true for some health problems.

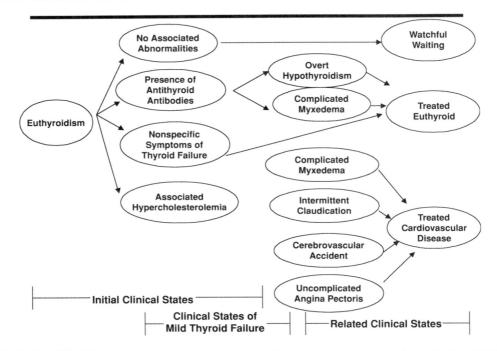

Fig. 2. Simplified Markov model to evaluate the cost-effectiveness of screening for mild thyroid failure (MTF). Screened individuals with MTF are treated with levothyroxine sodium, do not progress
to overt hypothyroidism, have a reduced risk of cardiovascular disease (CVD) from lowered cholesterol, and have symptoms relieved. Nonscreened individuals lower CVD risk through more expensive
lipid-lowering therapy but do experience progression and symptoms. Combinations of hypercholes-
terolemia, antithyroid antibody, and symptom states are possible, but not shown, are used for decision
analysis of screening for mild thyroid failure. (Reprinted with permission from: Danese MD, Powe
NR, Sawin CT, Landenson PW. Screening for mild thyroid failure at the periodic health examination:
a decision and cost-effectiveness analysis. JAMA 1996;276:285–292. Copyrighted © 1996, American
Medical Association. All rights reserved.)

Selecting Outcome Measures

One strength of the decision analysis process is that it may be used for a variety of
outcome measures. The outcome measure of interest determines the information needed
for analysis. For example, one may use *clinical measures* such as survival after bone
marrow transplant, preservation of vision after ophthalmic surgery, or meeting a target
level for serum cholesterol. *Economic measures* provide measures of cost and resource
use. When cost measures are included, it is important to consider whose perspective is
represented. Depending on the goals of the decision maker, analyses may reflect the
viewpoint of society, insurers, hospitals, or patients *(10)*. A detailed analysis of costs
may be used for *cost-effectiveness analysis* or *cost-utility analysis*, both of which will be
discussed further later in this chapter. *Utility* measures reflect quality of life preferences
(11,12). They are quantitative values used to summarize multiple dimensions, which
may be conflicting. For example, decision makers frequently choose between strategies
that have differing effects on length of life and quality of life. Utilities are traditionally
scored on a scale from 0 to 1. The ideal situation, often perfect health, is scored as a 1.
The worst situation, death, is scored as a 0, and this assumes that there are no utilities

worse than death. Intermediate states are assigned values between 0 and 1. For example, living with diabetes mellitus may receive a score of 0.80—less than perfect, but preferable to death. There are a number of important assumptions underlying this approach *(13)*. For example, estimates of utilities are assumed to be stable (i.e., the estimates obtained prior to experiencing an event will not change after the event has been experienced). The "it-does-not-matter-how-you-get-there assumption" also applies (i.e., death or other outcomes have the same utility regardless of the route a patient takes in getting there). In addition, utility units are assumed to be equal so that a unit difference is valued the same regardless of where it is on the scale, even including a unit that means the difference between being alive and being dead.

There are different ways to obtain utility values for different health states. One relatively simple method is the visual analog scale in which a subject is asked to rate a given health state on a scale from 0 to 100. There also are more specific ways of determining utility. The *standard gamble* approach was developed by von Neumann and Morganstern as a method for assessing utility. One advantage of this method is that it incorporates the participant's attitudes about risk taking, because the process involves consideration of a hypothetical gamble. As an example, we will consider Mr. P., a 74-yr-old diabetic with known coronary artery disease and a chronically infected lower extremity ulcer. His physicians have discussed treatment with antibiotics vs a below the knee amputation (BKA). Assume that antibiotics have a 10% cure rate, whereas BKA has a 95% cure rate. In order to assess utility from the patient's perspective, we (1) list all of the possible outcomes, (2) rank the outcome states in the order of preference, (3) assign a utility of 1 to the most preferred outcome and 0 to the least preferred outcome, and (4) formulate situations where a patient is indifferent about choosing between a gamble (between outcomes of known utility) and a sure thing (involving an outcome with unknown utility). This is how we determine the utility of each intermediate outcome. For example, Mr. P. decides that a cure with antibiotics is an appealing outcome. We compare this outcome to those with known utilities—perfect health and death. When asked to choose between a cure with antibiotics and a gamble in which he has a 90% chance of achieving perfect health and a 10% chance of dying, he is unable to choose (indifferent). Thus, the utility for the outcome of cure with antibiotics is 0.9. However, a surgical cure with BKA is a less appealing scenario. A utility score of 0.9 does not apply to this scenario because Mr. P. prefers gambling for a 90% chance at perfect health instead of receiving a BKA. For him to reach a point of indifference, the chance of receiving perfect health is reduced to 75%. The utility for BKA is 0.75. After going through this process, the estimated utilities of the intermediate outcomes are shown in Table 2. The utility score can then be incorporated into a decision tree (*see* Fig. 3).

The expected utility for each decision alternative may be obtained by adding each (utility × probability) value. The utility for each outcome is on the right. The probabilities are below the outcome branches.

The utility for antibiotic treatment = $(0.1 \times 0.9) + (0.9 \times 0.5) = 0.54$

The utility for below the knee amputation = $(0.95 \times 0.75) + (0.05 \times 0) = 0.71$

In terms of Mr. P.'s quality of life, the expected value of amputation is greater than the expected value of antibiotic treatment. Different utilities for these health states would alter the analyses.

Table 2
Estimated Utilities

Outcome	Initial utility	Estimated utility
Perfect health	1	1
Cure with antibiotics	?	0.9
Receive BKA and survive	?	0.75
Fail antibiotics. Need BKA later	?	0.5
Receive BKA. Operative death	0	0

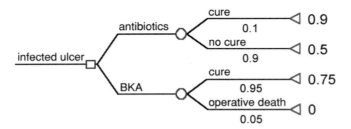

Fig. 3. Decision tree with probabilities and utilities.

The *time tradeoff method* is another way of determining utility. The utility may be described as a number between 0 and 1. For example, a subject may consider 10 yr with pain from chronic pancreatitis equivalent to 5 yr in perfect health. The utility of chronic pancreatitis is 0.5. Alternatively, the utility may be expressed in *quality-adjusted life-years (QALYs)*. To determine the number of QALYs associated with an outcome, the time horizon for the outcome state is specified. Often, this is a patient's life expectancy in a particular outcome state. The number of years in full health that the subject sees as equivalent to the specified time with that outcome is the corresponding number of QALYs.

Determine the Probability of Each Chance Event

Once the decision tree structure is formed, the probability of each chance event may be determined. In general this is best done with a systematic review of published, peer-reviewed literature *(14,15)*. However, this approach assumes that probabilities derived from a past period of time accurately reflect the probabilities in the future. Moreover, it assumes that the probabilities derived from other settings apply to your own. However, all these probabilities must reflect actual practice. For example, if using decision analysis to determine the best strategy for a specific individual then risk probabilities must be those of the site where the care is to be delivered. At times, not all of the information needed for the decision tree is available. This frequently occurs during analysis of a relatively new practice. If possible, primary data may be collected or secondary data may be analyzed. Expert opinion may be used in the absence of relevant data. At a given chance node, the sum of probabilities equals one.

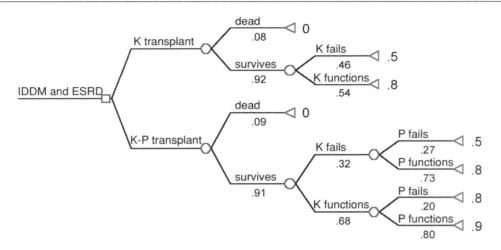

Fig. 4. Kidney transplant vs kidney–pancreas transplant as a treatment for end stage renal disease (ESRD) and insulin-dependent diabetes mellitus (IDDM). K, kidney; P, pancreas.

Deciding on a Strategy: Averaging Out and Folding Back the Tree

The goal of decision analysis is to identify the strategy that leads to the most favorable expected outcome. To calculate the expected outcome, one starts at the outcome measures (typically the far right). Each group of branches, which start at a single chance node, is reduced to a single numerical value by multiplying each outcome measure by the probability associated with that outcome and than adding all of the values. This is the process of *folding back* the decision tree. This process is repeated until there is a single numerical value for each strategy at the initial decision node. At this point, the expected outcome for each strategy has been calculated. The strategy with the more favorable outcome is the preferred strategy. Figure 4 compares kidney transplant with kidney–pancreas transplant as a treatment for end-stage renal disease (ESRD) and insulin-dependent diabetes mellitus (IDDM) in terms of utility based on quality of life.

The expected value for the kidney transplant strategy is:

$$0.92 \: [(0.46 \times 0.5) + (0.54 \times 0.8)] + (0.08 \times 0) = 0.46$$

The expected value for the kidney–pancreas transplant strategy is 0.75. This strategy has a higher utility based on quality of life and is the preferred strategy.

Discounting of Future Events

More value is placed on current events than future events. It is better to pay $100 in 10 yr rather than pay $100 now. Similarly, if one is to have a disease, it is preferable to have a disease in the future than to have it today. The value of a future event then depends on how far in the future it occurs. *Discounting* refers to calculating the present value of an outcome that occurs in the future. The *discount rate* is the annual rate at which costs are discounted, which is usually the rate of interest that money would bring if it were invested. The present value of a future expense is given by the formula:

$$P = \frac{S}{(1+r)^n}$$

where S = amount of future expense, P = present value of S, r = discount, and n = number of time periods until the expense is incurred rate (per time period).

For example: $100 is spent today on a screening test, and that test prevents an illness costing $1000 in 10 yr. If one accounts for a discount rate of 7%, the present value of a $1000 cost 10 yr from now is $508. The cost savings is $408.

Sensitivity Analysis

Sensitivity analysis is an important part of the decision analysis process that tests the stability or robustness of a conclusion over a range of structural assumptions, value judgments, and estimates of probability *(16,17)*. The initial analysis, or *base case analysis*, uses the best estimates for each part of the model. In sensitivity analysis a plausible range of values is determined for each portion of the model. Variables that have the most influence on the model are determined. Different time horizons or perspectives may be considered. The objective is to see whether conclusions change when possibilities within a reasonable range are included.

Cost-Effectiveness Analysis Using Decision Analysis

Cost-effectiveness analysis is the use of decision analysis to compare strategies in terms of their cost per unit of output *(18–20)*. Output is an outcome such as years of life, utility, or cases of disease prevented. Cost-effectiveness ratios are interpreted by comparing them to ratios for other strategies. An *incremental cost-effectiveness ratio* (IC-ER) indicates how much additional money needs to be spent for a better, but more expensive strategy to generate one additional unit of outcome. Of practical importance, there usually is a limit to the amount of money a policymaker is willing to spend to gain one QALY; this is termed the *willingness-to-pay threshold (21)*.

Cost-utility analysis is a specific type of cost-effectiveness analysis that uses QALYs (or other measures of utility) as the effectiveness endpoint. By convention, cost-utility analyses are often called cost-effectiveness analyses. However, not all cost-effectiveness studies use the cost-utility methodology. Because they use QALYs as an endpoint, cost-utility analyses generate information that may be compared across disease states *(22)*. An example is shown in Table 4. In addition to performing decision analysis oneself, published studies can be applied to ones own practice. Principles for assessing decision analysis have been developed by the EBM group are shown in Table 3 *(16,17)*. Representative decision analyses related to endocrine disorders are shown in Table 5.

AN APPLICATION OF DECISION ANALYSIS IN ENDOCRINOLOGY

Diagnosis and Treatment of Adrenal Incidentaloma

Clinically inapparent adrenal masses, commonly called adrenal incidentalomas, are those discovered inadvertently when patients receive abdominal diagnostic imaging for unrelated reasons. At autopsy, an adrenal mass is found in at least 3% of persons older than 50 yr of age *(23)*. Improvements in imaging techniques have increased detection of adrenal incidentalomas. A small proportion of incidentalomas are sources of clinically significant endocrine disorders, and approx 1 in 4000 adrenal tumors is malignant. Thus, the detection of an incidentaloma necessitates a management strategy. The challenge exists in developing strategies to optimize health outcomes at an acceptable cost *(24)*.

Table 3
Questions for Assessing Validity and Generalizability

Are the results valid?
- Were all important strategies and outcomes included?
- Was an explicit and sensible process used to identify, select, and combine the evidence into probabilities?
- Were the utilities obtained in an explicit and sensible way from credible sources?
- Was the potential impact of any uncertainty in the evidence determined?

What are the results?
- In the baseline analysis, does one strategy result in a clinically important gain for patients?
  If not, is the result a toss-up?
- How strong is the evidence used in the analysis?
- Could uncertainty in the evidence change the result?

Will the results help me in caring for my patients?
- Do the probability estimates fit my patients' clinical features?
- Do the utilities reflect how my patients would value the outcomes of the decision?

Adapted from Richardson and Detsky *(16,17)*.

Table 4
Comparison of Screening for Mild Thyroid Failure to Other Widely Accepted Medical Practices

Medical practices	*Cost per QALY* * *(1994 dollars)*
Women	
Breast cancer screening every 2 yr, age 50–70 yr	4836
Breast cancer screening every 2 yr, age 40–70 yr	6943
Mild thyroid failure screening every 5 yr, age 35–75yr	9223
Hypertension screening at age 40 yr	26,130
Men	
Exercise for preventing coronary heart disease at age 35 yr	13,508
Hypertension screening at age 40 yr	18,323
Mild thyroid failure screening every 5 yr, age 35–75 yr	22,595

From ref. *39*.
Note: *QALY indicates quality-adjusted life-year.

Quantitative Analysis and Decision Model

Kievit and Haak *(25)* performed a cost-effectiveness analysis of 70 different strategies for the diagnosis and treatment of adrenal incidentaloma that was updated in 2003. They performed a structured, quantitative literature review and collected information on patient symptoms, diameter of the adrenal incidentalomas, diagnostic tests used, and treatment outcomes.

Costs were calculated in US dollars and were determined using a societal perspective. Direct health care costs were recalculated to 1998 levels using a 3% discount rate.

Table 5
Representative Decision Analyses in Endocrinology

Study	Clinical problem and strategies	Time horizon	Outcome measures	Result
Diabetes				
DCCT (34)	Conventional vs intensive insulin therapy in approximately 120,000 persons with IDDM in the US who meet DCCT inclusion criteria	Lifetime	Years free from diabetic complications; Cost per life-year	Intensive insulin therapy results in a gain of 920,000 yr of sight, 691,000 yr free from ESRD, 678,000 yr free from lower extremity amputation, and 611,000 yr of life at a cost of $4 billion. Cost per life-year gained is $28,661.
CDC (35)	Screening for type 2 DM with routine medical contact at age 25 vs age 45	Lifetime	Cost per life-year; Cost per QALY	IC-ER for early screening was $236,449 per life-year gained and $56,649 per QALY gained. Early screening is more cost-effective in younger persons and African Americans.
Vijan (36)	Prevention of blindness and ESRD in patients with type 2 DM with lowering hemoglobin A1c by 2 percentage points to a lower limit of 7.	Lifetime	Risk of developing blindness and ESRD	Patients with early onset of type 2 diabetes benefit from near-normal glycemic control. Moderate control prevents most of the studied complications in patients with later onset of disease.
Hoerger (37)	Screening for type 2 DM in all people vs only screening those with hypertension	Lifetime	Cost per QALY	Screening in people with hypertension is more cost-effective. Targeted screening for people age 55–75 is most cost-effective.

Table 5 *(continued)*

Study	Clinical problem and strategies	Time horizon	Outcome measures	Result
Golan *(38)*	To preserve kidney function in patients with type 2 DM, strategies of treating all patients with ACE-inhibitors vs screening for microalbuminuria vs screening for gross proteinuria	Lifetime	Cost per QALY	Screening for gross proteinuria has the highest cost and lowest benefit. Compared with microalbuminuria, treating all patients with an ACE-inhibitor was beneficial with an IC-ER of $7500 per QALY gained.
Thyroid				
Danese *(39)*	In asymptomatic adults, screening for mild thyroid failure every 5 yr starting at age 35 vs no screening	Lifetime	Cost per QALY	Screening was cost-effective with a cost per QALY gained of $9223 for women and $22,595 for men
Vidal-Trecan *(40)*	Four strategies to treat solitary toxic thyroid adenoma in a 40-yr-old woman: (A) Primary radioactive iodine (B) Primary surgery after euthyroidism achieved by ATDs (C) ATDs followed by surgery or (D) ATDs followed by radioactive iodine. C and D were used if severe reaction to ATDs occurred.	Lifetime	Cost per QALY	Surgery was the most effective and least costly strategy. Primary radioactive iodine was more effective if surgical mortality exceeded 0.6%.
Nasuti *(41)*	Evaluation of FNA by a cytopathologist with on-site processing vs standard processing at the University of Pennsylvania M.C.	Short-term	Cost	By avoiding nondiagnostic specimens, an estimated cost savings of $404,525/yr may be achieved with on-site FNA review.

(continued)

Table 5 *(continued)*

Study	Clinical problem and strategies	Time horizon	Outcome measures	Result
Other				
King *(29)*	Four strategies to manage incidental pituitary microadenoma in an asymptomatic patient: 1. Expectant management 2. PRL screening 3. Screening for PRL, insulin-like growth factor 1, and 4. MRI follow-up	Lifetime	Cost per QALY	PRL test may be the most cost-effective strategy. Compared to expectant management, the IC-ER for PRL was $1,428. The IC-ER for the extended screening panel was $69,495. MRI follow-up was less effective and more expensive.
Sawka *(42)*	Three strategies to evaluate pheochromocytoma in patients with refractory hypertension, suspicious symptoms, adrenal mass, or history of pheochromocytoma: (A) Fractionated plasma metanephrines with imaging if abnormal (B) 24-h urinary metanephrines or catecholamines with imaging if abnormal (C) Plasma metanephrines. If modestly elevated, urine studies to decide on imaging	Short-term	Cost per pheochromocytoma detected	Strategy C is least costly and has reasonable sensitivity in patients with moderate pre-test probability for pheochromocytoma
Col *(43)*	For menopausal symptom relief in healthy, white, 50-yr-old women with intact uteri, use of hormone therapy vs no hormone therapy	2 yr	Survival; Quality-adjusted life expectancy (QALE)	Hormone therapy is associated with lower survival but gains in QALE. Benefits depend on severity of menopausal symptoms and CVD risk.

Table 5 *(continued)*

Study	Clinical problem and strategies	Time horizon	Outcome measures	Result
Smith *(44)*	For 60-yr-old men with erectile dysfunction, sildenafil vs no drug therapy	Lifetime	Cost per QALY gained	From the societal perspective, cost per QALY gained with sildenafil is less than $50,000 if treatment-related morbidity is less than 0.55% per year, treatment success rate is greater than 40.2%, or cost of sildenafil is less than $244/mo

Abbr: DCCT, Diabetes Control and Complications Trial; IDDM, insulin-dependent diabetes mellitus; ESRD, end-stage renal disease; DM, diabetes mellitus; QALY, quality-adjusted life-year; IC-ER, Incremental cost-effectiveness ratio; ACE, angiotensin-converting enzyme; CVD, cardiovascular disease; ATDs, anti-thyroid drugs; FNA, fine-needle aspiration; M.C., medical center; PRL, prolactin; MRI, magnetic resonance imaging; QALE, quality-adjusted life expectancy.

Costs outside health care were determined from the number of days off work multiplied by the US per capita per day gross national product. Each strategy was compared to a strategy of ignoring the incidentaloma. Each strategy was compared to the ignore strategy or the next best option to derive a "cost per QALY gain." The most efficient strategy was defined as the approach that provided the best outcome, given that its incremental cost-effectiveness ratio did not exceed a willingness-to-pay threshold of $40,000 QALY in comparison to the next best option.

In addition to the strategy used for comparison, ignoring the incidentaloma, they also analyzed strategies using one of eight single tests, various two-test sequences, and sequences suggested by Copeland *(26)* and Ross and Aron *(27)* (*see* Fig. 5). Primary outcomes were expressed in QALYs and others.

Study Results

When incidentalomas were ignored in the reference case, the discounted life expectancy decreased from 16.8 to 15.6 QALYs, a mean potential loss of –1.2 QALY or –7%. Most of the loss was caused by the potential presence of adrenocortical cancer (4.3% risk of losing 15.3 QALYs), metastasis from extra-adrenal cancer (2.4% risk of losing 15.5 QALYs), or pheochromocytoma (3.4% risk of losing 4.0 QALYs).

With respect to final outcomes, strategies differed strongly in costs (up to 10-fold) but only marginally in their health effects (up to 1.5%) as seen in Fig. 5. Lowest cost single strategies were adrenomedullary hormonal analysis and fine-needle aspiration cytology. Improvements in outcome, compared to ignoring the incidentaloma, occurred in all single strategies except surgery, CT scan, and NP59. The lowest cost per QALY improvement occurred with adrenomedullary hormonal analysis, which improved outcome with 0.07 QALY (equal to 25 quality-adjusted days [QADs]) at an incremental cost effectiveness ratio (IC-ER) of $22,400/QALY. This is compared to full hormonal

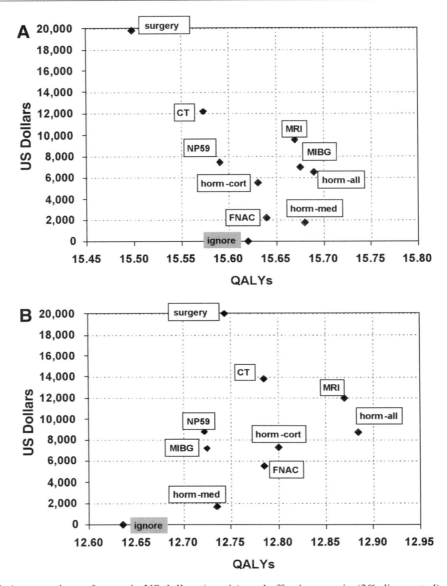

Fig. 5. A comparison of costs, in US dollars (y-axis), and effectiveness, in (3% discounted) quality-adjusted life-years (QALY; x-axis), of various single diagnostic strategies. (A,B) and two-step diagnostic strategies (C,D) for incidentaloma-based cases, with ignore as the least aggressive and surgery as the most aggressive strategy. Single strategies (A) and single strategies for large incidentalomas (6 cm) (B) demonstrate results in the reference case population. Results in two-step strategies (C) and two-step strategies for large incidentalomas (6 cm) (D). (C,D) Note strategies in the lower right quadrants offer better effectiveness at little additional cost; strategies in the upper left quadrants offer equal or lower effectiveness despite increasing costs. One-step strategies (A,B) QALYs = (3% discounted) quality-adjusted life-year. CT = computed tomography; FNAC = fine-needle aspiration cytology; horm-all = analysis of adrenal hormonal function, both cortical and medullary; horm-cor = analysis of adrenocortical hormonal function by 17-ketosteroids and overnight dexamethasone suppression test; horm-med = analysis of adrenomedullary hormonal function by urinary metanephrines; ignore = neither test nor treat, but ignore the incidentaloma; MIBG = metaiodobenzylguanidine [131] I-scan; MRI = magnetic resonance imaging; NP59 = iodomethyl-norcholesterol

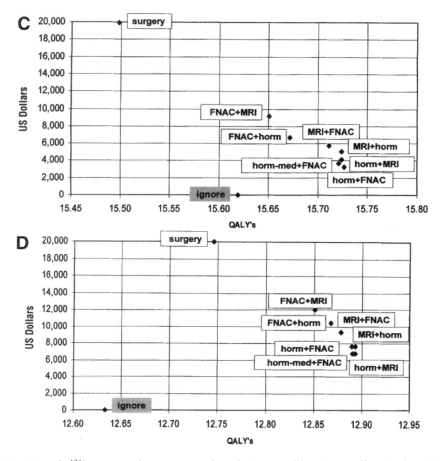

Fig. 5. *(continued)* ^{131}I-scan; and surgery = adrenalectomy without preceding testing. Two-step strategies **(C,D)** the second test follows a positive first test to increase specificity. horm = analysis of adrenal hormonal function, both cortical and medullary (i.e., has the same meaning as horm-all). All other abbreviations have the same meaning as explained for single strategies. (Reprinted from: Kievit J, Haak HR. Diagnosis and treatment of adrenal incidentaloma. A cost-effectiveness analysis. Endocrinol Metab Clin North Am, pp 78–79. Copyright 2000 with permission from Elsevier.

analysis, which resulted in slightly higher QALY (0.08 QALY), but its higher cost resulted in an excessive IC-ER of $1,366,100/QALY. Presence of the pheochromocytoma symptom triad did not change the preferred strategy. However, the presence of hypertension and hypokalemia, suggestive of Conn's disease, made full hormonal analysis the preferred strategy with an outcome improvement of 0.29 QALY at $27,700/QALY. Similarly when the incidentaloma diameter was ≥4 cm was full hormonal analysis the preferred strategy.

Discussion of Adrenal Incidentaloma Cost-Effectiveness Analysis Results

As shown by this study, the health risk of adrenal incidentalomas (in terms of potential QALY loss) mainly depends on characteristics of the patient and the incidentaloma. The choice of diagnostic-therapeutic strategy has far less impact because two of the three significant disorders (adrenocortical cancer and metastases) have a poor prognosis that is not drastically changed by treatment. There is no strategy that is clearly ideal. Strategies with low false-positive rates have higher false-negative rates. Studies with low false-negative rates cause more patients to receive unnecessary surgery.

Thus, the conclusions of this analysis have limitations. It is designed to evaluate strategies according to QALYs and cost. In clinical practice other factors that influence decisions include risk aversion, fear of liability, and varying tolerance for ambiguity *(28)*. Because of these motivators, physicians and patients are usually more aggressive in diagnosis and treatment than what is dictated by cost-effectiveness evaluations. In fact, in decision analysis of both adrenal and pituitary incidentalomas, the analysis is most sensitive to the degree of disutility (i.e., decrease in utility) associated with anxiety about harboring such a lesson *(29,30)*. However, given the growing rate at which incidentalomas, and for that matter incidental findings of all sorts, are being discovered, cost needs to be considered. For that reason, cost-effectiveness analysis is a valuable tool for both physicians and policymakers *(23,31–33)*.

REFERENCES

1. Hunink M, Glasziou P, Siegel J, Weeks J, Elstein A, Weinstein MC. Decision Making in Health and Medicine: Integrating Evidence and Values. Cambridge University Press, New York, NY, 2001.
2. Djulbegovic B, Hozo I, Lyman GH. Linking evidence-based medicine therapeutic summary measures to clinical decision analysis. MedGenMed 2000;2:E6.
3. Tunis SR, Stryer DB, Clancy CM. Practical clinical trials: increasing the value of clinical research for decision making in clinical and health policy. JAMA 2003;290:1624–1632.
4. Guyatt GH, Sinclair J, Cook DJ, Glasziou P. Users' guides to the medical literature: XVI. How to use a treatment recommendation. Evidence-Based Medicine Working Group and the Cochrane Applicability Methods Working Group. JAMA 1999;281:1836–1843.
5. Weinstein MC, Fineberg HV, Elstein AS, Frazier HS, Neuhauser D, Neutra RR. Clinical Decision Analysis. WB Saunders Co., Philadelphia, PA, 1980.
6. Sox HL, Blatt MA, Higgins MC, Marton KI. Medical Decision Making. Butterworths, Boston, MA, 1988.
7. Brand DA, Kliger AS. Planning for a didney transplant: is my doctor listening? JAMA 1999;282:691–694.
8. Beck JR, Pauker SG. The Markov process in medical prognosis. Med Decis Making 1983;3:411–458.
9. Sonnenberg FA, Beck JR. Markov models in medical decision making: a practical guide. Med Decis Making 1993;13:322–338.
10. Weinstein MC, Stason WB. Foundations of cost-effectiveness analysis for health and medical practices. N Engl J Med 1977;296:716–721.
11. Torrance GW. Utility approach to measuring health-related quality of life. J Chron Dis 1987;40:593.
12. Sackett DL, Torrance GW. The utility of different health states as perceived by the general public. J Chronic Dis 1978;31:697–704.
13. Riegelman RK. The Measures of Medicine. Benefits, Harms, and Costs. Oxford, UK, Blackwell Science, 1995.
14. Guyatt GH, Sinclair J, Cook DJ, Glasziou P. Users' guides to the medical literature: XVI. How to use a treatment recommendation. Evidence-Based Medicine Working Group and the Cochrane Applicability Methods Working Group. JAMA 1999;281:1836–1843.
15. Powe NR, Danese MD, Ladenson PW. Decision analysis in endocrinology and metabolism. Endocrinol Metab Clin North Am 1997;26:89–111.
16. Richardson WS, Detsky AS. Users' guides to the medical literature. VII. How to use a clinical decision analysis. A. Are the results of the study valid? Evidence-Based Medicine Working Group. JAMA 1995;273:1292–1295.
17. Richardson WS, Detsky AS. Users' guides to the medical literature. VII. How to use a clinical decision analysis. B. What are the results and will they help me in caring for my patients? Evidence Based Medicine Working Group. JAMA 1995;273:1610–1613.

18. MR, Siegel JE, Russell LB, Weinstein MC. Cost-effectiveness in Health and Medicine. Oxford, England, Oxford University Press, 1996.
19. Meltzer MI. Introduction to health economics for physicians. Lancet 2001;358:993–998.
20. Granata AV, Hillman AL. Competing practice guidelines: using cost-effectiveness analysis to make optimal decisions. Ann Intern Med 1998;128:56–63.
21. Shekelle PG, Woolf SH, Eccles M, Grimshaw J. Clinical guidelines: developing guidelines. BMJ 1999;318:593–596.
22. Johannesson M, O'Conor RM. Cost-utility analysis from a societal perspective. Health Policy 1997; 39:241–253.
23. Grumbach MM, Biller BM, Braunstein GD, et al. Management of the clinically inapparent adrenal mass ("incidentaloma"). Ann Intern Med 2003;138:424–429.
24. Siegel JE, Weinstein MC, Russell LB, Gold MR. Recommendations for reporting cost-effectiveness analyses. Panel on Cost-Effectiveness in Health and Medicine. JAMA 1996;276:1339–1341.
25. Kievit J, Haak HR. Diagnosis and treatment of adrenal incidentaloma. A cost-effectiveness analysis. Endocrinol Metab Clin North Am 2000;29:69–90.
26. Copeland PM. The incidentally discovered adrenal mass. Ann Intern Med 1983;98:940–945.
27. Ross NS, Aron DC. Hormonal evaluation of the patient with an incidentally discovered adrenal mass. N Engl J Med 1990;323:1401–1405.
28. Yates JF. Risk-taking Behaviour. Chichester, England, John Wiley and Sons, 1992.
29. King JT, Jr., Justice AC, Aron DC. Management of incidental pituitary microadenomas: a cost-effectiveness analysis. J Clin Endocrinol Metab 1997;82:3625–3632.
30. Aron DC, Kievit J. Adrenal Incidentalomas. In: Scwarz AE, Pertsemlidis D, Gagner M, eds. Endocrine Surgery. Marcel Dekker, New York, NY, 2004.
31. Detsky AS, Naglie IG. A clinician's guide to cost-effectiveness analysis. Ann Intern Med 1990;113: 147–154.
32. Drummond MF, Richardson WS, O'Brien BJ, Levine M, Heyland D. Users' guides to the medical literature. XIII. How to use an article on economic analysis of clinical practice. A. Are the results of the study valid? Evidence-Based Medicine Working Group. JAMA 1997;277:1552–1557.
33. O'Brien BJ, Heyland D, Richardson WS, Levine M, Drummond MF. Users' guides to the medical literature. XIII. How to use an article on economic analysis of clinical practice. B. What are the results and will they help me in caring for my patients? Evidence-Based Medicine Working Group. JAMA 1997;277:1802–1806.
34. Lifetime benefits and costs of intensive therapy as practiced in the diabetes control and complications trial. The Diabetes Control and Complications Trial Research Group. JAMA 1996;276:1409–1415.
35. The CDC Diabetes Cost-Effectiveness Study Group. The cost-effectiveness of screening for type 2 diabetes. JAMA 1998;280:1757–1763.
36. Vijan S, Hofer TP, Hayward RA. Estimated benefits of glycemic control in microvascular complications in type 2 diabetes. Ann Intern Med 1997;127:788–795.
37. Hoerger TJ, Harris R, Hicks KA, Donahue K, Sorensen S, Engelgau M. Screening for type 2 diabetes mellitus: a cost-effectiveness analysis. Ann Intern Med 2004;140:689–699.
38. Golan L, Birkmeyer JD, Welch HG. The cost-effectiveness of treating all patients with type 2 diabetes with angiotensin-converting enzyme inhibitors. Ann Intern Med 1999;131:660–667.
39. Danese MD, Powe NR, Sawin CT, Ladenson PW. Screening for mild thyroid failure at the periodic health examination: a decision and cost-effectiveness analysis. JAMA 1996;276:285–292.
40. Vidal-Trecan GM, Stahl JE, Durand-Zaleski I. Managing toxic thyroid adenoma: a cost-effectiveness analysis. Eur J Endocrinol 2002;146:283–294.
41. Nasuti JF, Gupta PK, Baloch ZW. Diagnostic value and cost-effectiveness of on-site evaluation of fine-needle aspiration specimens: review of 5,688 cases. Diagn Cytopathol 2002;27:1–4.
42. Sawka AM, Gafni A, Thabane L, Young WF, Jr. The economic implications of three biochemical screening algorithms for pheochromocytoma. J Clin Endocrinol Metab 2004;89:2859–2866.
43. Col NF, Weber G, Stiggelbout A, Chuo J, D'Agostino R, Corso P. Short-term menopausal hormone therapy for symptom relief: an updated decision model. Arch Intern Med 2004;164:1634–1640.
44. Smith KJ, Roberts MS. The Cost-Effectiveness of Sildenafil. Ann Intern Med 2000;132:933–937.

15 Clouded Thinking

The Misguided Use of Cost-Effectiveness Analysis and the Implications for Endocrine Interventions

Amiram Gafni, *PhD*

CONTENTS

INTRODUCTION

Rising health care costs are of concern to policymakers, employers, health care leaders, patients, and citizens all over the world. Health care decision makers struggle to satisfy the increasing demands for health care services associated with aging populations, increasing health care technologies, and changing population expectations using the resources available to the health care system. Notwithstanding, improvements in the level of health of the populations and increasing productivity of health care providers, there appears to be a continuous call for health care systems to do more and to do better. The economics discipline has been identified as providing relevant "toolbox" for dealing with these challenges and there is now over a quarter century of experience of applying an economics way of thinking as an input to health care decision processes. Until recently, this application occurred in an opportunistic, or at least nonsystematic way, within health care systems. In recent years there have been movements in both academic and policymaking environments to promote more systematic and standardized approaches to the use of economics as an input to decision making about the investment in health care programs.

From: *Contemporary Endocrinology: Evidence-Based Endocrinology*
Edited by: V. M. Montori © Mayo Foundation for Medical Education and Research

Endocrinology in general, and diabetes in particular, are large areas within health care that affect many individuals. Hence, decisions regarding how to use existing health care resources efficiently are of great importance. The purpose of this chapter is to review the methods used and assess their usefulness. In particular, it is argued that, although the proponents of the current methods have economic efficiency as their (often stated) goal, the proposed methods to pursue this goal are in several ways inconsistent with the economic principles on which the goal of economic efficiency is based. Current methods for economic evaluation can generate important information on production relationship (i.e., relationship between changes in the levels and types of services provided and changes in the health status of patients). But this is insufficient to determine whether changes in resources use or service provision under consideration are economically efficient. Although cost–benefit analysis (CBA) is the most commonly used method of economic evaluation in all other content areas (e.g., environment, transportation, safety, education), in health care, the most commonly used method of economic evaluation is cost-effectiveness analysis (CEA). Hence, this chapter will concentrate mainly on examining this method. Finally, the goal of this chapter is not to review the literature on economic evaluation in endocrinology but rather to provide the reader with an understanding of what the economic question is and how the proper use of economic tools can help decision makers use scarce health care resources efficiently. In other words, to enable the reader to better assess the value of such analyses. Whenever possible, examples from the literature on economic evaluation in endocrinology will be used to illustrate the different points made.

DOING THE BEST POSSIBLE: THE CONCEPT OF ECONOMIC EFFICIENCY

"Health economics as a discipline does not exist independently of economics as a discipline." (1)

The discipline of health economics is concerned primarily about maximizing some stated objective, such as the production of health-related well-being among a given population or patient group through the choice of which health care procedure to provide, and to whom, given the resources available. Economics in general is based on three fundamental but related concepts: *scarcity* (what ever resources are available they are insufficient to support all possible activities), *choices* (because resources are scarce, we must choose between different ways of using them), and *opportunity cost* (by choosing to use resources in one way, either in terms of which procedures to make available and/or which patients to treat, we forgo other opportunities to use the same resources). The goal of economics is than, in a way, analogous to the goal (or ethics) of medicine; to make choices in ways which do most good, that is ensuring that the *value* of what is gained from the use of resources exceeds the *value* of what is forgone by not using them in all other ways *(2)*.

Maximization of benefits from available resources, or the condition of economic efficiency, is a combination of both technical (i.e., objective) and value (i.e., subjective) considerations. The technical considerations concern using only those methods of production that minimize the quantity of resources used to produce a chosen level of service provision (i.e., avoiding the wasteful use of resources). Technical efficiency is a necessary, but not sufficient, condition for economic efficiency because any wasteful use of resources would necessarily increase the cost of inputs being used above what is needed to produce the chosen level of service. The value consideration, which under-lie economic efficiency, concerns the decision about what to produce from among all the possible mixes of services, each of which is to be produced in the most technically efficient way. In other words, because the advocated services compete for available health care resources with other possible services to the same, or other, clients of the health care system, choices have to be made about which service to provide and how much to provide, to whom, and in what quantities.

When the goal is to maximize benefits from available resources (i.e., economic effi-ciency) than choices concerning whether to provide a service and how much to provide (as distinct from the technical considerations of how to provide a service) are deter-mined by society's (or the decision maker's) values of the alternative mixes of the types and quantities of services that could be provided from the available resources. In par-ticular, to maximize benefits from available resources, a service should be provided (or extended) if, and only if, the value to society of providing (or extending) that service is greater that the value to society of the next best (i.e., highest valued) alternative use of the resources that are required to produce (or extend) the service. This is the condition of *allocative efficiency*.

Finally, it is often assumed that economic evaluation deals with the efficient deploy-ment of resources and equity being viewed at best as ". . . competing dimension upon which decisions are made in addition to that of efficient deployment of resources" *(3)*. The implication is that also equity considerations are important in the decision making process, they can be considered separately from considerations of efficiency. However, assuming that efficiency and equity are in some way separable is wrong *(4–7)*. Effi-ciency involves a maximization of an objective function that, by definition, already involves equity considerations, subject to a constraint. In other words, the evaluation of the alternative uses of health care resources is based upon the estimation and aggre-gation of individuals' *values* of the effects of those alternative uses, which necessarily involves attaching weights to the values of effects falling on different individuals or groups. Yet this is precisely what equity is concerned with—assumptions about the rel-ative values among individuals. Thus, equity considerations are "an intrinsic part of any evaluation; efficiency and equity are interdependent" *(7)*. Because equity consid-erations are all pervasive in economics, and the results of evaluations are in general dependent on the particular equity criteria adopted, it is important that the criteria used are recognized and their implications understood. For example, if the criteria used in the analysis do not reflect those of the decision maker (e.g., society and payers), the results of the analysis are of no use to this decision maker. Furthermore, equity criteria extend beyond identification of how programs effects are aggregated and compared; they also affect how those program effects are measured *(5)*.

FROM CONCEPT TO PRACTICE: COST-EFFECTIVENESS ANALYSIS

The literature on the methods of economic evaluation of health care interventions has focused primarily on the development and application of two techniques—CEA and cost-utility analysis (CUA). Both approaches involve the comparison of outcomes and costs between two (or more) alternative healthcare programs (e.g., different strategies to manage incidental pituitary microadenomas, different screening strategies for screening for mild thyroid failure, and different screening intervals for diabetic retinopathy). The difference between CEA and CUA lies in the way outcomes are measured. In CEA, measurement is in neutral units (e.g., life years saved, cases of retinopathy found, or improvement in functional status), and applications of CEA are therefore restricted to comparisons among programs that produce directly comparable outcomes measured in the same natural unit. Under CUA, measurement of outcomes encompasses both quantitative and qualitative aspects of changes in health status (i.e., effects on morbidity and mortality). Consequently, CUA enables comparison of programs producing different types of health outcomes (e.g., changes in survival and/or changes in functional status). Moreover, because CEA does not involve any assessment of the value of outcomes, it is unable to address those elements of economic efficiency condition that pertain to value, in particular the issue of allocative efficiency. Finally, many in the literature do not use different names for the two approaches (i.e., CEA and CUA). They call both CEA but describe the type of outcome used (i.e., natural units or a comprehensive measure of outcome like quality-adjusted life-years [QALYs]). The remainder of the paper uses CEA to describe both methods and I describe the type of outcome measured used when it is important.

CEA has, and is, presented in the research literature as a methodology to help decision makers allocate limited pool of resources. The underlying premise of CEA is that society or the decision maker wishes to maximize the total aggregate health benefit conferred for a given level of available resources (3,8–12). The economic question of how to maximize health improvements generated by a given level of resources has an obvious attraction for decision makers in health and, thus, it is not surprising to watch the growing number of papers reporting the results of such analyses. On the other hand, it has been argued that decision makers "should maintain a healthy skepticism about the results of cost-effectiveness analyses and the usefulness of those results in purchasing and planning decisions" (13). It has also been argued that "health funding is increasingly based on the results of economic evaluation. But current methods fail to consider all society's health objectives and are too complex for policymakers to use" (14).

The problem that economics tries to help us solve (i.e., maximization of health benefits from available health care resources) is a complex one because "reality is horrendously complicated" (15). But as Williams (15) recognizes that "the more complex the reality is, the more dangerous it is to rely on intuitive short-cuts rather than careful analysis." This paper addresses the question whether it is the flows in the economic methods themselves or the oversimplification and misapplication of these methods are responsible for the perceived (or real) lack of usefulness of this growing body of knowledge. Whereas not being able to cover all aspects of economic evaluation methodology because of a lack of space this chapter will demonstrate that economics provides valid methods for maximizing the health improvements that can be attained with a given allocation of resources. These methods can help decision makers to allocate health care resources efficiently under circumstances of fixed, shrinking, or increasing budgets. Although the data requirements for these methods might be substantial, the level and complexity of such analyses reflects the nature and complexity of the questions being addressed. The use of simple tools, as often is the case in many analyses, represents a departure from the economics discipline and typically fails to address the decision maker's problem. To illustrate the problem of oversimplification and misapplication of economic principles following areas will be discussed: how are health consequences being valued and how are the data used to make recommendations about economic efficiency.

HOW ARE HEALTH CONSEQUENCES BEING VALUED?

The most commonly used measure of the valuation of outcome in CEA is the QALYs, which combines morbidity (i.e., quality of life) and mortality aspects into one dimension. Also there is much agreement about the structure of the QALY measure (i.e., discounted duration weighted by a health-status score), there is no agreement about the methods used to measure the weights. Furthermore, as discussed below, the QALY has major limitations, which casts doubt on its usefulness as a measure of benefits for evaluations with maximization of benefits (or economic efficiency) as the goal. An alternative measure of outcome, the healthy years equivalent (HYE) that overcomes many of these limitations, will be briefly discussed.

When first introduced, QALYs were presented as a health-status index.

"The first approach to this problem falls under the rubric of health status indexes. A health-status index is essentially a weighting scheme. Each definable health status, ranging from death to coma to varying degrees of disability and discomfort to full health . . . is assigned a weight from zero to one and the number of years spent at a given health status is multiplied by the corresponding weight to yield a number that might be thought of as an equivalent number of years in full health–number of quality adjusted life years (QALYs)." (8)

In the policy content QALYs are used as follows:

"The policy objective underlying the QALY literature is the maximization of the community health. An individual's health is measured in terms of QALYs and the community's health is measured as the sum of QALYs." (16)

In economics the choice of measure of outcome is determined by the underlying welfare theory used to determine whether a change in resource allocation is worth implementing *(17)*. This also enables us to identify requirements of the measurement method. The most commonly used theory is the welfarist approach *(9,18)*. Under this approach an individual's preferences are embodied in that individual's utility function. Thus, for a measure to be consistent with the welfarist approach it must be consistent with a utility theory. Utility is defined in economics as the value of a function that represents an ordering—specifically a preference ordering of different combinations of goods and services consumed. One prospect is better than another if, and only if, it has greater utility. Different utility theories exist which are based on different fundamental axioms. The method for measuring utility is determined by the particular theory being followed. We might choose between alternative theories based on how we would like individuals to behave or based on how they really behave. If one follows the welfarist approach, one assumes that individuals are the best judges of their own welfare and hence we should chose a theory based on its accuracy in measuring individuals' true preferences (even if these are not the preferences we feel they should have).

Pliskin et al. *(19)* were the first to suggest an underlying utility model to QALY for an individual who is an expected utility maximizer. In doing so, the QALY measure was related to a formal economic theory of utility (a prerequisite of the welfarist approach) and related to a theory that describes behavior under conditions of uncertainty (coincides with the nature of decisions in health care). It is, however, widely recognized that the conditions under which the QALY measure is related to a formal utility theory are very restrictive. As explained elsewhere in more details *(18)*, both the underlying utility theory (vNM utility theory also known as expected utility theory) and the additional assumptions (i.e., in addition to those required by the vNM approach) required by the model are neither supported by empirical evidence nor are normatively appealing (mainly the additional assumptions). Hence this model violates the requirement in the welfarist approach of consumer sovereignty. In other words it assumes rather than measures individuals' preferences.

The implications of the limitations of the QALY concept are neither academic nor trivial. Misrepresentation of individuals' preferences can result in either preference reversal or biased estimates of the magnitude of the strength of preference, which can affect the results of an economic evaluation *(18)*. Notwithstanding the conceptual limitation of the QALY model as a method of measuring individuals' or societal (which is calculated as the sum of individuals' values) preferences, the use of alternative (and distinct) approaches to derive the "utility weights" generates further problems for the QALY approach. As a consequence, programs might be evaluated as being a "burden" or "bargain" depending on the particular methods of measurement chosen. Moreover, the criteria used to derive the weights might be related to the outcome of the evaluation. In so far as "utility weights" differ according to the particular method of measurement than the QALY scores, which are based on these weights, will also differ indicating that (1) QALY need not represent a common unit of measure that it was intended to represent and (2) invalidates comparisons between CE studies in which differing methods of measurement are used *(18)*.

Careful review of the following three studies illustrates the problem of incomparability of QALYs used in different studies. The study by Vijan et al. *(20)* examined the cost effectiveness of various screening intervals for eye in patients with type 2 diabetes. QALYs were used as the primary model outcome measure. The model predictions for overall life expectancy were adjusted for time spent blind based on a utility for blindness (i.e., QALY weight) of 0.69 that was taken from the literature (presumably an average value of the values in the three studies referenced). The study by the CDC Diabetes Cost Effectiveness Group *(21)*, estimated the incremental cost effectiveness of intensive glycemic control, intensified hypertension control and reduction in serum cholesterol level, relative to conventional control, for patients with type 2 diabetes. Remaining life years and the number of discounted QALYs were the primary model outcomes. Utility levels (i.e., QALY weights) were obtained from the literature for the main outcomes (blindness, end stage renal disease, lower extremity amputation, stroke, cardiac arrest/MI, and angina. "Utility levels for all other health states were set to one," (i.e., they were ignored). Finally the study by The Diabetes Prevention Program Research Group *(22)* compared within trial cost effectiveness of lifestyle interventions or metformin for the primary prevention of type 2 diabetes. QALYs were one of the outcomes measured. Utility weights were measured on participants in the trial using the self-administered Quality of Well-Being Index (QWB-SA). The QWB is a generic quality of life instrument that is used to derive the QALY weights. However, this instrument is not related to a utility theory that violates the requirement of the welfarist approach. It has not been verified whether all the QALY weights used in the other two studies were utility based.

Even though the three studies used QALYs as a measure of outcome it is clear that these three QALY measures are not comparable. Whereas the first two studies used "utility weights" obtained from the literature, the third study used a generic measure of quality of life to measure the utility weights. The use of weights obtained from different sources in the literature is problematic. For example, recent study *(23)* conducted a systematic review of quality of life weights in the literature elicited with the time tradeoff (TTO) method. Even though all these weights were obtained using the same measurement technique to eliminate the problem of between measurement technique variations (which is not the case in the above two studies), the authors concluded that there are major problems with using those values. For example, ranking of the weights found for 102 diagnostic groups had no apparent relationship to severity. One diagnostic group was assigned weights ranging from 0.39 to 0.84. The authors recommend that these weights should not be used for QALY calculations. Also, what constitutes an event that affects a patient's quality of life was different in the three studies. Whereas in the first study it was only being blind or not, in the second study it was a set of different events, blindness being one of them. Because both studies followed individuals over their remaining life span, it does not make sense that individuals in the first study did not suffer from any other event beside blindness. In the third study, the impact on quality of life was measured directly by asking individuals at preset intervals to assess their quality of life using a classification system that required them to rank their condition on several scales or attributes— mobility, physical activity, social activity, and symptom-problem complex. This was likely to result in different values than those obtained from the literature.

The HYE has been suggested as an alternative approach to QALYs. The intent was to provide a measure of outcome that preserved what was considered to be the intuitively appealing meaning of the QALY measure but without the need to subscribe, at the individual level, to the restrictive assumptions that underlie the QALY-utility model. Unlike the QALY, which means different things to different people (e.g., an index or a utility), the HYE means only one thing—it is a utility based concept, derived from the individual utility function by measuring the equivalent number of years in full health, holding other arguments in the utility function constant, that produced the same level of utility to the individual as produced by the potential lifetime health profiles following a given intervention. The definition of HYE is a general one and does not require an individual to subscribe to any specific utility theory (e.g., vNM utility theory). Any type of utility theory that reflects the individual's true preferences can be the basis for generating algorithms to measure HYEs and the choice of utility theory will determine the method of measurement. The only requirement is that preferences be measured under the condition of uncertainty in order to reflect the nature of decision making in health care. HYE is more complex to measure than QALYs but not prohibitive. Feasibility of measurement is important but it cannot justify measuring the wrong outcome just because it is feasible to do so. Future research in this area should concentrate on developing ways to simplify the measurement task without having to make restrictive assumptions. For more on the HYE measure *see* refs. *17* and *24*.

HOW ARE THE DATA USED TO MAKE RECOMMENDATION ABOUT ECONOMIC EFFICIENCY?

"To improve efficiency, decision makers need information on what economists call opportunity costs—the benefits forgone when scarce resources are used one way rather than another . . . In absence of any information about opportunity cost, however, they cannot attempt to achieve the efficient use of resources." (25)

The analytical tool of CEA is the incremental cost-effectiveness ratio (IC-ER). The IC-ER is given by the difference in costs between the two programs compared divided by the difference in outcome (typically measured by QALYs). According to the methods literature *(3,8–10)* the ratio of the net increase in costs to the net increase in effects is the appropriate way to analyze the data in order to determine if a program is worthwhile (i.e., helps achieve the stated goal of economic efficiency) with the recommended criterion being "the lower the value of this ratio, the higher the priority in terms of maximizing benefits derived from a given health expenditure" *(8)*. More specifically, two decision rules have been presented in the literature to determine whether a new program is worth implementing: the league table approach and the threshold approach.

Under the league table approach, the decision maker is only concerned with the relative value of the IC-ER for the program under consideration. Programs are adopted at a descending order of IC-ER until all available resources have been exhausted. In real life, IC-ER values are available only for those programs that have been studied, which are a small subset of all programs provided. As a result, the league tables presented to decision makers are incomplete and their use for the allocation of health care resources is incompatible with the maximization of health gains from those resources *(26,27)*. Under the threshold approach, the decision maker focuses on the absolute value of the program's IC-ER. If the program's IC-ER is lower than the threshold value (also known as lambda [λ]), it should be adopted. The application of the threshold value approach is much simpler than the league table approach once the threshold value is determined and thus it is not surprising that it is the approach most commonly used. Despite the central role of the threshold value, little attention has been given to determining the value of the threshold or evaluating the usefulness of this approach.

The theoretical foundation of the threshold IC-ER is described in Weinstein and Zeckhauser *(28)* and more recently in Birch and Gafni *(29,30)* identified the conditions required for these IC-ER decision rules to lead to benefit maximization subject to fixed budget. In particular, these include perfect divisibility, constant returns to scale for all programs under consideration, and constant marginal opportunity costs. Weinstein and Zeckhauser *(28)* showed that under the conditions of perfect divisibility and constant returns to scale the league table and the threshold approaches are identical in terms of the resource allocation recommended. Under these conditions the threshold value represent the "shadow price" of the budget or the opportunity cost of the resources at the margin. It is also equal to the IC-ER of the last program adopted if the league table approach was used. But these conditions mean that all programs can be purchased in incremental units (e.g., 1 min of dialysis machine) or provided to incremental patients (e.g., 2.3 type 2 diabetes patients or only to half of the patients who need this treatment). It also means that the rate of output produced by the program is constant no matter how many increments are purchased (e.g., if one dialysis machine would produce 50 QALYs/yr than one-tenth of a dialysis machine would produce five additional QALYs/yr). As already been shown, these conditions are not realistic and do not exist in the real world where such decisions are being made *(29–31)*.

Even if one is willing to accept the unrealistic assumptions underlying the required conditions for the CEA approach, the application of this model to real life decision making is not practical. For the threshold value to be consistent with the model the following properties also have to hold. According the model, the threshold value is inter alia, a function of the budget, and every change in the budget will generate a change in the threshold value *(30)*. In addition, as previously explained, the threshold value is equal to the IC-ER of the last program selected before the budget is exhausted. But the costs and effects of all programs including the last program selected for funding are subject to uncertainty. As a result the threshold value is stochastic *(31)*. Finally, new programs are being developed all the time. As new programs are funded, and others are replaced, the identification of the last program changes, implying that the value and distribution of the threshold value also changes *(31)*. Hence, a threshold value that is consistent with the model will be stochastic and dynamic (i.e., its value will change all the time even if the budget does not change). However, as previously explained, information on IC-ERs is not available for all programs; in fact, information is not available for the vast majority of programs being provided. Hence there is no way to allocate the system resources in a descending order of IC-ER and find out the threshold value even at a given point in time. As a result it is recognized that the threshold value cannot be determined endogenously and is thus being assumed *(9,15,26,27,32,33)*. No alternative approaches have been presented to determine the threshold value, either in ways that are consistent with the Weinstein–Zeckhauser *(28)* model, or based on any alternative model of health maximization from a constrained budget. However, this has not prevented researchers (including in the area of endocrinology) from claiming to identify the "cost-effectiveness" of new programs based on some "preferred" or assumed value for the threshold IC-ER.

For example, Laupacis et al. *(34)* justified their choice of $20,000 (Canadian) per QALY as a threshold value "following a review of available economic evaluations and previously suggested guidelines." They argued that programs with IC-ERs less than this "critical value" ". . . are almost universally accepted as being appropriate ways of using society's and the health care system's resources." No attempt is made by the authors to justify this figure in terms of it representing the shadow price of the health care expenditures in Canada in 1992. On the contrary, the ratio is derived from a 1982 US study, which suggested an arbitrary cut-off for programs at $20,000 per QALY. Far from helping decision makers identify efficient uses of available health care programs, use of similar arbitrary figures led to the allocation of unconstrained resources among programs without any evidence that overall health benefits were maximized *(27,35,36)*.

Elsewhere $50,000 and $100,000 per QALY is often presented as a range for the threshold value without any justification in terms of the shadow price of the budget or the compatibility of its use with the maximization of health benefits from available resources *(33)*. It is interesting to note that the lower limit of the range is based on the IC-ER for renal dialysis treatment for patients with chronic renal failure although as Winkelmayer et al. *(37)* note ". . . it was initially expressed in Canadian rather than US dollars." Because in the United States, Medicare is required by law to cover the cost of renal dialysis for all US citizens receiving the procedure, it has been argued that this represents a threshold that has been deemed to be an acceptable price for health improvements in the US population. Hence, all interventions with IC-ER value less than or equal to this should be funded. However, Medicare does not fund other programs for all US citizens irrespective of whether the IC-ER values are greater or less than this arbitrary figure. There may be many programs that meet this critical ratio, but to fund them all would imply that the opportunity cost of health care resources was constant over whatever range of expenditures were required to support all these programs. In other words, it implies that at the extreme, there is an infinite stream of resources available at constant marginal opportunity costs *(30)*.

This leads us to the question the usefulness of such decision rule in helping decision makers allocating scarce health care resources. A positive IC-ER represents a situation where the resources used by the current intervention for patients with a particular condition are not sufficient to cover the costs of providing the new intervention for the same patients. It is the most common result in existing CEA and the one, which requires further analysis before the implications for economic efficiency can be identified. Following the concept of opportunity cost, in order to determine whether adoption of the new program would increase health benefits to the population the following necessary, but not sufficient, conditions should be met: (1) consider the total costs of the new intervention in its proposed used, and (2) identify other programs that would need to be forgone to provide the additional resources to fund the new program and stay within the budget constraint. But total costs of the new intervention are eliminated from the typical CEA by calculating the IC-ER and making a value judgment, either explicitly or implicitly, whether this IC-ER represent a good value for money (i.e., is equal or less than the threshold). It is important to emphasize that even if we assume that new funds will be made available over time, the information provided by the IC-ER is insufficient to identify whether a proposed program represent an efficient use of even these additional resources (*see* ref. *36* for a numerical example).

Thus, the use of IC-ER and a threshold value as a decision rule ignores the simple reality that, if overall funds are fixed, the additional funds required for a new program must come from other uses, that is, cut to other programs. Furthermore, funding new technologies that have "acceptable IC-ERs" requires and, hence, leads to continuous increase in program expenditures because the new, more costly, technologies are added without other programs being cut to generate sufficient resources for the new program *(27,36)*. Furthermore, without explicitly considering the source of the additional funds required to support new, more costly, programs (i.e., the opportunity costs of these additional resources), we do not know if the adoption of a new intervention will lead to an overall increase in health improvements. This is because there is no way to judge if the added health benefits are greater than the health benefits forgone by the elimination of other programs. As Cookson et al. *(25)* conclude, based on the experience in the United Kingdom of mandating the use of new technologies if their IC-ER fall under a given threshold, such recommendations have resulted in inappropriate allocation of resources by ". . . diverting funding away from more cost-effective services that lack politically powerful advocates," and "by cutting (or by diluting, delaying, deterring, or deflecting) other services."

The use of an IC-ER and comparing it to a threshold value is also common in cost effectiveness analyses performed for endocrinology interventions. The following examples illustrate the points made above. King et al. *(38)* compared the cost effectiveness of four management strategies for a patient with an incidentally discovered asymptomatic pituitary microadenoma. They used a threshold value of $50,000 per QALY to determine if an intervention was cost-effective (i.e., should be adopted). They reported that "[A]t a quality of life value for anxiety about having an asymptomatic microadenoma of 0.99 only the PRL strategy meets the $50,000/QALY threshold. At a quality of life value of 0.97 all three strategies, including MRI follow-up strategy, meet the $50,000/QALY threshold." Their final recommendation was that "a single PRL test may be the most cost-effective management strategy." There is no consideration in this paper of (1) the total costs of the different strategies in their proposed use and (2) where the required additional funds would come from (i.e., which potential programs will be cut), and what would the opportunity cost be for these additional resources.

The study by the CDC Diabetes Cost Effectiveness Group *(21)* is another interesting example. This study compares the cost effectiveness of different treatment interventions to reduce complications of type 2 diabetes. These authors probably read more carefully the recommendations by the US Panel on cost effectiveness in health and medicine *(9)*. They stated that "[T]he US Panel on cost-effectiveness in health and medicine notes that no absolute standard exist for deciding whether an intervention's cost effectiveness ratio is 'cost-effective' or 'not cost-effective.' Instead, the panel recommends describing interventions as more or less cost-effective than other interventions." The authors proceeded with such comparisons and concluded that "[I]ntensive glycemic control and reduction in serum cholesterol level increase costs and improve health outcomes. The cost-effectiveness ratio for these two interventions are comparable with those of several other frequently adopted health care interventions." However, the fact that the CE ratio of "these two interventions are comparable with those of several other frequently adopted health care interventions" does not tell us (1) what the total cost to implement these two strategies for example nationwide would be and (2) where the required additional funds would come from, and what the opportunity costs of these funds would be. As Crookson et al. *(25)* state "in absence of any information about opportunity cost, however, they (i.e., decision makers) cannot attempt to achieve the efficient use of resources."

ECONOMIC SOLUTIONS

Elsewhere it was explained that economics provide valid methods for identifying the maximization of health improvements for a given allocation of resources (e.g., Integer Programming) *(29,30,39)*. Although the data requirements for these methods may be substantial, this reflects the complexity of the question being addressed. As mentioned earlier, the data requirements identified by the Weinstein–Zeckhause *(28)* model for the proper use of CEA are also substantial in spite of the unrealistic assumptions underlying this model.

An alternative practical approach is available, which involves modifying the objective from maximizing the health improvements produced from available resources to one of producing unambiguous increases in health improvements *(29,39)*. This approach requires that the health improvements of the proposed program be compared with the health improvements produced by that combination of programs that have to be given up to generate sufficient funds in order to support the proposed program. It is only when the health improvements of the proposed program exceed the health improvements of the combination of programs to be given up that the new technology represents an improvement in the efficiency of the resource utilization. This approach has been extended to deal with the uncertain nature of costs and outcomes associated with health care intervention and to replace current approaches (e.g., cost-effectiveness acceptability curves, net health benefit approach, and probabilistic modeling), which are all dependent on knowing the threshold value or its range *(31)*.

This approach provides unambiguous improvement in efficiency because it results in an overall increase in the total health improvements without using additional resources. It does not rely on choosing a subjective threshold value to determine the desirability of the program, without any considerations where the additional resources (funds) will come from. In this approach the source of the additional funds has to be identified and the implications of the cancellation of a program are part of the analysis. Further, this approach does not involve IC-ERs, so the results do not require unrealistic assumptions such as perfect divisibility and constant returns to scale with respect to programs.

Under this approach, more than one program (or set of programs) might satisfy the condition. In this situation, maximization of health improvements from available resources requires that the new program be funded by reduction in the least productive (i.e., that producing least health improvements) of all possible combinations of programs. Because data constraints are likely to prevent this from being identified, the approach will identify a "second best" solution of unambiguous improvement of health gains from available resources. However, as more data become available, an iterative process can be used to identify further improvements until optimization is reached. This concept does not tell us how to find a potential program (or programs) that can be candidates for cancellation. A practical approach to identifying such programs was suggested by Gafni (40). The idea is to first look for such programs in the same therapeutic area. For example, when introducing a new, more effective but more expensive, intervention in the area of diabetes, one can ask the question, "are all programs to treat diabetic patients as efficient as the new intervention?" If the answer is yes, one can start to look at other therapeutic areas. This policy of "first clean your own budget" does not guarantee that the least productive program will be eliminated first. However, it assumes that administrators and clinicians (and possibly researchers) are more familiar with inefficiencies in their own area; this makes it easier to identify candidate programs for cancellation. It also help in preventing departments from looking first for inefficiency in other areas without making sure that their own operation meets similar standards.

WITHER OR WHITHER ECONOMIC EVALUATION?

This chapter has described the economic question and demonstrated some major problems with the methods currently recommended for economic evaluations (more specifically CEA and CUA) of health care programs. These problems, as well as others not addressed here, demonstrate that CEA and CUA, as currently recommended and practiced, are unable to address the economic efficiency question. Moreover, it has been shown elsewhere (27,36) that the use of these methods has led to (1) uncontrolled rises in health expenditures without any evidence of any increase in total health improvements, (2) increased inequalities in the availability of services, and (3) concerns about the sustainability of funding for new technologies. But this does not mean that the discipline of economics is useless. On the contrary, methods for economic evaluations, which adhere to the basic concepts of economics, as outlined in the first section of this chapter, overcome these limitations and provide the information needed by decision makers aiming to maximize benefits produced from available resources.

Culyer (1) noted that health economics as a discipline does not exist independently of economics as a discipline. Thus, when the discipline of economics is chosen as the "mode of thinking" for resource allocation in health, the principle of the discipline must be followed. Culyer *(1)* went on to note that, "economics is not the only discipline applicable to this topic (i.e., resource allocation), nor topics within the general topic of health." However, only economics through the use of opportunity cost concepts provide valid approaches to maximizing health improvements from available resources. It is not surprising that simple tools—such as the IC-ER criterion as currently used, which represents departure from the concept of opportunity costs—fails to address the problem at hand. As others *(41)* have already noted, "health economists, while seeking to colonize the clinical mind may have lost their disciplinary head."

Although it is not the purpose of this chapter to review in detail these approaches (those interested should consult the references and even go beyond) it is worth acknowledging that applications of the proper techniques are not without challenges and the methods for these applications are under continuous development. Proper execution of an economic evaluation might result in a more complex study as compared with current methods. Although simplified methods might be a method of reducing the costs of the analyses, it is not believed that such simplification is justified where it might result in wrong solutions or recommendations, something that the methods alone would be unable to determine. As H. L. Mencken has said, "[T]o every complex question there is a simple answer . . . and it is wrong." A model is only as good as its assumptions, and the use of unrealistic assumptions (i.e., assumptions that are known to be empirically invalid) or strong assumptions (i.e., assumptions that have no normative appeal) will not help us solve real life problems. Also, one should not attempt to change the problem to fit it to the solution. The following are exampled of such attempts: recognizing the limitation of the IC-ER and the threshold value approach there are those who claim that CEA is not about affordability and the threshold value approach is only meant to determine value for money. It is interesting to quote Williams *(15)* who recently acknowledged that "[T]he third cheer still has to be withheld because NICE still insists that this benchmark zone has nothing to do with affordability or with the rationing of health care, despite the fact that such considerations are the only justification there is for having a benchmark!"

CONCLUSION

In summary, questions about how to maximize the benefits produced from given resources (i.e., economic efficiency) are in many ways similar to questions about how to maximize the outcome for individual patients. Both types of decisions involve a mixture of technical and value judgment and neither can be reflected adequately in a small number of simple questions. Economics provides useful (but not simple) methods to help sort out resource allocation to optimize benefits. When reading an economic evaluation, readers should check if they follow sound economic principles.

REFERENCES

1. Culyer AJ. Economics and Health Economics. In: VanderGang J, Perlman M, eds. Health, Economics, and Health Economics. North Holland, Amsterdam, 1981, pp 3–11.
2. Williams A. The economic role of health indicators. In: Teeling SG, ed. Measuring the Social Benefit of Medicine. Office of Health Economics, London, 1983, pp. 63–67.
3. Drummond M, Stoddart G, Torrance G. Methods for the Economic Evaluation of Health Care Programmes. Oxford University Press, Oxford, 1987.

4. Birch S, Gafni A. On being NICE in the UK: guidelines for technology appraisal for the NHS in England and Wales. Health Econ. 2002;11:185–191.

5. Gafni A, Birch S. Equity considerations in utility-based measures of health outcomes in economic appraisals: an adjustment algorithm. J Health Econ 1991;10:329–342.

6. LeGrand J. Equity and Choice: An Essay in Economics and Applied Philosophy. Harper Collins, London, 1991.

7. Mooney G. Economics, Medicine, and Health Care. Wheatsheaf, Brighton, 1986.

8. Weinstein MC, Stason WB. Foundations of cost-effectiveness analysis for health and medical practices. N Engl J Med 1977; 296:716–721.

9. Gold MR, Siegel JE, Russel LB, Weinstein MC. Cost-Effectiveness in Health and Medicine. Oxford University Press, New York, 1996.

10. Drummond M, O'Brien B, Stoddart G, Torrance G. Methods for the Economic Evaluations of Health Care Programmes. Oxford University Press, Oxford, 1997.

11. National Institute for Clinical Excellence. Riluzole for Motor Neurone Disease–Full Guidance. London, 2001.

12. National Institute for Clinical Excellence, Guide to the Methods of Technology Appraisal (reference N0515). National Institute of Clinical Excellence, London. Available at http://www.nice.org.uk/pdf/brdnov03item3b-pdf. Accessed 2004.

13. Naylor D. Cost-effectiveness analysis: are the outputs worth the inputs? ACP J Club 1996;124:A12–14.

14. Coast J. Is economic evaluation in touch with society's health values? BMJ 2004;329:1233–1236.

15. Williams A. What Could Be Nicer Than NICE? Office of Health Economics, London, 2004.

16. Wagstaff A. QALYs and the equity-efficiency trade-off. J Health Econ 1991;10:21–41.

17. Gafni A. Proper preference-based outcome measures in economic evaluations of pharmaceutical interventions. Med Care 1996;34:DS48–DS58.

18. Gafni A, Birch S. Preferences for outcomes in economic evaluation: an economic approach to addressing economic problems. Soc Sci Med 1995;40:767–776.

19. Pliskin JS, Shepard DS, Winstein MC. Utility functions for life year and health status. Oper Res 1980;28:206–224.

20. Vijan S, Hofer TP, Hayward, RA. Cost-utility analysis of screening intervals for diabetic retinopathy in patients with type 2 diabetes mellitus. JAMA 2000;283:889–896.

21. CDC Diabetes Cost Effectiveness Group. Cost-effectiveness of intensive glycemic control, intensified hypertension control, and serum cholesterol level reduction for type 2 diabetes. JAMA 2002;287:2542–2551.

22. Diabetes Prevention Program Research Group. Within-trial cost-effectiveness of lifestyle intervention or metformin for the primary prevention of type 2 diabetes. Diabetes Care 2003;26:2518–2523.

23. Arnesen T, Trommald M. Roughly right or precisely wrong? Systematic review of quality-of-life weights elicited with the time trade-off method. J Health Serv Res Policy 2004;9:43–50.

24. Ried W. QALYs versus HYEs: what's right and what's wrong. A review of the controversy. J Health Econ 1998;17:607–625.

25. Cookson R, McDaid D, Maynard A. Wrong SIGN, NICE mess: is national guidance distorting allocation of resources? BMJ 2001;323:743–745.

26. Devlin N. An introduction to the use of cost-effectiveness thresholds in decision making: what are the issues? In: Towse A, Pritchard C, Devlin N, eds. Cost Effectiveness Thresholds: Economics and Ethical Issues. Kings Fund and Office of Health Economics, London, 2002, pp. 16–21.

27. Gafni A and Birch S. NICE methodological guidelines and decision making in the National Health Service in England and Wales. Pharmacoeconomics 2003;21:149–157.

28. Weinstein M, Zeckhauser R. Critical ratios and efficient allocation. J Public Econ 1973;2:147–157.

29. Birch S, Gafni A. Cost effectiveness/utility analyses. Do current decision rules lead us to where we want to be? J Health Econ 1992;11:279–296.

30. Birch S, Gafni A. Changing the problem to fit the solution: Johannesson and Weinstein's (mis) application of economics to real world problems. J Health Econ 1993;12:469–476.

31. Sendi P, Gafni A, Birch S. Opportunity costs and uncertainty in the economic evaluation of health care interventions. Health Econ 2002;11:23–31.

32. Devlin N, Parkin D, Gold M. WHO evaluates NICE. BMJ 2003;327:1061–1062.

33. Ubel PA, Hirth RA, Chernew ME, Fendrick AM. What is the price of life and why doesn't it increase at the rate of inflation? Arch Intern Med 2003;163:1637–1641.

34. Laupacis A, Feeny D, Detsky AS, Tugwell PX. How attractive does a new technology have to be to warrant adoption and utilization? Tentative guidelines for using clinical and economic evaluations. CMAJ 1992;146:473–581.
35. Laupacis A. Inclusion of drugs in provincial drug benefit programs: who is making these decisions, and are they the right ones? CMAJ 2002;166:44–47.
36. Gafni A, Birch S. Inclusion of drugs in provincial drug benefit programs: Should "reasonable decisions" lead to uncontrolled growth in expenditures? CMAJ 2003;168:849–851.
37. Winkelmayer WC, Weinstein MC, Mittleman MA, Glynn RJ, Pliskin JS. Health economic evaluations: the special case of end-stage renal disease treatment. Med Decis Making 2002;22:417–430.
38. King JT, Jr., Justice AC, Aron DC. Management of incidental pituitary microadenomas: a cost-effectiveness analysis. J Clin Endocrinol Metab 1997;82:3625–3632.
39. Gafni A, Birch S. Guidelines for the adoption of new technologies: a prescription for uncontrolled growth in expenditures and how to avoid the problem. CMAJ 1993;148:913–97.
40. Gafni A. Economic evaluation of health care interventions: an economist's perspective. ACP J Club 1996;124:A12–A14.
41. Maynard A, Sheldon T. Health economics: has it fulfilled its promise? In: Maynard A, Chalmers I, eds. Non-random Reflection on Health Services Research. BMJ Press, London, 1977.

16 Translation Research in Diabetes
Asking Broader Questions

Russell E. Glasgow, PhD,
Elizabeth Bayliss, MD, MSPH,
and Paul A. Estabrooks, PhD

CONTENTS

INTRODUCTION
ISSUES IN AND CHALLENGES FOR TRANSLATION
FOCAL POINTS FOR TRANSLATIONAL WORK IN DIABETES
CONCEPTUAL AND EVALUATION FRAMEWORKS
    FOR TRANSLATIONAL RESEARCH
KEY DIABETES TRANSLATIONAL EFFORTS
CONCLUSIONS: COMPLEXITIES AND CHALLENGES
REFERENCES

"If we want more evidence-based practice;
then we need more practice-based evidence,"
Larry Green, 2004

INTRODUCTION

The burden of diabetes is well documented. Adverse health conditions, disability, reduced quality of life, and heightened risk of premature death characterize the progression of this disease *(1–3)*. The considerable personal burden of diabetes is magnified by the penetration of the disease into the American population. By the age of 60, approx 1 in 10 Caucasians, 1 in 6 Latinos, and 1 in 5 African Americans, have type 2 diabetes *(4)*. Further, the prevalence of diabetes is projected to increase by almost 40% by 2010 *(5)*. An unfortunate sidebar to these statistics is the increasing prevalence of type 2 diabetes or its precursor, impaired glucose tolerance, among American children *(6)*. In clinic-based studies, the proportion of diagnosed pediatric type 2 diabetes (i.e., type 2 vs type 1) has risen from less than 5% prior to 1994 to 30–50% in recent years *(6)*. Similar to adults, the disease is disproportionately high among youth with minority ethnic and racial backgrounds *(6)*. In addition to the considerable burden on personal

From: *Contemporary Endocrinology: Evidence-Based Endocrinology*
Edited by: V. M. Montori © Mayo Foundation for Medical Education and Research

health, it is estimated that the annual direct and indirect economic costs of diabetes in the Unites States are approx \$132 billion *(7)*.

This information is probably not new to the audience reading this chapter, but our point here is to illustrate breadth of the impact of diabetes across age groups, cultures, and the economy in the United States *(1)*. This context highlights the importance of identifying strategies to address the personal and societal costs of diabetes. Fortunately, the health outcomes and cost of managing diabetes can be strongly influenced by integrated care management that includes self-management support *(8,9)*. However, individuals with diabetes often find it difficult to sustain healthy self-management behaviors. Although there is research support for the efficacy of behavioral programs to improve maintenance of self-management behaviors, there is little evidence that these programs or strategies are being adopted and offered within typical health care or health-education settings. Similarly, there are compelling data that appropriate management of glucose levels, blood pressure, and other risk factors can substantially reduce diabetes complications, but evidence-based guidelines for diabetes are seldom implemented at anything approaching recommended levels *(10)*.

Based on the impact of diabetes on health and economic outcomes, the current high prevalence and projected proliferation of diabetes, and the lack of dissemination of efficacious interventions into regular practice, it is clear that there is a need to understand and address the issues and challenges of translating promising findings into regular practice. The purpose of our chapter is to investigate the issues associated with how to successfully translate diabetes management research into regular practice. We have organized the chapter to (1) identify the issues and challenges related to translation, (2) highlight priority areas for translational work, (3) present possible solutions to addressing translational issues and challenges, and finally (4) provide some conclusions regarding the effective translation of research into practice.

ISSUES IN AND CHALLENGES FOR TRANSLATION

The current medical practice environment is characterized by limitations and demands that differ substantially from the controlled setting of a research environment. Patients with diabetes rarely, if ever, carry a single diagnosis. Caring for persons with diabetes mandates that the provider think about multiple potential comorbidities: hyperlipidemia, coronary artery disease, renal disease, and the potential for other endocrinopathies, to name a few. As previously discussed, the US population with diabetes is both aging and becoming more sociodemographically diverse, requiring individualized adaptations of treatment recommendations. Patients with diabetes also participate in unhealthy eating patterns, sedentary behavior, and cigarette smoking, all of which further increase their risk for cardiovascular disease and premature death. Therefore, disease management in diabetes is not simply about managing a single disease or encouraging one behavior change. Given the comprehensive nature of diabetes care, brief clinical visits can feel inadequate and frustrating to both patients and providers. Finally, collaboration between specialty and primary care, sometimes across entirely different health care systems, puts a premium on effective professional communication.

In the face of these competing demands, the amount of clinical evidence and guidelines is skyrocketing. It behooves the clinician to carefully assess the quality and practicality of the evidence before translating it into practice *(11)*. Or, put another way, to

use evidence without "teaching to the test" (practicing to the single outcome) and optimize the care of the patient, not the care of the single disease or risk factor.

In the 21st century, translating evidence-based strategies into practice is not limited
to the exam room. Available technologies permit (and the volume of evidence encourages) population-based interventions that can be delivered by additional and innovative
channels (12,13). Clinicians are now held accountable for their entire panel of patients,
not just those who are regular attendees at office visits. Research investigations are
often conducted using disease registries, interactive voice technologies, and interactive
computer programs—both office-based and available to remote sites. Such interventions are appropriate for translation into practice as well.

Regardless of whether the intervention is office-, patient-, or population-based, and
pharmacological, behavioral, or health systems-based, there are multiple potential barriers to translation (or dissemination) of an evidence-based intervention that should be
considered in translating it into practice: these barriers include the general issues of
the quality of the data and results, the clinical relevance of the outcome, the generalizability of the results to a clinical population, and the feasibility of the intervention in the
practice setting (Table 1). The results of the intervention must be clinically relevant
and should address the following questions:

- Is the outcome important to patient care?
- Is the margin of improvement in the outcome owing to the intervention truly clinically
  relevant?
- Does the intervention "fit" into a clinical setting like mine?
- Is the intervention cost-effective and how many start-up resources does it require?
- Is the intervention acceptable to patients, providers, other office staff, and administrators—
  both in the practice setting and of the relevant health systems?

Finally, in making decisions about translation of evidence into practice, the specialty
provider has the additional responsibility of having to look downstream as well:

- Will the intervention that was efficacious in a randomized clinical trial and effective in
  the endocrinology practice continue to be effective when the patient returns to the world
  of primary care?

Any real or perceived problems with any of these issues can present a barrier to translation. Specific barriers to translation can be categorized into four categories: (1) characteristics of the intervention, (2) characteristics of the research design, (3) characteristics
of potential adoption settings, and (4) interactions among the first three categories (14).
These are listed in Table 1.

Overcoming barriers to the translation of research into practice begins where the
evidence is generated—at the level of study planning and design. The *sine qua non* of
evidence-based medical treatment has historically been the randomized clinical trial
(RCT). Results from a well-designed RCT are considered Level I evidence in assessing
the potential translation of research into practice (15). However, the majority of RCTs
are designed to assess a single aspect of care in a controlled environment—often with
a carefully selected study population. It is often difficult to determine whether the
results of an RCT will generalize to a broader population in a "real-world" setting and
additionally be relevant to the patients for whom it is intended. In Practical Clinical
Trial Models, we discuss an alternative type of RCT: the practical clinical trial. This
latter study design is specifically designed with translation in mind.

Table 1
Barriers to Dissemination

Characteristics of the intervention	Characteristics of the research design
High cost	Not relevant or representative:
Intensive time demands	• Sample of patients
High level of staff expertise required	• Sample of settings
Difficult to learn or understand	• Sample of clinicians
Not packaged or "manualized"	Failure to evaluate cost
Not developed considering user needs	Failure to assess implementation
Not designed to be self-sustaining	Failure to evaluate maintenance
Highly specific to particular setting	Failure to evaluate sustainability
Not modularized or customizable	

Characteristics of potential adopting "settings"	Interactions among the three other barrier "types"
Competing demands occur	Because of barriers, the program reach or participation is low
Program imposed from outside	Intervention is not flexible
Finance or organizations are unstable	Intervention is not appropriate for the target population
Clients and setting have specific needs	
Resources are limited	Staffing pattern does not match intervention requirements
Time is limited	
Organizational support is limited	Inconsistent organization and intervention philosophies
Prevailing practices that work against innovation	
Prevailing practices that work against innovation	Inability to implement intervention adequately
Perverse incentives or regulations that oppose change	

FOCAL POINTS FOR TRANSLATIONAL WORK IN DIABETES

There is obviously much that needs to be done to translate the results of controlled trials into diabetes practice. We suggest that this translation might best be focused in three important and crosscutting areas or "focal points (16)." Rakowski et al. (17) defines a focal point as "the simultaneous combination of the target population, the health practice, the intervention setting, and the eventual setting for implementing the behavior as a regular practice in daily life." We suggest that attention to the three issues below will be most likely to help close the "chasm" (18) between research and practice. This will be true especially when combined into research on and translation of interventions that can (1) reach a large and representative proportion of high-risk patients, (2) be consistently implemented by different staff members found in most health care settings, and (3) be maintained or integrated into ongoing usual care procedures.

Populations Reached

The past decade has seen substantial improvement in the diversity of patients who have participated in clinical trials (19). Additional work is still needed, however, to make sure that research includes the complex, multi-morbid patients seen in everyday primary and specialty care. Some of these population issues are biological—such as stage of disease and micro- and macrovascular health—others are psychosocial in nature and include making sure that our interventions work for those who are less privileged, reside in medically underserved areas, have few economic resources, and have low-health literacy *(20,21)*.

Implementation

One of the key challenges in translation is consistent implementation of a program. One of the most common reasons that evidence-based interventions do not work in clinical practice is that the interventions are not delivered as in the original research. This issue is so pervasive that the term "type 3 error" has been used to refer to the error of concluding that an intervention or program is not effective when it was in fact not delivered *(22)*. There has been much recent and appropriate focus on fidelity of intervention and many interventions have certainly failed because implementers have delivered only parts of a program or modified it so substantially that it was no longer efficacious *(23)*. However, this fidelity approach assumes that any deviation from the original intervention is detrimental, and we know from community-based participatory research *(24,25)*, that tailoring and customization of behavioral interventions are often necessary for successful application. In fact, "reinvention" of certain aspects of an intervention may actually make it more effective for a given setting *(26)*. What is needed is: (1) recognition by program developers that adaptations *will* be made, (2) specification of what program components are essential and must not be changed and what aspects of the program can be adapted, (3) identification of the principles that underlie intervention effectiveness, and (4) new approaches that will help to better evaluate what adaptations of evidence-based programs are appropriate.

Institutionalization

Successful translation of evidence-based research findings into practice is highly dependent on institutional support. This is true whether the institution is a private office, a multi-specialty clinic, a health maintenance organization, or a VA hospital. Bradley et al. report that the successful adoption of evidence-based innovations in health care depends on:

> *"[T]he roles of senior management and clinical leadership; the generation of credible supportive data; an infrastructure dedicated to translating the innovation from research into practice; the extent to which changes in organizational culture are required; and the amount of coordination needed across departments or disciplines." (27)*

Commenting on the successful translation of research findings into practice, Lomas *(28)* identifies institutional support (of both clinically relevant research and its translation) as instrumental in improving clinical outcomes. As examples, he credits support for both initiation and translation of relevant health services research by the Veterans Administration and Kaiser Permanente in improving diabetes control, improving screening for cervical cancer and use of β-blockers after myocardial infarction *(28)*. Needless to say, the level of institutional support will depend on the congruence between the interventions and the goals of the organization. Furthermore, members of the administration of the organization may need to be educated on the importance of their role in

(1) defining and (2) visibly supporting the role of evidence-based health care in their organization.

CONCEPTUAL AND EVALUATION FRAMEWORKS FOR TRANSLATIONAL RESEARCH

It would help to have a concise, convenient way to summarize the various issues previously discussed, and to classify the status of interventions along the dimensions important for translation to practice. That is why the RE-AIM framework was developed: to help in the planning and evaluation of interventions intended to produce broad-based effects *(29,30)*. Table 2 briefly summarizes the five RE-AIM dimensions (Reach, Effectiveness, Adoption, Implementation, and Maintenance), provides a brief definition, questions to ask related to that dimension, and strategies that may help to enhance results on that dimension (*see* www.re-aim.org for more detail). *Reach* refers to the breadth of a program in terms of the percent and representativeness of potential patients that will participate in a given intervention. *Effectiveness* is the impact of an intervention on important outcomes, including potential negative effects, quality of life, and economic outcomes. There are also three less often studied, but equally important factors, which concern impact at the level of the organizational setting. These "AIM" dimensions are: *adoption*, or the percent and representativeness of settings, and clinicians within these settings, that are willing to adopt or try a health promotion program; *implementation*, or how consistently various elements of a program are delivered as intended by different staff, and the time/cost requirements of intervention; and *maintenance*, or the extent to which a program or policy becomes institutionalized or part of the routine practices and policies of an organization. Maintenance in the RE-AIM framework also has referents at the individual level. At the individual level, Maintenance refers to the long-term effects of a program on outcomes 6 mo or more following the most recent intervention contact. The RE-AIM framework can be applied in several capacities including planning studies to maximize understanding of both internal and external validity characteristics, comparing the effectiveness of several interventions for policy decisions, and judging the level of "transferability" of findings to other settings and populations *(29,31,32)* (www.re-aim.org).

Examples of RE-AIM Application

It may seem impossible or idealistic to address all the issues in the RE-AIM framework, while still conducting an internally valid study. Admittedly, this way of thinking, with an equal emphasis on internal and external validity, is different than that in which most medical investigators have been trained. However, as illustrated in the two studies described next and summarized in Table 3, it is quite feasible to address all or most of the RE-AIM dimensions in a moderate sized study.

The first study, by Glasgow et al. *(33)* is similar to a traditional randomized controlled trial (RCT). Two-hundred-and-six adult diabetes patients (62% female, average age 63, moderate income and education levels) participated in this 12-mo RCT designed to test the effect of a brief, primary care-based, dietary, self-management program. The program took place in a primary care office with two participating internal medicine physicians. However, with the exception of the physicians, the primary interventionists were research staff employees as opposed to clinical staff members. Intervention group

Table 2
RE-AIM Questions to Ask and Ways to Enhance Overall Impact

Key RE-AIM dimensions for dissemination	Questions to ask of potential programs	Possible ways to enhance translation and dissemination
Reach (Individual Level)	1. What percent of the target population will participate? 2. Does program reach a representative sample and those most in need?	Formative evaluation with users and nonusers Small scale recruitment experiments Identify and reduce barriers Use multiple channels
Effectiveness (Individual Level)	1. Does program achieve key targeted outcomes? 2. Does it produce unintended adverse consequences? 3. What is the impact on quality of life?	Incorporate more tailoring to individual Reinforce via multiple staff modalities and levels Add components to address shortcomings Use stepped care approach
Adoption (Setting/ Organizational Level)	1. What percent of target settings and organizations will use? 2. Will organizations having underserved or high-risk populations use it? 3. Does program help the organization address its primary mission?	Provide different cost options Allow for customization Encourage flexibility and optional modules Formative evaluation with adoptees and nonadoptees
Implementation (Setting/ Organizational Level)	1. What percent of staff within a setting will try this? 2. Can different types of staff members implement the program successfully? 3. Are different components delivered as intended?	Clear intervention protocols Can part of the program be automated? Monitor and provide staff feedback and recognition for implementation
Maintenance (Individual and Setting Level)	1. Does the program produce lasting effects at individual level? 2. Can organizations sustain the program over time? 3. Are those persons and settings that show maintenance, those most in need?	Reduce level of resources required Incorporate "natural environmental" and community supports Conduct follow-up assessments and interviews to learn from those successful and those not Institute incentives and policy supports

Table 3
Results Summary Using RE-AIM Framework

RE-AIM dimension	Results of study	
	Glasgow et al. 2004 (33)	Glasgow et al. 2004 (34)
REACH (Patient participation)	60% of those with a scheduled visit participated. Representative on all measures collected.	75% participation representative on most of measures compared to state BRFSS data.
EFFECTIVENESS (Positive and negative outcomes)	Meaningful improvements. Intervention significantly > computer comparison condition on dietary behavior and cholesterol. Not on A_{1C}.	Significantly improved both laboratory assay and behavioral counseling processes of care, with no decrement in QoL.
ADOPTION (Setting and staff participation)	Only approached and conducted with two clinicians in one clinic.	Only 5% of primary care providers throughout Colorado participated, but surprisingly they were comparable on numerous measures of practice characteristics to a statewide survey of over 1000 PCPs.
IMPLEMENTATION (Intervention delivery)	Consistent implementation but mostly by research staff.	99% received touchscreen computer. 92% discussed with physician. 99% met with care manager. 86% received follow-up call.
MAINTENANCE (Sustainability)	Results on dietary behavior change and cholesterol as strong at 12 mo as 3 mo. No setting level data.	Results on effectiveness measures maintained well at 12-mo follow-up. Setting level sustainability data now being collected.

patients received tailored printouts on their dietary barriers, brief physician reinforcement of the importance of working on managing their diet, and 20-min interventionist counseling that included patient-centered dietary goal setting, problem-solving, and self-help materials. The patient's goals were reinforced at intervals by the interventionist via telephone follow-up calls, and patients returned for a follow-up office visit at 3 mo. Control group patients received the same computer-based assessments as the intervention group, followed by usual care.

Reach for the study was good, with 60% of those who scheduled an outpatient visit participating in the study, and participants being similar to nonparticipants on all measures collected. However, representation was limited resulting from the use of only one clinic, and patients with a scheduled visit. The authors suggested that participation rates could be improved by including the program as part of a routine office visit. *Effectiveness* was evidenced by the long-term impact on dietary behaviors (2.2% less calories from fat, $p = .023$) and serum cholesterol levels (15 mg/dL: $p = .002$) compared to the control condition. HbA_{1c} and body mass index (BMI) were not significantly affected, possibly resulting from the inclusion of both type 1 and type 2 patients, and the fact that a majority of subjects used insulin. Possibly because of these factors, baseline glycemic and weight control were already good. Following intervention, patient satisfaction with their visit was significantly higher for intervention patients compared with controls ($p < .02$). *Adoption* of this cost-effective, simple intervention seems feasible; however, this would need to be tested with clinic staff delivering the intervention vs research staff. *Implementation* of the intervention was consistent, but again it was largely conducted by research staff with the exception of physician advice. *Implementation* of the intervention was also relatively low cost (i.e., $137/patient/yr over usual care). *Maintenance* of individual level results was quite good, with 12-mo results on both dietary patterns and cholesterol being essentially the same as at the 3-mo visit. Information on setting level maintenance is only anecdotal. The clinic staff reported still using the touch-screen computer to set goals after the conclusion of the project, but they were not systematically conducting the follow-up phone calls.

A more recent study illustrates the use of RE-AIM to design and evaluate a broader study that is closer to dissemination, because it was conducted in a variety of clinical settings by usual medical staff. This project by Glasgow et al. *(34)* used results from a computer-assisted, patient-centered intervention to help both patients and clinicians to improve the level of diabetes care. Eight hundred and eighty-six patients with type 2 diabetes under the care of 52 primary care physicians in mixed-payer settings across Colorado participated. Physicians were stratified and randomized to intervention or control conditions and evaluated on two primary outcomes: number of NCQA/ADA recommended laboratory screenings and recommended patient-centered care activities completed (*see* Provider Recognition Program). Secondary outcomes were evaluated using the PAID Quality of Life scale and the PHQ-9 depression scale. Seventy-five percent of eligible patients participated in the project *(reach)*; however, only 5% of physicians approached were willing to participate *(adoption)*. The program was well *implemented* by regular clinical staff having many competing demands (Table 3) and significantly improved both laboratory assays and patient-centered aspects of diabetes care patients received compared to those in randomized control practices that received an alternative touch-screen computer health-risk appraisal program *(effectiveness)*. Both conditions improved in quality of life, but there were no between condition differences on quality of life or depression. These results were *maintained* at a 12-mo follow-up assessment. In summary, patients are very willing to participate in a brief computer-assisted intervention that is effective in enhancing quality of diabetes care. Staff in primary care offices can consistently deliver an intervention of this nature, but most physicians were unwilling to participate in this translation research study.

Practical Clinical Trial Models

As the quote at the beginning of this chapter indicates, one of the best ways to convince practicing clinicians to adopt evidence-based practices is to conduct research that they feel is more relevant to their concerns and setting. In particular, clinicians and administrative decision makers often feel that the results of the "best science" from RCTs and from evidence-based reviews do not apply to their practice setting, the types of patients they see, or the level of resources, time, and expertise they have available.

Table 4
Key Characteristics of Practical Clinical Trials (35,36)

Includes heterogeneous patients, representative of usual care.

Conducted in multiple settings (and by multiple interventionists) to increase
generalizability.

Compares clinical or policy—relevant alternatives (not just comparisons to no treatment
or placebo).

Includes multiple outcomes. Recommended for diabetes are measures of:
1. Representativeness and generalization.
2. Intervention implementation.
3. Cost and economic support.
4. Behavior change of patients and clinicians.
5. Quality of life or possible negative outcomes.
6. Biological outcomes.

Tunis et al. (35) proposed in a seminal article, a solution to this dilemma—namely, a
series of practical clinical trials that would retain the rigor and methodological advantages of RCTs but include characteristics that make them more relevant to target audi-
ences of clinicians and policymakers. As summarized in Table 4, they identify four
characteristics of practical clinical trials. The first is that such studies reach a broad,
diverse, and representative population. Key strategies to achieve this goal are to drastically reduce the exclusion criteria often employed in RCTs, especially those that
exclude patients having other chronic illnesses, psychiatric problems (especially
depression), or that are not sufficiently motivated (e.g., run in periods). The second
characteristic of a practical clinical trial is that it is conducted in multiple and heterogeneous settings. Too often, RCTs have been conducted only in university settings or
in clinics having the greatest resources, staff time, and most advanced technology;
and practitioners legitimately question whether interventions can be implemented (the
first RE-AIM study previously summarized would not meet the criteria for a practical
clinical trial, but the second one would).

The third characteristic of a practical clinical trial is that it evaluates a new intervention, drug, or program against a practical alternative. In many areas of medicine, this
would involve using the current standard of care as a comparison condition rather than
a placebo or no treatment. The rationale is that if a new (and almost always) more
expensive intervention is worthy of adoption, it should be superior to currently available
(and usually less expensive) alternatives—unless it can be demonstrated to be more
cost effective.

The final characteristic is that a practical clinical trial includes multiple outcomes of
interest to key stakeholders. Glasgow (36) has suggested that for diabetes, researchers
wishing to contribute practical clinical trials consider six types of measures (Table 4).
This does not preclude investigators from also collecting other measures central to their
specific aims. The first three types of measures—representativeness, implementation,
and cost (and/or economic outcomes)—can be collected with little or no burden on
participating patients. Representativeness, as in the RE-AIM framework, refers to the
similarity—or lack of comparability—of both participants and settings/clinicians in a

given program compared to those in that geographic area (or the nation), with emphasis on factors such as patient risk level and health disparities. Characteristics of participants can either be directly compared to those who decline participation or to those of the larger population in that region using secondary data such as census or Behavioral Risk Factor Survey data (*see* www.re-aim.org for more detail). Implementation can often be quantified from intervention checklists or contact logs. It is important to assess the extent to which different intervention components are delivered as intended, and the extent to which staff and clinicians of different levels of training and types of expertise can deliver these components. Entire books have been written on economic analysis and detailed discussion is beyond the scope of this chapter *(37)*. However, it is possible to collect the intervention costs and to estimate what it would cost to replicate the intervention in other types of settings *(38,39)* without the complexity and costs of conducting a full economic analysis.

The final two types of measures, behavior change and quality of life, do require moderate amounts of patient time to complete, but there are no alternatives for obtaining the patient perspective on intervention effects. Although "gold standard" measures of patient self-management are sometimes very lengthy and impractical for applied settings, there are brief measures feasible for real-world setting on patient behaviors such as healthy eating and physical activity *(40,41)*. For interventions targeting clinician or system change, it is also important to collect measures of staff and system behaviors. Finally, patient quality of life (and staff quality of work life measures if studying a staff or system change project) is important both as a patient-centered, bottom-line outcome, and also as a method to assess whether inadvertent harm is done. There is a variety of quality-of-life measures available, and a description and discussion of the strengths and limitations of several leading diabetes-related instruments is presented by Polonsky *(42)*.

KEY DIABETES TRANSLATIONAL EFFORTS

It is well documented in almost all representative or national reports of quality of diabetes care that there is a substantial gap between what research tells us (and evidence-based guidelines) and the care most patients receive *(43)*. However, progress is being made, and the teams and institutions reviewed in this section have been among the leaders in enhancing evidence-based care of diabetes care in real-world settings.

The Centers for Disease Control

The Centers for Disease Control (CDC) National Diabetes Prevention and Control Program (NDPCP) was established in 1975 as a small demonstration project and has since grown into a major coordinating force in diabetes translation. The NDPCP now has programs in all 50 states and the District of Columbia and 8 US jurisdictions. At present, the program primarily uses an "influence model" to work with state health departments and other partners *(44)*. The NDPCP has established goals congruent with the Healthy People 2010 public health objectives, and focuses on three "levers for change" (as opposed to conducting or supporting direct clinical or education programs). These levers or foci are: community interventions, health communications, and health systems change. The CDC is explicitly concerned with population health and also monitors the nation's progress on diabetes through surveillance, and reports on both quality of care and patient behavior over time.

The CDC is also currently funding two large programs that are providing important information about real-world systems and multi-level interventions. Project DIRECT is being conducted in poor, largely African American communities in South Carolina and is evaluating a joint community organization and health care system approach to managing diabetes on a community level *(45)*. The more recently funded TRIAD project is evaluating quality of diabetes care and factors related to both care and outcomes in a number of participating managed care organizations throughout the country *(46)*.

NCQA/ADA Provider Recognition Program

Several years ago the American Diabetes Association developed a system to recognize physicians who were providing high levels of diabetes care to their entire panel of patients. The fundamental idea behind this program is to recognize physicians and clinics that are providing excellent care and to make this information widely available. The Provider Recognition Program measures involve a combination of laboratory checks and patient-centered counseling *(47)* (www.ncqa.org/dprp) and thus can be considered "HEDIS Plus" measures because they go beyond the minimal data elements reported in HEDIS. More recently, the National Committee on Quality Assurance has partnered with the ADA in this endeavor, adding increased visibility and prestige to the program. The specific criteria for recognition will continue to change somewhat over time in ways that are congruent with HEDIS and emerging evidence-based practices, but this is one important effort to quantify the level of care being provided and to publicize this information. As of this writing, almost 500 physicians and clinics throughout the United States have achieved recognition status.

The Veterans Administration–Department of Veterans Affairs

The Veterans Administration (VA) has aggressively pursued quality improvement, especially through their research to practice mechanism entitled QUERI *(48,49)*. This ongoing program conducts practical research that is broadly applicable across VA settings. One indication of the success of this program is the recent report by the TRIAD group *(50)* providing evidence that the quality of care conducted in the five VA settings studied was higher than in managed care settings. This report controlled for numerous potential confounding variables including case-mix, and found that the VA settings consistently received higher quality scores.

Breakthrough Series

As in other areas of health care, the Institute for Health care Improvement has conducted a number of quality improvement "collaboratives" (www.ihi.org/IHI/topics/chronicconditions/diabetes). In diabetes, they have partnered with the Group Health Cooperative and their improvement collaboratives have featured content based on the Chronic Care Model of Wagner and colleagues *(18,51,52)*. The process in these collaboratives is for a number of teams, usually around 15–30, but sometimes as large as 100, to define specific goals, and to work with a group of faculty experts and other teams over a 6- to 14-mo period to improve care. Longitudinal data are collected on a registry or panel of patients and a variety of rapid cycle quality improvement "tests" are conducted to evaluate their impact *(53)*. The results of these collaborations, although largely uncontrolled have been impressive in terms of the breadth and consistency of improvement shown by a wide range of different health care systems *(54,55)* (www.rand.icice.org/health/ICICE).

HRSA Health Disparities

A spin-off of these collaboratives has been conducted for diabetes and several other illnesses by the Bureau of Primary Care in a series of "train the trainer" collaboratives conducted in community health and migrant health centers across the country *(56)* (http://bphc.hrsa.gov/programs). The magnitude of improvements produced by these health centers—which serve low-income, frequently uninsured patients and have some of the lowest levels of resources per patient—have been impressive. In terms of the RE-AIM model, both the Health Disparities program and the VA system improvements have been some of the most promising diabetes translation stories in terms of reaching high-risk populations with practical and replicable interventions.

We do not mean to imply that these are the only real-world translational efforts being conducted: for example, several group model health maintenance organization systems and the World Health Organization have active programs to improve diabetes care. The examples above are simply programs that have been widely published and replicated, or about which we have first-hand knowledge. The successes of these programs demonstrate that it is possible to translate research into practice, and to overcome the numerous challenges discussed above to improve care on a system-wide basis for all patients.

CONCLUSIONS: COMPLEXITIES AND CHALLENGES

If the 20th century was characterized by an explosion of biomedical research that elucidated the etiologies and treatments for multiple diseases; then the 21st century may be characterized by efforts to put relevant clinical research into practice in caring for a growing and heterogeneous population. Physicians work in a variety of practice settings with increased administrative obligations. They are under increasing pressure to manage populations (panels) as well as patients, under the scrutiny of observers who measure "quality" by quantifiable outcomes. Evidence-based practice offers one potential solution to the desire to improve both the quality and efficiency of medical care. One step in the process of implementing high-quality, evidence-based changes is the translation of research-based evidence for improving health care outcomes into practice.

As we have seen in this chapter, the process of effective translation of evidence into practice depends on several factors: awareness of one's own practice needs and patient population; an ability to identify high-quality evidence and, equally important, an ability to assess the "translatability" of this evidence (as illustrated by the application of RE-AIM principles); and recognition of the potential benefit of translation by all stakeholders: patients, clinicians, administrators, and overseers. Researchers need to design their interventions and their evaluations with translation in mind.

There have been recent calls for increased recognition of translation by funding agencies as well as commentary designed to bring national attention to this need *(57,58)*. However, not all translation needs to be on a grand, federally funded scale *(57)*. Small-scale trial implementations of evidence-based interventions can be effective. For example, the Plan Do Study Act method *(53)* is an iterative process of trying an intervention in the setting in which it will be used and fine-tuning and adapting it for that setting as it is being implemented *(39,53)*. This sort of small-scale translation and local adaptation can be successful for either making a change in a small practice, or gradually introducing a systematic practice change to a large organization.

Practice change has the highest likelihood of being effective if stakeholders choose from a menu of options to overcome potential barriers in their particular setting *(59)*. Careful work up front to evaluate the potential of a translation effort, coupled with active data collection and revision as needed during the translation process, can result in successful changes in practice and associated improvement in health and quality-of-life outcomes for patients.

ACKNOWLEDGMENTS

Preparation of this manuscript was supported by Grant number 35524 from the NIDDK and HS10123 from the AHRQ.

REFERENCES

1. Centers for Disease Control and Prevention. National Diabetes Fact Sheet: National Estimates and Information on Diabetes in the United States. Department of Health and Human Services, Centers for Disease Control and Prevention, Division of Diabetes Translation, Atlanta, GA, 1997.
2. Nelson RG, Knowler WC, Pettitt DJ, Bennett PH. Kidney disease in diabetes. In: Nelson RG, Knowler WC, Pettitt DJ, Bennett PH, eds. Diabetes in America. National Institutes of Health, Rockville, MD, 1995, pp. 349–400.
3. Wingard DL, Barrett-Connor E. Heart disease and diabetes. In: Harris MI, Cowie CC, Stern M.P., Boyko EJ, Reiber GE, Bennett PH, eds. Diabetes in America. National Institutes of Health, Rockville MD, 2004, pp. 429–448.
4. American Diabetes Association. Economic Costs of Diabetes in the US in 2002. Diabetes Care 2003; 26:917–932.
5. Boyle JP, Honeycutt AA, Narayan KMV, et al. Projection of diabetes burden through 2050: Impact of changing demography and disease prevalence in the U.S. Diabetes Care 2001;24:1936–1940.
6. Diabetes in Children Adolescents Work Group of the National Diabetes Education Program. An update on type 2 diabetes in youth from the national diabetes education program. Pediatrics 2004;114: 259–263.
7. Hogan P, Dall T, Nikolov P. American Diabetes Association. Economic costs of diabetes in the US in 2002. Diabetes Care 2003;26:917–932.
8. Glasgow RE, Hiss RG, Anderson RM, et al. Report of the health care delivery work group: Behavioral research related to the establishment of a chronic disease model for diabetes care. Diabetes Care 2001;24:124–130.
9. Lorig KR, Holman HR. Self-management education: history, definition, outcomes, and mechanisms. Ann Behav Med 2003;26:1–7.
10. McGlynn EA, Asch SM, Adams J, et al. The quality of health care delivered to adults in the United States. N Eng J Med 2003;348:2635–2645.
11. Sackett DL, Straus SE, Richardson WS, Rosenberg W, Haynes R. Evidence-based medicine: How to practice and teach EBM. 2nd ed. Churchill Livingstone, Edinburgh, New York, 2000.
12. Bodenheimer TS, Grumbach K. Electronic technology: a spark to revolutionize primary care? JAMA 2003;290:259–264.
13. Glasgow RE, Bull SS, Piette JD, Steiner J. Interactive behavior change technology: A partial solution to the competing demands of primary care. Am J Prev Med 2004;27:80–87.
14. Glasgow RE, Marcus A, Bull SS, Wilson K. Disseminating effective cancer screening interventions. Cancer 2004;101:1239–1250.
15. U.S. Preventive Services Task Force. Guide to clinical preventive services (2nd ed.). 2nd ed. Williams and Wilkins, Baltimore, MD, 1996.
16. Rakowski W. The potential variances of tailoring in health behavior interventions. Ann Behav Med 1999;21:284–289.

17. Rakowski WR, Breslau E. Perspectives on behavioral science research in cancer screening. Cancer 2004;101:1118–1130.
18. Institute of Medicine, Committee on Quality of Health Care in America. Crossing the quality chasm: A new health system for the 21st Century. National Academy Press, Washington, DC, 2001.
19. Knowler WC, Barrett-Connor E, Fowler SE, et al. Reduction in the incidence of type 2 diabetes with lifestyle intervention or metformin. N Engl J Med 2002;346:393–403.
20. Schillinger D, Piette JD, Bindman A. Closing the loop: missed opportunities in communicating with diabetes patients who have health literacy problems. Arch Intern Med 2003;163:83–90.
21. Schillinger D, Grumbach K, Piette JD, et al. Association of health literacy with diabetes outcomes. JAMA 2002;288:475–482.
22. Basch CE, Sliepcevich EM, Gold RS. Avoiding Type III errors in health education program evaluations. Health Educ Q 1985;12:315–331.
23. Bellg AJ, Borrelli B, Resnick B, et al. Enhancing treatment fidelity in health behavior change studies: best practices and recommendations from the Behavior Change Consortium. Health Psychol 2004;23: 443–451.
24. Mercer SL, MacDonald G, Green LW. Participatory research and evaluation: From best practices for all states to achievable practices within each state in the context of the Master Settlement Agreement. Health Promot Pract 2004;5:167S–178S.
25. Leung MW, Yen IH, Minkler M. Community-based participatory research: A promising approach for increasing epidemiology's relevance in the 21st century. Int J Epidemiol 2004;33499–506.
26. Rogers EM. Diffusion of innovations. 5th ed. Free Press, New York, NY, 2003.
27. Bradley EH, Webster TR, Baker D. Translating research into practice: Speeding the adoption of innovative health care programs. The Commonwealth Fund. Publication no. 724, July, 2004.
28. Lomas J. More lessons from Kaiser Permanente and Veterans' Affairs health care system. Br Med J 2003;327:1301–1302.
29. Glasgow RE, Vogt TM, Boles SM. Evaluating the public health impact of health promotion interventions: The RE-AIM framework. Am J Public Health 1999;89:1322–1327.
30. Glasgow RE. Evaluation of theory-based interventions: The RE-AIM model. In: Glanz K, Lewis FM, Rimer BK, eds. Health behavior and health education. John Wiley and Sons, San Francisco, 2002, pp. 531–544.
31. Glasgow RE, McKay HG, Piette JD, Reynolds KD. The RE-AIM framework for evaluating interventions: what can it tell us about approaches to chronic illness management? Patient Educ Couns 2001;44:119–127.
32. Glasgow RE, Funnell MM, Bonomi AE, Davis C, Beckham V, Wagner EH. Self-management aspects of the improving chronic illness care Breakthrough Series: Implementation with diabetes and heart failure teams. Ann Behav Med 2002;24:80–87.
33. Glasgow RE, La Chance P, Toobert DJ, Brown J, Hampson SE, Riddle MC. Long term effects and costs of brief behavioral dietary intervention for patients with diabetes delivered from the medical office. Patient Educ Couns 1997;32:175–184.
34. Glasgow RE, Nutting PA, King DK, et al. A practical randomized trial to improve diabetes care. J Gen Intern Med, 2005;19:1167–1174.
35. Tunis SR, Stryer DB, Clancey CM. Practical clinical trials. Increasing the value of clinical research for decision making in clinical and health policy. JAMA 2003;290:1624–1632.
36. Glasgow RE. Translating research to practice: lessons learned, areas for improvement, and future directions. Diabetes Care 2003;26:2451–2456.
37. Gold MR, Siegel JE, Russell LB, Weinstein MC. Cost-effectiveness in health and medicine. Oxford University Press, New York, NY, 2003.
38. Meenan RT, Stevens VJ, Hornbrook MC, et al. Cost-effectiveness of a hospital-based smoking cessation intervention. Med Care 1998;36:670–678.
39. Glasgow RE, Magid DJ, Beck A, Ritzwoller D, Estabrooks PA. Practical clinical trials for ranslating research to practice: Design and measurement recommendations. Med Care 2005;43:551–557.
40. Toobert DJ, Hampson SE, Glasgow RE. The summary of diabetes self-care activities measure: results from 7 studies and a revised scale. Diabetes Care 2000;23:943–950.
41. Glasgow RE, Ory MG, Klesges LM, Cifuentes M, Fernald DH, Green LA. Practical and relevant self-report measures of patient health behaviors for primary care research. Ann Fam Med. 2005;3: 73–81.
42. Polonsky W. Emotional and quality-of-life aspects of diabetes management. Current Diabetes Reports 2002;2:153–159.

43. Narayan KMV, Gregg EW, Englegau MM, et al. Translation research for chronic disease: the case of diabetes. Diabetes Care 2000;23:1794–1798.
44. Murphy D, Chapel T, Clark C. Moving diabetes care from science to practice: the evolution of the National Diabetes Prevention and Control Program. Ann Intern Med 2004;140:978–984.
45. Engelgau MM, Narayan KM, Geiss LS, et al. A project to reduce the burden of diabetes in the African-American Community: Project DIRECT. J Natl Med Assoc 1998;90:605–613.
46. Kim C, Williamson DF, Mangione CM, et al. Managed care organization and quality of diabetes care: The Translating Research into Action for Diabetes (TRIAD) study. Diabetes Care 2004;27:1529–1534.
47. Joyner L, McNeeley S, Kahn R. ADA's provider recognition program. HMO Practice 1997;11: 168–170.
48. Reiber GE, Boyko EJ. Diabaetes research in Department of Veterans Affairs. Diabetes Care 2004;27: B95–B98.
49. Sawin CT, Walder DJ, Bross DS, Pogach LM. Diabetes process and outcome measures of the Department of Veterans Affairs. Diabetes Care 2004;27:B90–B94.
50. Kerr EA, Gerzoff RB, Krein SL, et al. Diabetes care quality in the Veterans Affairs Health Care System and commercial managed care: the TRIAD study. Ann Intern Med 2004;141:272–281.
51. Bodenheimer TS, Wagner EH, Grumbach K. Improving primary care for patients with chronic illness. JAMA 2002;288:1775–1779.
52. Wagner EH, Austin BT, Davis C, Hindmarsh M, Schaefer J. Improving chronic illness care: translating evidence into action. Health Affairs 2001;20:64–78.
53. Langley GJ, Nolan KM, Nolan TW, Norman CL, Provost LP. The improvement guide: A practical approach to enhancing organizational performance. Jossey-Bass, San Francisco, CA, 1996.
54. Wagner EH, Glasgow RE, Davis C, et al. Quality improvement in chronic illness care: A collaborative approach. Jt Comm J Qual Improv 2001;27:63–80.
55. Glasgow RE, Davis CL, Funnell MM, Beck A. Implementing practical interventions to support chronic illness self-management in health care settings: lessons learned and recommendations. Jt Comm J Qual Improv 2003;29:563–574.
56. Chin MH, Cook S, Drum ML, et al. Improving diabetes care in Midwest community health centers with the Health Disparities Collaborative. Diabetes Care 2004;27:2–8.
57. Lenfant C. Clinical research to clinical practice—lost in translation? N Engl J Med 2003;349:868–874.
58. Garfield SA, Malozowski S, Chin MH, et al. Considerations for diabetes translational research in real-world settings. Diabetes Care 2003;26:2670–2674.
59. Grol R, Grimshaw J. From best evidence to best practice: effective implmentation of change in patients' care. Lancet 2003;362:1225–1230.

IV CASE STUDIES IN EVIDENCE-BASED PRACTICE

17 The Patient With Type 1 Diabetes and Hypoglycemia

Yogish C. Kudva, MBBS, Teck-Kim Khoo, MD, and Peter J. Tebben, MD

CONTENTS

INTRODUCTION
PATIENT EDUCATION
TARGET BLOOD GLUCOSE
INSULIN PREPARATIONS
CONCLUSION
REFERENCES

INTRODUCTION

Type 1 diabetes (T1D) was fatal prior to the discovery of insulin in 1921. Insulin injections saved the lives of patients with T1D with a dramatic improvement in the symptoms of hyperglycemia and diabetic ketoacidosis *(1)*. Vascular and neuropathic complications of T1D became apparent by the 1950s *(2)*.

Development of technology enabling self-management facilitated the conduct of the Diabetes Control and Complications Trial (DCCT) *(3)*. The DCCT showed a substantive decrease in the risk of microvascular complications and neuropathy with intensive diabetes management. However, intensive diabetes management in the DCCT was associated with a significant increase in the risk of hypoglycemic events including severe hypoglycemia *(4,5)*.

The resources expended in the DCCT to achieve near normal glycemia were formidable and have been difficult to implement in clinical practice. Eleven years after the first report of the DCCT, translation of intensive diabetes management to a significant percentage of the population with T1D in the United States remains a challenge *(6)*. In patients on intensive diabetes management, achieving glycemic goals long term and minimizing hypoglycemia remain formidable challenges *(6a)*.

Soon after the therapeutic use of insulin in patients with T1D, hypoglycemia was recognized as a side effect of such therapy. Even though hypoglycemia continued to be described, the diabetes community had to wait until the DCCT for an accurate

From: *Contemporary Endocrinology: Evidence-Based Endocrinology*
Edited by: V. M. Montori © Mayo Foundation for Medical Education and Research

epidemiologic description. Hypoglycemia in clinical practice may be mild or severe. Mild hypoglycemia is associated with one or more hyperadrenergic symptoms such as sweating, tremor, palpitations, hunger, and prompt relief with ingestion of easily absorbed carbohydrate. Hereafter, severe hypoglycemia is defined as an episode of hypoglycemia requiring third party intervention.

In the following case studies, we illustrate the challenges of hypoglycemia confronting endocrinologists and their patients with T1D attempting to decrease the long-term morbidity of T1D by achieving near normal glycemic status.

Case 1: Frequent, Severe Hypoglycemia in a Patient on Multiple Daily Injection Refusing to Consider Other Therapeutic Options

Our patient is a 58-yr-old male with T1D for 51 yr. Complications include coronary artery disease requiring a coronary artery bypass graft, mild neuropathy, proteinuria, and erectile dysfunction.

Initial treatment of multiple daily injection insulin (MDI) consisted of boluses of regular insulin, with Ultralente for basal needs. He switched to Lispro insulin as bolus insulin when it became available. He continued to experience frequent episodes of mild and occasional severe hypoglycemia. Our patient participated in a randomized clinical trial comparing Ultralente and Glargine as basal insulin in T1D, with a target blood glucose of 80–120 mg/dL. At every stage, multiple treatment options including the external insulin pump and pancreas transplantation were discussed but declined by our patient. He experienced at least one episode of severe hypoglycemia every month necessitating a modification of target blood glucose from 80–120 to 120–180 mg/dL in stages. At the current target, he experiences mild hypoglycemia one to three times per week but severe episodes have decreased in frequency to once every 6–12 mo.

Clinical Question

IN A PATIENT WITH SEVERE HYPOGLYCEMIA ON MULTIPLE DAILY INJECTION REFUSING OTHER OPTIONS, WHAT INNOVATIONS IN MULTIPLE DAILY INJECTION INSULIN ARE AVAILABLE TO DECREASE THE RISK?

In normal subjects, the body continuously secrets insulin in a pulsatile manner. Meals result in an increase in the frequency and amplitude of the secretory pulses. Traditionally, insulin therapies attempt to mimic this by using NPH insulin or Ultralente once or twice a day as basal, and regular insulin at mealtime as bolus. However, even modern insulin preparations are unable to reproduce the physiologic pattern of insulin secretion. The advent of rapid and long-acting insulin analogs in the 1990s has provided a more physiologic means of insulin replacement therapy. Insulin therapy in patients with T1D is intended to maintain near normal glycemia while minimizing hypoglycemia.

The best available data regarding the long-term benefits of normoglycemia, as well as incidence of hypoglycemia in patients with T1D, is found in the DCCT. This was a large multicenter randomized controlled trial (RCT) designed to assess the relationship between glycemic control and development of diabetic vascular complications. The pilot and feasibility trial based on 278 enrollees, conducted in 1986, showed that a large multi-centered randomized study of the relationship between glycemic control and complications could be performed. The risk of hypoglycemia was found to be threefold higher in the intensive control group (7,8). This was followed by the long-term study that provided data regarding long-term benefits of excellent glycemic control. Exclusion criteria included two or more hypoglycemia seizures or comas within the previous 5 yr, although this was changed to all-cause seizures or comas in the previous 2 yr. Enrollment involved 1441 subjects including the patients from the feasibility study. The DCCT found that patients treated with intensive insulin therapy had an increased risk of hypoglycemia (61.2 events/100 patient-years vs 18.7 events/100 patient-years in the intensive-therapy group and the standard-therapy group, respectively $p < 0.001$). This occurred most often during sleep. Risk factors for hypoglycemia in both the intensive and conventional therapy group include male gender, adolescence, no residual C-peptide, or a history of hypoglycemia. This risk was greater in the intensive therapy group *(4,5)*.

In our patient, there are several intervention options to improve glycemic status and minimize large deviations from target blood glucose. These include better patient education programs, adjusting the target blood glucose range, and alternate insulin formulations.

PATIENT EDUCATION

Prior to the DCCT, physicians managed diabetes with less input from the patient. With data from the DCCT regarding excellent glycemic control, as well as the changing role of physicians from a paternalistic to a partnership role, patients now hold a greater responsibility in their own healthcare and management of disease. Hence, it is only logical that education be the primary step in improving glycemic control.

This education includes teaching patients to identify symptoms of hypoglycemia and hyperglycemia, appropriate self-blood glucose monitoring, and accurate record keeping. Cox et al. *(9)* initially performed a RCT evaluating whether blood glucose awareness training (BGAT) could improve the accuracy of patients estimations of blood glucose values. Subjects in the BGAT group improved both their accuracy of blood glucose estimation and hemoglobin A1c. However, subjects did not consistently improve their ability to detect low blood sugars.

Follow-up studies were designed to determine whether an updated BGAT program (BGAT II) could improve hypoglycemia awareness and if this effect could be sustained over a 12-mo period *(10)*. This multicenter study compared patients' ability to estimate blood glucose concentrations before and after the awareness training program. This involved seven training sessions that were based on a standardized training manual that had been updated and expanded since the original BGAT trial. Topics taught included internal cues of hypoglycemia, such as autonomic and neuroglycopenic symptoms, as well as external cues such as timing, amount, and type of insulin, and the effects of exercise. After training, all subjects improved their ability to estimate their blood glucose concentration. However, only subjects with reduced hypoglycemic awareness at baseline were able to improve their ability to detect blood glucose values less than 70 mg/dL. A more recent trial employing BGAT II demonstrated an improved ability of subjects to detect both high and lowblood sugars up to 12 mo after training *(11)*. Despite a reduction in severe hypoglycemia, there was no increase in HbA$_1$C. These studies clearly demonstrate the importance of intensive patient education in the management of T1D. However, because there were no control groups in the BGAT II trials it is difficult to determine whether these reductions in adverse events (DKA, severe hypoglycemia, and motor vehicle violations) were a result of specific training in blood glucose awareness or if it is related to enhanced diabetes education in general.

TARGET BLOOD GLUCOSE

In the DCCT, patients on intensive insulin therapy were found to have an increased risk of hypoglycemia. These patients had a target preprandial blood glucose of 70–120 mg/dL, postprandial of <180 mg/dL, and a 3:00 AM target of >60 mg/dL. With the subgroup analysis showing an increased risk of hypoglycemia in male adolescents with no C-peptide and a history of severe hypoglycemia, one method of minimizing this occurrence would be to increase the target blood glucose. Although this approach has not been tested in clinical studies, the rationale is logical.

INSULIN PREPARATIONS

In 1921, insulin was discovered in Toronto, Canada. Early treatments consisted of multiple injections daily of regular insulin, leading to the quest for longer-acting agents. This resulted in the development of NPH in 1950 and Lente in 1951. Previous insulin regimens consisting of multiple injections of a longer-acting agent such as NPH and a more rapid-acting insulin such as regular are poor mimics of the body's endogenous secretions of insulin and frequently associated with hypoglycemia. With the development of analogs of insulin, several studies are now available comparing these analogs with recombinant insulin preparations.

Newer, rapid-acting insulin analogs have also been introduced in an attempt to more closely mimic the rapid rise and subsequent decline in insulin concentrations after a meal in normal subjects. Little long-term data is available regarding the incidence of severe hypoglycemia in patients treated with rapid acting insulin analogs compared with regular insulin treatment. A meta-analysis of eight studies comparing Lispro insulin to regular insulin was performed by Brunelle et al. *(12)*. A total of 2576 patients with T1D were included among the eight studies. Severe hypoglycemia was defined as coma, the need for an intravenous glucose infusion, or treatment with glucagon. None of the individual studies demonstrated a significant difference in severe hypoglycemia between Lispro and regular insulin treatment. However, when all studies were combined, there was a small but statistically significant decrease in the frequency of severe hypoglycemia associated with the use of Lispro insulin (3.1 vs 4.4% in the Lispro and regular insulin groups respectively; $p = 0.024$) *(12)*.

The introduction of Glargine insulin heralded a significant change in long-acting insulin with no obvious peaks in serum concentrations after an injection. Ratner et al. *(13)* performed a 28-wk multicenter randomized parallel group trial comparing MDI with Glargine at bedtime to NPH insulin one to two times daily, depending on the patients' pre-trial regimen (Table 1). Results showed no significant difference in glycosylated hemoglobin (7.54 vs 7.49% in the Glargine and NPH insulin groups, respectively, $p = 0.44$) or symptomatic hypoglycemia. However, a statistically significant decrease in severe hypoglycemia was observed in the group using Glargine (7.9 episodes per 100 patients/yr vs 16.7 episodes per 100 patients/yr; $p = 0.03$) *(13)*.

In a similar multicenter randomized study of 619 patients followed for 16 wk, a decrease in the variability of fasting blood glucose was found with no difference in the incidence of severe hypoglycemia (5.2 vs 4.6% in the Glargine and NPH insulin groups respectively; $p = 0.67$) *(14)* (Table 1).

In contrast, Rosenstock et al. conducted a shorter 4-wk randomized trial comparing NPH insulin and Glargine (Table 1). The investigators used a dosage for the Glargine

Table 1
Studies Comparing MDI With Glargine to NPH in Patients With Type 1 Diabetes

Author and year	Type of study	Subjects	Duration (week)	Glycemic control	Hypoglycemia
Ratner R et al. 2000 (13)	Multi-centered randomized NPH vs Glargine MDI	534	28	Decreased FBG	Decreased severe hypoglycemia
Rosenstock J et al. 2000 (15)	Multi-center randomized, partially-blinded NPH vs Glargine	256	4	Decreased FBG	Slightly increased hypoglycemia
Raskin P et al. 2000 (14)	Multi-center randomized NPH vs Glargine	619	16	Decreased variability in FBG	No difference

263

group that was equal to the total daily dose of the subjects' pre-study NPH dose. Insulin was titrated to maintain a fasting blood glucose of 72–126 mg/dL. The authors found that Glargine demonstrated a significant benefit in lowering fasting plasma glucose but was associated with a higher rate of hypoglycemia compared to NPH (93.2 vs 97.6–100% of patients reported an episode of hypoglycemia in the NPH and Glargine groups, respectively; $p = 0.03$). This was attributed to an inappropriate starting dose and the relatively short duration of the study, as demonstrated by a decreasing rate of hypoglycemia as the study progressed *(15)*. These studies suggest that, with appropriate usage, Glargine may reduce the frequency of hypoglycemia compared to NPH insulin.

As hypoglycemia still remains an issue, the quest for better insulin preparations continues. For example, insulin detemir appears to have a greater predictability of response compared to NPH *(16)*.

Case 2: Patient on Multiple Daily Injections With Severe Hypoglycemia Interested in Continuous Subcutaneous Insulin Infusion

A 28-yr-old female with a 15-yr history of T1D has frequent hypoglycemia. She has had surgery for cataracts and mild background diabetic retinopathy, but no other complications of diabetes. She was prescribed an MDI program with basal and bolus insulin initially consisting of NPH and regular, and subsequently changed to Lispro and Ultralente.

She experienced one to two episodes of severe hypoglycemia/yr. The option of an insulin pump was discussed, but the patient declined citing concerns with comfort and scarring, and preferred continuing with the MDI program. In 2003, she became pregnant. During her pregnancy, episodes of severe hypoglycemia increased and she experienced three episodes within 2 mo. Several months after delivery of a healthy, term, appropriate for gestational age infant, she opted to begin therapy with continuous subcutaneous insulin infusion (CSII).

Clinical Question

In a Patient With Frequent Severe Hypoglycemia, How Does Continuous Subcutaneous Insulin Infusion Therapy Compare with Multiple Daily Injection in Terms of Preventing Hypoglycemia?

With the availability of techniques to measure urine and blood glucose, the increased glycemic variability in patients with T1D compared to patients with type 2 diabetes was recognized *(17)*. The most significant perturbation of glucose concentration was seen with food intake and attempts were made to normalize both fasting and postprandial glucose concentrations. Various combinations have been studied with intermediate and long-acting preparations to provide basal insulin and short-acting preparations to minimize excursions of blood glucose associated with meals. The best glucose control was achieved with intravenous insulin infusion. Therefore, in the late 1970s efforts started to provide exogenous continuous insulin and, hence, the idea of the insulin pump was conceived.

The CSII, or insulin pump, has been used for over 20 yr and delivers one single, rapid-acting insulin dose subcutaneously. The pump provides a basal infusion throughout the day with user-controlled boluses given before meals *(18)*.

Limited data are available regarding the complications of CSII compared to modern MDI programs. Rapid advances in technology have resulted in continually evolving insulin preparations and pump devices rendering data in the literature irrelevant to current state-of-the-art practice. The primary outcomes of clinical investigation have been based on achieving near normal glycemia rather than minimizing hypoglycemia. Therefore, data regarding a decrease in severe hypoglycemia when comparing MDI to CSII is limited. Several early smaller studies suggest that CSII is associated with a decreased incidence of mild and severe hypoglycemia (19). In the largest series reported to date, Bode et al. (20) published an observational study of 55 patients switching from MDI to CSII (Table 2). Of 255 patients using insulin pumps, 55 were studied since they had been on an MDI program for at least 1 yr and used CSII for at least 1 yr. Patients were followed for a mean of 3.1 yr with quarterly routine visits and 24-h telephone support. The rate of severe hypoglycemia declined significantly in the CSII group without a detrimental effect on HbA_1C values. This effect was sustained for the duration of the study period. Subgroup analysis revealed that patients with baseline HbA_1C greater than 8% had a significant reduction after 1 yr (20). In another prospective case-controlled study of 75 adolescents who chose their insulin program (MDI vs CSII), patients who chose CSII had significantly fewer (approx 50% fewer) episodes of severe hypoglycemia, had lower HbA^1C values, and had lower daily insulin requirements (Table 2). However, this study was performed on subjects without frequent severe hypoglycemia at baseline (21). Meta-analyses comparing the CSII to the MDI suggest that CSII is superior to MDI therapy with improved mean glucose concentrations and HbA_1C (22,23). Several meta-analysis suggest that the CSII use is associated with a decreased frequency of mild and severe hypoglycemia. However, studies prior to 1993 suggested that CSII use was associated with an increased risk of diabetic ketoacidosis and hypoglycemia (24). Because this has not been demonstrated in later studies, this may have been a reflection of less reliable, early model insulin pumps.

CSII offers an attractive alternative to patients with complex T1D suffering from hypoglycemic episodes and has been shown to decrease the incidence of hypoglycemia compared to the MDI. However, the majority of studies did not use Glargine or even Ultralente. Therefore, comparative data between CSII and current MDI programs are still lacking.

Case 3: Patient Recently Started on the Multiple Daily Injection Program and Doing Relatively Well Considering Changing to Continuous Subcutaneous Insulin Infusion

An 18-yr-old woman was diagnosed with T1D 1 yr prior when she presented with diabetic ketoacidosis, a blood glucose concentration of 835 mg/dL, and a HbA_1C of 15.0%. Insulin treatment was initiated with formal instruction in an MDI program shortly after diagnosis.

She did well on her MDI program consisting of Glargine once daily with a rapid acting analogue with meals. Her current HbA_1C was 5.6%. She would only rarely be out of her target blood glucose range of 80–120 mg/dL.

She would infrequently have mild hypoglycemic episodes, usually occurring preprandial or after strenuous physical activity. At follow-up, she expressed satisfaction with her diabetes management, but was interested in learning more about CSII.

Table 2
Studies Comparing Rate of Hypoglycemia in MDI vs CSII

| Author, year of publication | Type of study | N MDI | N CSII | Duration | Rate of severe hypoglycemia (per 100 patient-yr) | | | | |
| | | | | | MDI | CSII | | | |
						1 yr	2 yr	3 yr	4 yr
Boland E et al. 1999 (21)	Prospective case-controlled	50	25	1 yr	46	24	N/A	N/A	N/A
Bode BW et al. 1996 (20)	Prospective crossover	55	55	3.1 yr (mean)	138	22	26	39	36

Note: Rate of severe hypoglycemia in the DCCT; 62/100 patients/yr with intensive treatment and 19/100 patient/yr with standard treatment.

Clinical Question

In Uncomplicated Type 1 Diabetes, Does Continuous Subcutaneous Insulin Infusion Provide Additional Benefit as Compared With the Multiple Daily Injection?

In this patient with recently diagnosed diabetes who was doing relatively well on her MDI insulin regimen, the decision to convert to CSII becomes more challenging. Several studies have been published comparing the two in terms of HbA₁C, hypoglycemia, glycemic variability, and DKA.

Boland et al. *(21)* reported an observational, parallel study evaluating 75 nonrandomized patients with no more than two severe hypoglycemic episodes in the last 6 mo (CSII *n* = 25; MDI *n* = 50). The authors reported significant reductions in severe hypoglycemia by nearly 50% in the CSII group compared to the MDI group despite a lower HbA₁C level *(21)*. More recently, several authors have published randomized, controlled trials. Hanaire-Broutin et al. *(18)* conducted a randomized crossover study of 41 patients with T1D. Patients were assigned to CSII or MDI, both using lispro insulin, for two crossover periods of 16 wk. The investigators reported that HbA₁C levels at the end of each treatment period were significantly lower with CSII compared to the MDI group (7.89% with CSII and 8.24% with MDI, *p* < 0.001) but there was no significant difference in the frequency of mild and severe hypoglycemia between groups *(18)*. However, hypoglycemic events were reported only in the last 14 d of each treatment period, possibly introducing a source of bias owing to increased patient compliance right before the follow-up visit.

Tsui et al. *(25)* reported a 9-mo randomized parallel trial of 27 patients using either CSII or MDI with Lispro, which showed no differences in hypoglycemia (8.0 vs 7.4 hypoglycemic events over 9 mo in the CSII and MDI groups, respectively; *p* > 0.10) or HbA₁C between groups (7.73% for CSII and 8.16% for MDI; *p* > 0.10) *(25)*.

In a more recent 16-wk randomized controlled trial comparing CSII to MDI using Glargine insulin in youth with T1D, a significant reduction in HbA₁C was observed in the group randomized to CSII (*see* Fig. 1). The CSII patients in this study had a baseline HbA₁C of 8.1%. This is consistent with the study by Bode et al., which demonstrates improvement in glycemic control in patients with a baseline HbA₁C greater than 8%, which was not seen in patients with a baseline HbA₁C less than 8%. However, because of the limited duration of the study and small number of patients, limited conclusions can be made regarding the complications of each treatment regimen. This is the only published randomized controlled trial comparing MDI using Glargine insulin to CSII.

Whereas larger randomized controlled studies are needed to document the incidence of severe hypoglycemia in each treatment regimen, data thus far appear to show greater efficacy of CSII in reducing hypoglycemic episodes compared to MDI. In patients with a baseline HbA₁C greater than 8%, there appears to be an improvement in HbA₁C in CSII treated patients compared to those on MDI. As previously mentioned, it must be kept in mind that the majority of studies comparing CSII to MDI have used NPH one to two times daily as the basal insulin, which is not consistent with most intensive insulin programs currently being prescribed to patients with T1D.

Therefore, in patients with few hypoglycemic events on MDI programs and lower HbA₁C values, there is insufficient evidence to support switching to CSII to improve

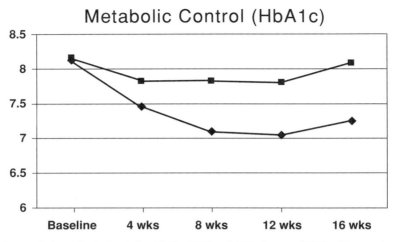

Fig. 1. HbA1c trends in patients treated with the CSII vs MDI. Square: MDI with aspart and glargine, Diamond: CSII with aspart. Doyle et al. Diabetes Care July 2004.

glycemic control. Other factors would need to be considered in the decision-making process include patient preference, cost, and available resources regarding insulin pump training and management.

Case 4: Patient With Severe Hypoglycemia While on Continuous Subcutaneous Insulin Infusion, Wishing to Consider Islet Transplantation

A 34-yr-old male with T1D for 31 yr, had been on the MDI with poor control prior to starting CSII therapy 9 yr ago. Even on CSII, he experiences frequent hypoglycemia, with up to one severe episode every 4–6 mo.

He enjoys good health although he has had laser surgery for retinopathy. The patient is very interested in islet transplantation.

Clinical Question

HOW DOES ISLET TRANSPLANTATION COMPARE TO CONTINUOUS SUBCUTANEOUS INSULIN INFUSION IN TERMS OF HYPOGLYCEMIC RISK AND GLYCEMIC PROFILE?

Soon after the discovery of insulin, the idea of transplanting isolated islets was conceived. However, islets were successfully isolated from rodent models only by 1967. Early human trials yielded poor results, with only about 8% providing sustained insulin independence. Goals of islet transplantation in patients with T1D not tolerating intensive diabetes management include elimination of hypoglycemia, and restorations of insulin secretion.

In a landmark paper, Shapiro et al. (26) described sustained insulin independence in seven patients treated with glucocorticoid-free immunosuppression, a program referred to as the Edmonton protocol. All seven patients had a history of metabolic instability and frequent severe hypoglycemia. Induction immunosuppression was achieved by daclizumab and sirolimus. Maintenance therapy consisted of sirolimus and low-dose tacrolimus. All patients required islets from at least two cadaveric pancreas.

Ryan et al. (27) later published an update with 17 recipients of islet transplant with the Edmonton protocol. Median follow-up was 20.4 mo. Twelve of fifteen (80%) patients

---

Factors in the Consideration of SCII vs MDI for Type I Diabetes

Patient Factors:
- Comfort
- Ease of use of treatment regimen
- Esthetics
- Financial reasons
- Medical suitability

Physician Factors:
- Unfamiliarity
- More experience in traditional injection symptoms
- Lack of educator support
- Lack of infrastructure for follow-up of device

Healthcare System Factors:
- Expense of wide-scale introduction of infusion systems
- Multidisciplinary approach implementation
- Infrastructure

---

were insulin independent 1 yr after islet transplantation. At the time of article submission, 11 patients were insulin independent *(27)*.

Hirshberg et al. *(28)* report a cohort of six patients undergoing islet transplantation with less promising results. All were women with at least 5 yr of diabetes and undetectable C-peptide, who were experiencing severe hypoglycemia. They were otherwise free of other significant medical conditions. The follow-up period ranged from 17 to 22 mo. Following the procedure, three patients remained insulin independent for greater than 18 mo once adequate islet numbers were infused. One patient resumed insulin therapy after immunosuppression was discontinued secondary to adverse effects, and two patients required oral hypoglycemic agents to maintain optimal glucose levels. None of their patients suffered a repeat episode of severe hypoglycemia. Explanations for the lower success rate offered by the authors included that the protocol used limited patients to islets from only two donors, and that of the six patients, one patient suffered a complication that resulted in her receiving only one islet dose. The authors concluded that although islet transplantation can bring insulin independence, the procedure is not yet perfected and that glycemic profile is often imperfect and deteriorates in time. These studies used islets procured by more than one donor, which makes clinical application difficult in view of the lack of donors.

Single center experiences described above indicate a need for a multi-center effort in islet transplantation. The Immune Tolerance Network funded a multi-center trial of Islet transplantation alone (ITA) (ITN trial) to replicate the results from Edmonton *(26,27)*. Four patients underwent islet transplantation alone at each of nine centers. Enrollment was completed by January 2003. Primary end point is insulin independence at 3 yr after ITA. Results will be available after January 2006. Preliminary results reveal 52% success after ITA from two cadaver donors *(29,30)*. Centers with more extensive experience achieved 90% insulin independence compared to centers with less experience (23%). Peer-reviewed publication of results is eagerly awaited.

In an attempt to compare the glycemic profiles of diabetes patients treated with different therapies, Kessler et al. *(31)* conducted a short study using continuous glucose monitoring systems. Twenty-six patients with T1D were monitored over 72 h; 10 patients were on CSII therapy, 9 patients with simultaneous pancreas–kidney transplantation (SPK), and 7 patients with pancreatic islet transplantation after kidney grafting (IT). In the IT group, four patients were totally insulin independent while the remaining three had decreased exogenous insulin needs. The authors found that the mean glucose concentration and variability in the PK and IT groups were significantly lower than the CSII group. The mean concentration in the IT group was 104.9 ± 14.6 mg/dL compared to CSII of 140.6 ± 27.9, with a variability of 23.8 ± 9.5 vs 62.5 ± 29.9. No hypoglycemia was noted in the SPK and insulin-independent IT groups.

In previous studies, more than one islet donor was required to result in insulin independence. This poses a problem in the clinical setting, as deceased donor organs are in scant supply. Recently, Hering et al. *(32)* conducted a study of six patients with T1D who received single-donor islet transplantation. These were done with optimized pancreas preservation, islet processing and induction immunosuppression. Four of the six patients maintained insulin independence and freedom from hypoglycemia 1 yr after islet transplant. One patient had reduced graft function requiring exogenous insulin whereas one had graft failure 2 wk after transplantation. This study provides exciting evidence, that with optimal preparation and procedure, single donor transplantation resulting in insulin independence is feasible *(32)*.

In summary, islet transplant can be performed successfully. However, this field is in its infancy. Long-term data on islet function and outcomes while on chronic immune suppression is unknown. Two significant factors affecting clinical success include skill in preparing high-quality and high-yield islets, as well as keeping immunosuppressant levels within a specified target range *(29)*. Adverse effects including gastrointestinal morbidity, nephrotoxicity, hypertension, and hyperlipidemia have been reported. So far, however, islet transplant shows great promise in reducing hypoglycemia faced by patients with brittle type 1 T1D on intensive diabetes management.

Case 5: Pancreas Transplant Alone While on Pump

A 59-yr-old female has a history of T1D for 48 yr. She had been on MDI for 11 yr before switching to CSII because of frequent, severe hypoglycemia. In spite of good medical continuing care, she experienced over 10 episodes of severe hypoglycemia per year, resulting in a referral for pancreatic transplantation. She was in good health. She had hypertension and mild background retinopathy but was otherwise in good health.

The patient underwent a pancreatic transplant alone (PTA) more than 2 yr ago without complications. Because of recurrent episodes of urinary tract infections, she underwent an enteric conversion of her PTA more than 1 yr ago.

Clinical Question

IN A PATIENT WITH TYPE 1 DIABETES AND INTACT RENAL FUNCTION, HOW DOES PANCREATIC TRANSPLANTATION COMPARE TO STANDARD MEDICAL THERAPY?

Pancreatic transplantation has been in use for treatment of diabetes in humans since 1966. This invasive procedure was associated with a high degree of morbidity and mortality before newer techniques and advances in immunosuppression led to improved survival and increasing popularity of this procedure. The pancreas may be transplanted alone (PTA), simultaneously with a kidney (SPK), or after kidney transplantation (PAK).

The International Pancreas Transplant Registry 2002 report recorded 18,909 pancreas transplants performed as of October 2002 *(33)*. This number increased to 19,600 in the 2003 mid-year report, with 14,300 performed in the United States alone, and 5300 elsewhere. From 1988 to 2002, most transplants were simultaneous pancreas–kidney transplants whereas pancreas transplantation alone contributed to about 6%.

Using much of this data, Venstrom et al. *(34)* conducted a retrospective observational multi-center cohort study of 11,572 patients on the waiting list for PTA or PKA. The main outcome was all-cause mortality within 4 yr following transplantation compared with similar patients not undergoing transplantation. The authors found that patients who underwent a PTA had an increased risk of mortality of 1.57%. Although patient selection might have played a role in these results (that patients who were able to wait were likely doing better), they were nonetheless startling. The authors concluded that patients with preserved renal function undergoing a pancreas transplant alone had significantly worse outcome than those awaiting transplantation. This subject is still hotly debated.

Based on clinical experience, it is generally accepted that PTA, when successful, would result in freedom from hypoglycemia, although mild hypoglycemia has been reported before. There is a lack of large-scale data on the prevalence of hypoglycemia in PTA because of the characteristics of the patient cohort. Redmon et al. *(35)* did conduct a case–control study on 27 patients, 10 of whom had symptoms of hypoglycemia after transplant, 9 asymptomatic transplant patients, and 8 healthy subjects. These patients were given a mixed-meal and then underwent a modified 24-h fast during which only sugar-free gelatin, diet soda, and bouillon were given. Blood glucose, insulin, C-peptide, and glucagons levels were measured at various times. The authors found that transplant patients who reported frequent hypoglycemia tended to have lower glucose values after an overnight fast. After 24 h they had significantly lower blood glucose concentrations (71 vs 81 mg/dL). However, patients in this study did not find these glucose levels disabling.

CONCLUSION

PTA remains a viable alternative for T1D patients and is associated with improved glycemic profile and decreased incidence of severe hypoglycemic events. However, limited data exists regarding application to a population of patients with T1D. Most patients may be self-selected and follow-up is frequently of short duration or incomplete in the longer term. Because of the surgical morbidity and mortality, patients should be carefully selected for suitability.

REFERENCES

1. Clarke B. Historical perspective. Hypoglycaemie and Diabetes: Clinical and Physiological Aspects. Edward Arnold, London, 1993, pp.1–16.
2. Nathan DM. Long-term complications of diabetes mellitus. N Engl J Med 1993;328:1676–1685.
3. The Diabetes Control and Complications Trial Research Group. The effect of intensive treatment of diabetes on the development and progression of long-term complications in insulin-dependent diabetes mellitus. N Engl J Med 1993;329:977–986.

4. The Diabetes Control and Complications Trial Research Group. Epidemiology of severe hypoglycemia in the diabetes control and complications trial. Am J Med 1991;90:450–459.
5. The Diabetes Control and Complications Trial Research Group. Hypoglycemia in the Diabetes Control and Complications Trial. Diabetes 1997;46:271–286.
6. Tabak AG, Tamas G, Zgibor J, et al. Targets and reality: a comparison of health care indicators in the U.S. (Pittsburgh Epidemiology of Diabetes Complications Study) and Hungary (DiabCare Hungary). Diabetes Care 2000;23:1284–1289.
6a. Barr CC. Retinopathy and nephropathy in patients with type I diabetes four years after a trial of intensive insulin therapy, by the Diabetes Control and Complications Trial/Epidemiology of Diabetes Interventions and Complications Research Group. N Engl J Med 2000;342:381–389.
7. The Diabetes Control and Complications Trial (DCCT). Design and methodologic considerations for the feasibility phase. The DCCT Research Group. Diabetes 1986;35:530–345.
8. Diabetes Control and Complications Trial (DCCT): results of feasibility study. The DCCT Research Group. Diabetes Care 1987;10:1–19.
9. Cox DJ, Gonder-Frederick L, Julian D, et al. Intensive versus standard blood glucose awareness training (BGAT) with insulin-dependent diabetes: mechanisms and ancillary effects. Psychosom Med 1991;53:453–462.
10. Cox D, Gonder-Frederick L, Polonsky W, Schlundt D, Julian D, Clarke W. A multicenter evaluation of blood glucose awareness training-II. Diabetes Care 1995;18:523–528.
11. Cox DJ, Gonder-Frederick L, Polonsky W, Schlundt D, Kovatchev B, Clarke W. Blood glucose awareness training (BGAT-2): long-term benefits. Diabetes Care April 2001;24:637–642.
12. Brunelle BL, Llewelyn J, Anderson JH, Jr., Gale EA, Koivisto VA. Meta-analysis of the effect of insulin lispro on severe hypoglycemia in patients with type 1 diabetes. Diabetes Care 1998;21:1726–1731.
13. Ratner RE, Hirsch IB, Neifing JL, Garg SK, Mecca TE, Wilson CA. Less hypoglycemia with insulin glargine in intensive insulin therapy for type 1 diabetes. U.S. Study Group of Insulin Glargine in Type 1 Diabetes. Diabetes Care 2000;23:639–643.
14. Raskin P, Klaff L, Bergenstal R, Halle JP, Donley D, Mecca T. A 16-week comparison of the novel insulin analog insulin glargine (HOE 901) and NPH human insulin used with insulin lispro in patients with type 1 diabetes. Diabetes Care 2000;23:1666–1671.
15. Rosenstock J, Park G, Zimmerman J, Group USIGTDI. Basal insulin glargine (HOE 901) versus NPH insulin in patients with type 1 diabetes on multiple daily insulin regimens. U.S. Insulin Glargine (HOE 901) Type 1 Diabetes Investigator Group. Diabetes Care 2000;23:1137–1142.
16. Danne T, Lupke K, Walte K, Von Schuetz W, Gall MA. Insulin detemir is characterized by a consistent pharmacokinetic profile across age-groups in children, adolescents, and adults with type 1 diabetes. Diabetes Care 2003;26:3087–3092.
17. Service FJ, Molnar GD, Rosevear JW, Ackerman E, Gatewood LC, Taylor WF. Mean amplitude of glycemic excursions, a measure of diabetic instability. Diabetes 1970;19:644–55.
18. Hanaire-Broutin H, Melki V, Bessieres-Lacombe S, Tauber JP. Comparison of continuous subcutaneous insulin infusion and multiple daily injection regimens using insulin lispro in type 1 diabetic patients on intensified treatment: a randomized study. The Study Group for the Development of Pump Therapy in Diabetes. Diabetes Care 2000;23:1232–1235.
19. Eichner HL, Selam JL, Holleman CB, Worcester BR, Turner DS, Charles MA. Reduction of severe hypoglycemic events in type I (insulin dependent) diabetic patients using continuous subcutaneous insulin infusion. Diabetes Research 1988;8:189–193.
20. Bode BW, Steed RD, Davidson PC. Reduction in severe hypoglycemia with long-term continuous subcutaneous insulin infusion in type I diabetes. Diabetes Care 1996;19:324–327.
21. Boland EA, Grey M, Oesterle A, Fredrickson L, Tamborlane WV. Continuous subcutaneous insulin infusion. A new way to lower risk of severe hypoglycemia, improve metabolic control, and enhance coping in adolescents with type 1 diabetes. Diabetes Care 1999;22:1779–1784.
22. Pickup J, Mattock M, Kerry S. Glycaemic control with continuous subcutaneous insulin infusion compared with intensive insulin injections in patients with type 1 diabetes: meta-analysis of randomised controlled trials. BMJ 2002;324:705.
23. Weissberg-Benchell J, Antisdel-Lomaglio J, Seshadri R. Insulin pump therapy: a meta-analysis. Diabetes Care 2003;26:1079–1087.
24. Anonymous. Implementation of treatment protocols in the Diabetes Control and Complications Trial. Diabetes Care 1995;18:361–676.

25. Tsui E, Barnie A, Ross S, Parkes R, Zinman B. Intensive insulin therapy with insulin lispro: a randomized trial of continuous subcutaneous insulin infusion versus multiple daily insulin injection. Diabetes Care 2001;24:1722–1727.
26. Shapiro AM, Lakey JR, Ryan EA, et al. Islet transplantation in seven patients with type 1 diabetes mellitus using a glucocorticoid-free immunosuppressive regimen. N Engl J Med 2000;343:230–238.
27. Ryan EA, Lakey JR, Rajotte RV, et al. Clinical outcomes and insulin secretion after islet transplantation with the Edmonton protocol. Diabetes 2001;50:710–719.
28. Hirshberg B, Rother KI, Digon BJ, 3rd, et al. Benefits and risks of solitary islet transplantation for type 1 diabetes using steroid-sparing immunosuppression: the National Institutes of Health experience. Diabetes Care 2003;26:3288–3295.
29. Shapiro AM, Ricordi C, Hering B. Edmonton's islet success has indeed been replicated elsewhere. Lancet 2003;362:1242.
30. Shapiro AM, Ricordi C. Unraveling the secrets of single donor success in islet transplantation. Am J Transplant 2004;4:295–298.
31. Kessler L, Passemard R, Oberholzer J, et al. Reduction of blood glucose variability in type 1 diabetic patients treated by pancreatic islet transplantation: interest of continuous glucose monitoring. Diabetes Care 2002;25:2256–2562.
32. Hering B, Kandasamy R, Harmon J, et al. Transplantation of cultured islets from two-layer preserved pancreases in type 1 diabetes with anti-CD3 antibody. Am J Transplant 2004;4:390–401.
33. Gruessner AC, Sutherland DE. Pancreas transplant outcomes for United States (US) and non-US cases as reported to the United Network for Organ Sharing (UNOS) and the International Pancreas Transplant Registry (IPTR) as of October 2002. Clin Transpl 2003;21–51.
34. Venstrom JM, McBride MA, Rother KI, Hirshberg B, Orchard TJ, Harlan DM. Survival after pancreas transplantation in patients with diabetes and preserved kidney function. JAMA 2003;290:2817–2823.
35. Redmon JB, Teuscher AU, Robertson RP. Hypoglycemia after pancreas transplantation. Diabetes Care 1998;21:1944–1950.

18 The Patient With Medically Complicated Obesity

Kurt A. Kennel, MD

CONTENTS

INTRODUCTION

Obesity is a worldwide epidemic as evidenced by the number of overweight and obese individuals and the magnitude of their obesity *(1)*. At the end of the last millennium, nearly one-third of all adults in the United States were classified as obese *(2)*. The prevalence of severe obesity (body mass index [BMI] >40 kg/m^2), which is associated with the highest health risk, doubled between 1990 and 2000 *(3)*. Given the prevalence of overweight among children and teens aged 6–19 yr tripled between 1980 and 2000 *(4)* and that overweight children often become overweight adults *(5)* the problem is likely to persist for some time *(6)*. Obesity in adults is associated with excess morbidity most notably excess risk of coronary heart disease, hypertension, hyperlipidemia, diabetes, gallbladder disease, certain cancers, and osteoarthritis *(7,8)*. Beyond morbidity, strong evidence links obesity to increased mortality. For example, young men and women with severe obesity may lose as much as 13 and 8 yr of life, respectively, as compared to peers of a healthy weight *(9)*.

Although the negative impact of overweight and obesity on morbidity and mortality is well documented, the evidence that weight loss is effective in the long-term treatment of disease and prolonging life is not. Most studies investigating the effect of weight loss on mortality to date are inadequately powered, uncontrolled for confounding variables or of insufficient duration *(10)*. Despite the availability of clinical guidelines and admonitions from multiple organizations (8), rates of diagnosis and treatment of obesity by physicians are low and increase only after moderate to severe obesity or co-morbidity have developed *(11–14)*. Equally important are patients' perceptions of weight and their

From: *Contemporary Endocrinology: Evidence-Based Endocrinology*
Edited by: V. M. Montori © Mayo Foundation for Medical Education and Research

goals for weight loss, which may be unrealistic. For example, Foster et al. *(15)* polled overweight patients regarding their perception of desirable weight loss. Study participants considered an average weight reduction of 25–32% as "desirable" or "acceptable," whereas a 17% weight loss was only considered "disappointing." Therefore, it is important for both physicians and patients considering treatment options for obesity to appreciate the data from a number of studies showing that even modest weight loss (losing up to 10% of body weight) improves quality of life and important disease risk factors such as blood pressure, cholesterol, and blood glucose *(8,16,17)*. The goal of this article is to demonstrate how a physician–patient encounter for obesity treatment can utilize the values and characteristics of the patient, clinical judgment of the physician and use of the available evidence to provide optimal care of the patient *(12)*.

CLINICAL ASSESSMENT OF THE OBESE PATIENT

A detailed history and examination focused on obesity may seem beyond the scope of a time-limited consultation or a chapter on an evidenced-based approach to the treatment of medically complicated obesity. Nothing could be further from the truth. Given the complexity of the problem and diversity of the obesity treatment literature, an in-depth understanding of each patient's obesity and co-morbid conditions is essential to be able to analyze and apply data from the literature and guidelines to their care *(19,20)*. Although uncommon, secondary causes of obesity, such as hypothalamic injury or thyroid dysfunction, may be missed without a systematic assessment of the obese patient. Not to be forgotten in the process is further assessment and treatment of co-morbid conditions independent of recommendations for obesity treatment. Examples include pain management for degenerative joint disease or clarification of the etiology of dysfunctional uterine bleeding. Ignoring the responsibility to treat the whole patient leads to a common complaint by obese patients that they are told "you just need to lose weight" when treatment, independent of weight loss, is available to improve health and quality of life *(21)*. Evidence-based practice must also consider that data evaluating the use of diagnostic tests and treatments may need to be interpreted differently in an obese population. The treatment of essential hypertension in the severely obese patient is a representative example *(22)*. Ultimately, the most important product of this comprehensive assessment is an understanding of the patient's insight, goals, and expectations for the treatment of their obesity, which is essential for the application of evidence to their care.

Severe Medically Complicated Obesity Case Presentation

A 60-yr-old male is self-referred for treatment of his obesity. He reports being overweight as a child and further weight gain as an adult. He recalls weight gain associated with smoking cessation and initiation of insulin therapy but he attributes much of his weight gain to declining physical activity as he aged. He is currently at his maximum weight of 159 kg.

He has several poorly controlled obesity co-morbidities including type 2 diabetes mellitus, hypertriglyceridemia, hypertension, advanced degenerative joint disease of the knees, gout, and gastroesophageal reflux disease. He has coronary artery disease with bypass grafting and a recent negative stress test. Medical treatment includes: insulin glargine (44 U daily), rosiglitazone, simvastatin, gemfibrozil, atenolol, amlodipine, furosemide, omeprazole, allopurinol, fluoxetine, and aspirin. There is no relevant surgical history.

As a small business owner he works long hours and, until now, prioritized work over healthy living. He wished to lose weight as he was concerned he would loose his business because of his health. Playing with his grandchildren and "just being around for them" was a motivating factor as well. His wife, who was formerly obese, was present and supportive. She expressed concern about his libido and erectile function. A cursory lifestyle history revealed that he is sedentary and feels unable to pursue physical activity because of knee pain and daily fatigue. Dietary patterns were unstructured including liberal use of convenience foods, skipping meals, and eating away from home. He had no psychiatric history but volunteered that he ate to manage stress. His wife observed that other triggers for eating included low blood glucose and watching television. He did not use tobacco or alcohol but drank soda regularly. Several first degree relatives were obese.

Physical examination revealed a height of 170 cm and weight of 159 kg (BMI 55 kg/m^2), blood pressure 150/88, and regular pulse of 80 beats/min. Truncal obesity without cushingoid features, a large abdominal pannus with intertriginous candidal infection, penile retraction, antalgic gait, pitting edema in both legs, and somnolence were notable findings. A summary of his laboratory data included normal thyroid, renal, and hepatic function tests. Triglycerides, plasma glucose, and HbA1c are elevated. Serum total testosterone was low with luteinizing hormone (LH) and follicle-stimulating hormone (FSH) in the lower half of the reference range.

His prior attempts at weight loss were revealing. He had met with a registered dietitian as part of diabetes education. A meal plan was provided but the patient felt hungry and "deprived" and abandoned the diet before any significant weight loss or follow-up. He attended a weight loss program in a residential setting away from home that instructed him in a low-fat diet and daily physical activity. He lost weight but did not maintain the new lifestyle when he returned to his home and eventually regained to his baseline weight. He had frequently initiated diets on his own but these attempts were unstructured, unsupervised, and short-lived. Treatment with amphetamines for obesity as a young adult was temporarily successful and associated with adverse effects.

This patient has severe obesity leading to medical complications that were motivating him to seek assistance with weight loss given past failed attempts (23). Observations made during the assessment relevant to the final recommendations included poor lifestyle behaviors, secondary hypogonadism, a question of a sleep-related breathing disorder, and the possible contribution of medications to weight gain and edema. Secondary causes of obesity were largely excluded. Although he had lost weight in the past, it was not sustained. How should his physician counsel him now that he was ready to take further action to manage his weight?

SEARCHING, EVALUATING, AND APPLYING THE EVIDENCE FOR WEIGHT LOSS TREATMENT

Lifestyle changes are the most common recommendation received by obese patients seeking assistance with losing weight. In addition to promoting healthy nutrition and fitness, diet therapy aims to decrease calorie intake while exercise therapy seeks to increase energy expenditure. A more intensive approach to effecting lifestyle change may involve behavior therapy. This intervention is performed under the guidance of psychologist or a workbook, in a group or individual setting, and may incorporate techniques to self-monitor eating and activity behavior, reduce eating cues, manage mood nonpharmacologically, and avoid relapse. These basic components of lifestyle change are used variably by clinicians and may be recommended singly or as additive measures for patients not meeting weight-loss goals. Although patients may report having tried to change lifestyle on their own, application of these interventions in a medically supervised program is the first step in most guidelines for the treatment of obesity *(8)*.

For a 60-yr-old man with severe medically complicated obesity who has failed to lose weight on his own, does medical nutrition therapy alone or in combination with other treatments such as exercise or behavior therapy result in modest (10%) weight loss?

Searching Medline using terms "diet therapy" or "medical nutrition therapy" and "obesity" yielded a large number of citations, which is not unexpected given the plethora of studies on the topic. However, limiting results using methodological filters that identify studies most likely to yield valid results eliminated all citations or yielded citations that were too focused for the question. A search of Medline using the National Library of Medicine's PubMed and its Systematic Reviews filter (under the Clinical Queries section) using the search terms "medical nutrition therapy" *AND* "obesity" yielded 77 citations. Two systematic reviews of randomized controlled trials (RCTs), which are part of a larger report commissioned by the National Health Service Research and Development Health Technology Assessment Programm *(24)* in the United Kingdom, are reviewed in abstract form. Whereas the first *(25)* focuses on the efficacy of medical nutrition therapy alone, the second investigates the utility of adding exercise, behavior therapy, drug therapy, or combinations thereof to weight reducing diets *(26)*. As the articles were part of a larger review, the search methods, inclusion and exclusion criteria, assessment of study quality, selection of outcomes, and methods of analysis were identical. Supporting the validity of these analyses is a prespecified protocol patterned after the methods of the Cochrane Collaboration. This included attention to study validity noting studies chosen ensured similar baseline characteristics, complete followup, a control group, and randomization—although subjects and investigators generally were not "blind" to treatment allocation.

The analysis of medical nutrition therapy for weight loss included low-fat diets, low-calorie diets of varying degrees, and protein-sparing modified fasts (liquid protein diets). The limited data available for analysis is readily apparent in the small fraction (26 out of 2163) of studies screened that qualified for inclusion. Of those included, most enrolled few participants, lasted just 12 mo, did not conceal randomization, and did not use an intention-to-treat analysis. About half of the recruited subjects with metabolic complications of obesity included men and were located in the United States. Only one study included subjects with severe obesity. Limiting inclusion to trials lasting at least 1 yr is a strength that influenced the inquiring practitioner to review the article but limited the number and scope of studies included considerably. Both studies intended to study dichotomous outcomes such as mortality, and surrogate endpoints such as cardiovascular risk factors, adverse events, and cost, in the final analysis the number and size of the trials yielded results with limited precision. Therefore, weight change is the only meaningful outcome reported.

Overall the weight change associated with a low-fat and low-calorie diet favored the treatment over the control with a mean weight change of –5 kg (–3.5 to –6 kg) at 12 mo. Significant statistical heterogeneity was noted but the direction of effect was consistent across all studies. Although only three studies included data beyond 12 mo, the average weight loss at 12, 24, 36, and 60 mo was consistently less and/or nonsignificant than at 12 mo implying regain of weight as is seen in most long-term studies of obesity treatment. Interestingly, subjects in the two studies with the least mean change in weight had the largest mean BMI (34 kg/m^2). When reported, weight loss resulting from low fat diet in this analysis was associated with small improvements in blood pressure, lipids, and plasma glucose at 12 mo consistent with other studies (27–29).

The efficacy of co-interventions with weight reducing diets in adults with obesity is of a similar magnitude (26). Compared to diet alone, the addition of exercise to diet is associated with a –2 kg (–3.2 to –0.7 kg) weight change at 12 mo. Data at 18 mo (–7.6 kg, –10.3 to –5.0 kg) and 36 mo (–8.2 kg, –15.3 to –1.2 kg) show still greater weight change but come from only two studies and the confidence intervals are wide. Four studies adding behavior therapy to diet therapy were notable for no randomization and only one intention-to-treat analysis. Weight reduction at 12 mo of –7.7 kg (–12.0 to –3.4) was reported with nonsignificant differences between groups beyond 12 mo and up to 60 mo. Combining diet, exercise, and behavior therapy yielded inconsistent results and overall suggested no additive benefit over diet therapy alone but was limited to two studies.

There are several limitations specific to the study of additive effects of interventions for weight loss. There are variations between methods of dietary, exercise, and behavior therapy. For example, for the exercise interventions previously analyzed, all but one study used supervised exercise. Furthermore, there may be overlaps between therapies intentionally or because therapists may be used to provide exercise counseling, diet recommendations may include behavioral advice. It may be difficult to replicate these interventions in clinical practice. Finally, weight change in the control groups, who were generally following a low-fat diet, were often less than reported for diet-therapy-only trials as discussed in the dietary therapy only study (25). This finding, and wide confidence intervals around the mean, raises the possibility that the actual differences between diet therapy compared with diet with co-interventions could be even less significant in clinical practice than suggested by this systematic review.

Ultimately, the quality of the trials available for review in both analyses raise questions about the validity of the results, even though the methods of the reviews are sound. Although it is possible that the efficacy of these treatments was underestimated as a result, applicability of the results to this heavier, older male patient is also in question. For example, the severely obese patient may represent a different or more extreme pathophysiological condition (30) and might respond differently to interventions such as medical nutrition therapy. The additional 2 kg weight loss reported with the addition of exercise to diet therapy may not be anticipated for this patient if he cannot match the intensity and duration of exercise of a motivated, younger, lighter, and relatively healthier study volunteer. Finally, adverse events were rarely reported in the trials included in the analysis limiting assessment of treatment benefit vs harm.

Treatment recommendations should consider which outcomes and what magnitude of effect are of significance to the patient and physician. What if a 10% weight loss at 12 mo was acceptable to the patient and physician? It is possible they could be persuaded of this by reminding them there would be some impact on the patient's metabolic co-morbidity and because this would be a greater weight loss than he had ever achieved on his own. If one takes this most optimistic view of the patient's dilemma and applies it to the interpretation efficacy of diet therapy alone or diet therapy plus exercise (–6.0 kg and –9.2 kg representing the upper end of the confidence intervals), this patient might lose 4 and 6%, respectively, of his total body weight at 12 mo. However, taking the most pessimistic view of the evidence, if the patient were to experience a weight loss at the lower end of the confidence intervals (–3.5 kg and –4.2 kg) compared to the subjects studied, he would only lose about 3% of his body weight at 12 mo.

Either way, both physician and patient chose to pursue diet therapy and exercise as part of a healthy lifestyle but neither is confident that these interventions alone or in combination are sufficient to treat his obesity. The physician then considers the role of pharmacotherapy thinking that appetite suppression or malabsorption of nutrients will augment the potential for weight loss with lifestyle changes. Side effects and long-term safety are the clinician's anticipated concerns when considering this approach.

For a 60-yr-old man with severe medically complicated obesity who has failed to lose weight with medical nutrition therapy and exercise counseling, does pharmacotherapy improve the chances for modest (10%) weight loss with an acceptable risk?

A search in Medline limiting results to Evidence-Based Medicine Reviews in the OVID interface (selects articles highlighted by the ACP Journal Club and Cochrane Reviews) with the terms "obesity" and "pharmacotherapy" yields three citations. Two systematic reviews specifically address pharmacotherapeutic interventions for obesity using meta-analysis. Review of the abstracts reveals that one article analyzes several medications that are no longer available for clinical use with limited information on the currently approved medications. The other, the Cochrane Review *(10)* "Long-term pharmacotherapy for obesity and overweight" by Padwal and Lau, seems pertinent for review in full text.

Several strengths of the article are notable when considering the application of the results to the clinical question. First is the detailed description of the methods of the review including quality assessment of the RCTs screened for inclusion. Concise descriptions of the studies included and excluded from the analysis are helpful for applying the results of the analysis to the treatment of the patient. The rationale for the medications and outcomes analyzed is supported by background information on the health hazards associated with obesity, the potential benefits of weight loss, and the availability of the agents for clinicians to prescribe them. Given the frequency of relapse in obesity treatment *(31)*, the inclusion and separate analysis of both weight loss and weight maintenance studies as well as the exclusion of studies of short duration is laudable.

All studies included were of similar quality but they also shared two ubiquitous problems in obesity trials. The first was high attrition rates in both treatment and control arms, which affected the validity of the studies including the results of this analysis. Even with the use of last-observation-carried-forward intention-to-treat analyses, high attrition rates in treatment and control groups may introduce considerable bias in favor or against treatments. The other weakness was the inclusion of weight loss during a "run-in" phase prior to randomization in the reported results, which inflates the absolute amount of weight loss in each study arm. However, the authors meticulously analyzed the results with this in mind and, as such, this did not affect the relative difference between treatment and controls which was how the results were presented in the review. Even so, the number of subjects who dropped out or who were excluded from randomization for noncompliance during the "run-in" phase was usually not reported. Thus, the pool of subjects studied was even more enriched than the average study population, further limiting the applicability of the results to patients in usual care. As expected, 15 of 16 studies included were supported by the drug manufacturer with employees listed as authors in half.

The subjects studied were younger (late 40s), lighter (BMI upper 30s), and mostly female (about 80%). Most studies included subjects with obesity co-morbid conditions and utilized standardized low-fat, hypocaloric diet (500–600 kcal/d deficit) recommendations. Although groups within a study were compared equally, co-interventions—such as exercise counseling and intensity of follow-up—varied across studies, which may affect inter-study comparisons and extrapolation to patient care. As included studies were not designed to measure hard outcomes, weight change was the primary outcome of the analysis. With the clinician in mind the authors had intended to analyze subgroups by BMI quartile but outcomes stratifying by baseline BMI was not available for analysis. Discussion of the clinical significance of the weight change results was supplemented with analysis of secondary endpoints as available from selected trials.

The results from studies of sibutramine excluded this drug for consideration in this patient. Although sibutramine therapy did produce a −4.3 kg (−3.6 to −4.9 kg) weight change relative to placebo at 1 yr in weight loss trials, patients using selective serotonin reuptake inhibitors were excluded because of the risk of serotonin syndrome (32). Uncontrolled hypertension was also an exclusion criterion. Sibutramine therapy was associated with an increase in systolic blood pressure of 1.9 mm Hg (0.2–3.6 mm Hg) and a heterogenous but consistent increase in diastolic blood pressure (range 1–4 mm Hg). Even for normotensive obese patients, these findings raise important questions about the effects of sibutramine therapy on mortality and cardiovascular morbidity as compared to the effects of weight loss.

Analysis of weight loss with orlistat vs placebo showed −2.7 kg (−2.3 to −3.1 kg) greater loss in favor of orlistat at 1 yr. In studies reporting percent weight change, orlistat therapy was associated with a −2.9% (−2.3 to −3.4%) weight change. Three of the studies analyzed exclusively enrolled subjects with type 2 diabetes and showed similar greater weight change and a 0.2% (0.2–0.3%) greater reduction in HbA1c with orlistat. Small changes in blood pressure and lipid parameters and fasting plasma glucose in favor of orlistat were observed. When the outcome of 5 or 10% weight loss at 1 yr (as opposed to absolute weight loss was analyzed), an average of 21% (19–24%) and 12% (8–16%), respectively, more subjects receiving orlistat achieved this goal than those on placebo. Weight maintenance was significantly improved with orlistat in as much as the differences in weight between the orlistat group and placebo group were preserved. However, both groups were regaining weight at essentially the same rate. Adverse effects were limited to readily reversible gastrointestinal symptoms. However, the heterogeneity of these effects, ranging from incontinence to transient loose stools, is difficult to predict in standard clinical practice in part as a result of the interaction of the several variables (orlistat, fat content of diet, current bowel habit). Variable reporting of these adverse events allows only a summary of individual study findings. However, in all studies there was a consistent, significant increase (16–40%) in the rate of gastrointestinal events in orlistat treated subjects as compared with placebo.

Although the overall effect of orlistat on weight loss was small compared to placebo, the magnitude and direction of effect was consistent across studies. It does somewhat increase the chance of achieving a 10% weight loss and has small but positive effects on glycemia, lipids, and blood pressure, which were the outcomes sought in the clinical question. Both by study data and the known mechanism of action of the drug, it appears that risk of harm is low, especially if a multivitamin is taken. Although higher risk study subjects seemed to lose slightly less weight with orlistat vs lower risk subjects, and noting the differences between the patient and the population represented in the study, a trial of orlistat appears reasonable to discuss with the patient for his consideration.

After the recommendation was discussed, the patient stated he was unwilling to use medications of any type in the treatment of his obesity. Not appreciated in the initial assessment was that his wife was found to have valvular heart disease after using the combination fenfluramine and phentermine (fen-phen) *(33)*. The patient also had negative memories about the physician-recommended use of amphetamines to treat his obesity in his youth. Additional discussion regarding the mechanism of action of orlistat differentiating it from centrally acting agents and the safety data gleaned from the systematic review did not change his perspective. This unexpected development exemplifies the importance of assessing and considering patients' values, expectations, and preferences in evidence-based practice *(18,20)*.

At this point the patient expressed that he was skeptical that medical therapies were likely to assist him in reaching his goals for health. Although he appreciated the potential impact of modest weight loss on his metabolic complications, he restated the degree of disability he experienced in performing activities of daily living such as personal hygiene, use of public transportation, and physical intimacy with his spouse resulting from his severe obesity. Even the best possible response suggested by the evidence to the treatment options previously presented was unlikely to satisfactorily improve these concerns. In contrast to the question of drug therapy for weight loss where the patient is the sole decision maker because of his fixed beliefs, he tentatively asks the physician's opinion regarding surgery for weight loss. He admitted he was overwhelmed by the positive and negative information he had received about bariatric procedures, but after the discussion of medical options he wondered if he should consider a more aggressive approach to treatment of his obesity.

What is the efficacy and safety of bariatric surgery in achieving weight loss and improving health in a 60-yr-old man with severe medically complicated obesity?

A search of the National Library of Medicine's PubMed using the clinical queries sensitive (broad) filter for treatment studies and the search terms "bariatric" or "obesity surgery" yielded 302 citations. Restricting the search to be specific (narrow) reduced this to 19 citations none of which appear useful. Applying the same search using the systematic reviews filter yields 36 citations. Two systematic reviews using meta-analysis focusing on medical outcomes after weight loss surgery are reviewed in abstract form. Whereas one focuses on the outcome of diabetes mellitus, the other, "Bariatric Surgery: a systematic review and meta-analysis" by Buchwald et al. in JAMA

(34) was selected as it considered the outcomes of four diseases which pertained to the clinical case.

This systematic review included a detailed description of study retrieval, inclusion and exclusion criteria, and analytic methods. Both meta-analyses and weighted means of outcomes were performed and reported. Strengths of interest to the clinical question included the separate analysis of four distinct bariatric procedures, clear definitions of the measured outcomes, and large pooled sample size of about 22,000 subjects. The authors took great care to avoid double counting patients given a number of "kin" publications (91 of the 136 fully extracted studies). Weaknesses included the lack of randomized or controlled trials, with three of every four subjects analyzed representing an uncontrolled single-center case series. However, when the data from five randomized controlled trials were examined separately, the results were within the range of values and trends found in the overall meta-analysis.

As in almost all weight loss studies, the patients included were predominantly women and were relatively young, with a mean age of 39 yr (range 16–63 yr). Unlike most studies, the mean BMI at baseline was 47 kg/m^2, thus characterizing these patients as severely obese. Outcomes reported represented an average of 2 yr of follow-up. In keeping with the usual reporting of outcomes in the bariatric surgery literature, the analysis reported change in body weight as percentage of excess body weight lost. Other criteria often cited as guidelines as to whom should and should not have bariatric surgery *(35,36)* were not reported in the baseline characteristics of the study subjects. Although the validity of some of the individual studies analyzed could be questioned, the magnitude of the effect on weight change, rates of improvement or resolution of four co-morbid conditions, and dose-response to the degree of restriction/malabsorption all argued against random chance or bias as an explanation for results.

Relative to the efficacy of medical treatments for obesity, all four categories of bariatric procedures studied consistently resulted in a large weight loss with an overall percentage of excess weight loss for all type of procedures of 61% (58–64%). This is of particular relevance to the severely obese patient who has a poor chance or achieving a healthy weight even with a large weight loss. When defined as the ability to discontinue diabetes medications and achieve normal blood glucose, 77% (71–83%) of subjects had complete resolution of their diabetes. Improvement in glycemia or resolution of diabetes increased this rate to 86% (78–94%). The risk reduction was proportional to weight loss achieved. As such, procedures with a greater malabsorptive component (biliopancreatic diversion or duodenal switch) had higher rates of resolution than purely restrictive procedures (gastric banding). Improvement in hyperlipidemia was demonstrated in 70% with variation in the results depending on the measure used and degree of malabsorption of the procedure. Considering all procedures as a total population showed continuous measures such as total cholesterol decreased an average of 33 mg/dL (23–44 mg/dL) and triglycerides 80 mg/dL (65–96 mg/dL). Hypertension resolved in 62% (56–68%) and improved or resolved in 76% (71–86%) of the total population with variable efficacy of the four procedures. Similarly, obstructive sleep apnea and other obesity-related sleep-disordered breathing resolved in 86% (79–92%) and improved or resolved in 84% (72–95%). Most of this data came from gastric bypass trials.

This second part of the question is related to the risks of a bariatric procedure in this patient. This review was able to report operative mortality, 30 d or less after surgery, in a large subset of subjects. Operative mortality ranged from 0.1% for purely restrictive procedures to 1.1% for biliopancreatic diversion. Although this provides a starting point for consideration of harm, analysis of co-variables such as age, cardiopulmonary status, or volume of procedures performed is not available. In this patient, age might be an important co-variable given the range of age of subjects in the analysis by Buchwald et al. *(39)* was 16–64 yr. Data regarding complications of bariatric surgery are available but do not constitute a systematic assessment of harm vs benefit *(37–41)*. Variability in surgical technique, bariatric procedure recommended, support systems and facilities, and rigor of follow-up in addition to the multifaceted complications (psychological, medical, or surgical) of such procedures add to the uncertainty. Therefore, a physician recommending bariatric surgery would need to be aware of the performance of the bariatric surgery program being considered. The perception of risk by the patient may ultimately be influenced more by their current health status and their observations of individuals within their community who have undergone a bariatric or other major abdominal surgery.

The physician discussed these data and the role of a bariatric procedure to treat the patient's obesity and co-morbidity and recommended that the patient consider this approach further. The patient was impressed at the potential magnitude and rapidity of weight loss with bariatric surgery, noting he was advised by his orthopedic surgeon to lose weight to reduce joint pain, and in anticipation that joint replacement would be needed in the future. The large amount of weight lost with a bariatric procedure relative to medical treatments is associated with a significant decline in reported joint pain and improved fitness for joint replacement *(42)*. Although not totally committed to this approach yet, he trusted the recommendation and requested a referral to a bariatric surgery program. He was referred to an informational meeting presented by a local bariatric surgery program to gather further information.

Independent of the obesity treatment plan, his physician recommended evaluation and treatment for the patient's co-morbid conditions. Consultation with a sleep specialist was requested to assess for a sleep-related breathing disorder noting his complaints of fatigue and observation of somnolence during the examination. As both insulin and thiazolidine-dione therapy were associated with edema and weight gain *(43,44)*, a trial of metformin in place of rosiglitazone while continuing insulin therapy was recommended *(45)*. However, this change was deferred for action until the presence and severity of a sleep-related breathing disorder was clarified and treated. Substitution of an alternative antihypertensive was recommended, noting worsening of edema after initiation of amlodipine for hypertension. The patient was encouraged to continue to consult with his orthopedist for joint injection and water-based physical therapy to ameliorate his joint pain. He was encouraged to continue to assess his work-life balance and lifestyle patterns and seek to make practical changes to improve his nutrition, fitness, and stress level. He was offered resources to assist him in making these changes. A follow-up appointment was scheduled to discuss his progress with these recommendations and additional clinical questions that may arise as a result of the bariatric informational meeting.

CONCLUSIONS

Current evidence about medical approaches for the treatment of obesity are largely inadequate mostly as a result of the lack of long-term efficacy and focus on patient-important hard outcomes. This is particularly true of options for the management of severe obesity. Even though short-term modest weight loss can improve cardiovascular risk factors and can be demonstrated with lifestyle modification or pharmacotherapy alone or in combination, the durability, effect on hard outcomes, and magnitude of this weight loss is unsatisfactory to obese patients *(15)*. Given the potential for some medical interventions for weight loss to cause harm, clinicians must judiciously apply less robust evidence when making recommendations. It is clear that the complexity of the problem will require more study and new strategies to find an effective solution *(46)*. Important data regarding the effects weight loss on cardiovascular events in patients with type 2 diabetes are expected from a large, long term, randomized-controlled trial *(47)*. This study and others will add to the evidence available for treatments and systems of care for the prevention and treatment of obesity.

Although an evidence-based treatment plan is in place for the patient presented in this article, a final review of the clinical case and critique of the investigation of treatment options exposes many other clinical questions that could have been considered in determining clinical recommendations. How does the presence of a normal weight (actually "reduced obese") supportive partner impact the efficacy of a weight loss treatment? How does the presence or absence of stress-eating behaviors influence the response to a treatment for obesity? Can genotype predict the efficacy of a weight loss intervention? Even after considering the methods used to apply evidence to the patient with endocrine disease, the clinical judgment of the physician remains central to evidence-based practice as exemplified by the matter of which questions to ask on behalf of the patient.

REFERENCES

1. Obesity: preventing and managing the global epidemic. Report of a WHO consultation. World Health Organ Tech Rep Ser 2000;894:i–xii,1–253.
2. Flegal KM, Carroll MD, Ogden CL, Johnson CL. Prevalence and trends in obesity among US adults, 1999–2000. JAMA 2002;288:1723–1727.
3. Freedman DS, Khan LK, Serdula MK, Galuska DA, Dietz WH. Trends and correlates of class 3 obesity in the United States from 1990 through 2000. JAMA 2002;288:1758–1761.
4. Ogden CL, Flegal KM, Carroll MD, Johnson CL. Prevalence and trends in overweight among US children and adolescents, 1999–2000. JAMA 2002;288:1728–1732.
5. Serdula MK, Ivery D, Coates RJ, Freedman DS, Williamson DF, Byers T. Do obese children become obese adults? A review of the literature. Prev Med 1993;22:167–177.
6. Hedley AA, Ogden CL, Johnson CL, Carroll MD, Curtin LR, Flegal KM. Prevalence of overweight and obesity among US children, adolescents, and adults, 1999–2002. JAMA 2004;291:2847–2450.
7. Mokdad AH, Ford ES, Bowman BA, et al. Prevalence of obesity, diabetes, and obesity-related health risk factors, 2001. JAMA 2003;289:76–79.
8. National Institutes of Health. Clinical guidelines on the identification, evaluation, and treatment of overweight and obesity in adults—the evidence report. Obes Res 1998;6:51S–209S.
9. Fontaine KR, Redden DT, Wang C, Westfall AO, Allison DB. Years of life lost due to obesity. JAMA 2003;289:187–193.
10. Padwal R, Li SK, Lau DC. Long-term pharmacotherapy for obesity and overweight. Cochrane Database Syst Rev 2004:CD004094.
11. Galuska DA, Will JC, Serdula MK, Ford ES. Are health care professionals advising obese patients to lose weight? JAMA 1999;282:1576–1578.
12. Sciamanna CN, Tate DF, Lang W, Wing RR. Who reports receiving advice to lose weight? Results from a multistate survey. Arch Intern Med 2000;160:2334–2349.
13. Stafford RS, Farhat JH, Misra B, Schoenfeld DA. National patterns of physician activities related to obesity management. Arch Fam Med 2000;9:631–638.
14. Wadden TA, Anderson DA, Foster GD, Bennett A, Steinberg C, Sarwer DB. Obese women's perceptions of their physicians' weight management attitudes and practices. Arch Fam Med 2000;9:854–860.

15. Foster GD, Wadden TA, Phelan S, Sarwer DB, Sanderson RS. Obese patients' perceptions of treatment outcomes and the factors that influence them. Arch Intern Med 2001;161:2133–2139.
16. Kushner RF, Foster GD. Obesity and quality of life. Nutrition 2000;16:947–952.
17. Blackburn G. Effect of degree of weight loss on health benefits. Obes Res 1995;3:211s–216s.
18. Montori VM, Guyatt GH. What is evidence-based medicine? Endocrinol Metab Clin North Am 2002;31:521–526, vii.
19. Expert Panel on the Identification, Evaluation, and Treatment of Overweight in Adults. Clinical guidelines on the identification, evaluation, and treatment of overweight and obesity in adults: executive summary. Am J Clin Nutr 1998;68:899–917.
20. Kushner RF, Roth JL. Assessment of the obese patient. Endocrinol Metab Clin North Am 2003;32: 915–933.
21. Collazo-Clavell ML. Safe and effective management of the obese patient. Mayo Clin Proc 1999;74: 1255–1259; quiz 1259–1260.
22. Hall J. Obesity, hypertension and renal disease. In: Eckel RH, ed. Obesity : Mechanisms and Clinical Management. Lippincott Williams Wilkins, Philadelphia, PA, 2003, pp. 273–300.
23. Gorin AA, Phelan S, Hill JO, Wing RR. Medical triggers are associated with better short- and long-term weight loss outcomes. Prev Med 2004;39:612–616.
24. Avenell A, Broom J, Brown TJ, et al. Systematic review of the long-term effects and economic consequences of treatments for obesity and implications for health improvement. Health Technol Assess 2004;8:iii–iv, 1–182.
25. Avenell A, Brown TJ, McGee MA, et al. What are the long-term benefits of weight reducing diets in adults? A systematic review of randomized controlled trials. J Hum Nutr Diet 2004;17:317–335.
26. Avenell A, Brown TJ, McGee MA, et al. What interventions should we add to weight reducing diets in adults with obesity? A systematic review of randomized controlled trials of adding drug therapy, exercise, behaviour therapy or combinations of these interventions. J Hum Nutr Diet 2004;17: 293–316.
27. Sacks FM, Svetkey LP, Vollmer WM, et al. Effects on Blood Pressure of Reduced Dietary Sodium and the Dietary Approaches to Stop Hypertension (DASH) Diet. N Engl J Med 2001;344:3–10.
28. Appel LJ, Champagne CM, Harsha DW; Writing Group of the PREMIER Collaborative Research Group. Effects of comprehensive lifestyle modification on blood pressure control: main results of the PREMIER clinical trial. JAMA 2003;289:2083–2093.
29. Diabetes Prevention Program Research Group. Reduction in the incidence of type 2 diabetes with lifestyle intervention or metformin. N Engl J Med 2002;346:393–403.
30. Eckell R. Obesity: disease or physiologic adaptation? In: Eckel RH, ed. Obesity: Mechanisms and Clinical Management. Lippincott Williams Wilkins, Philadelphia, PA, 2003, pp. 3–30.
31. McGuire MT, Wing RR, Klem ML, Hill JO. Behavioral strategies of individuals who have maintained long-term weight losses. Obes Res 1999;7:334–341.
32. Product Information: Meridia(R). Abbott Laboratories, North Chicago, IL, 2004.
33. Wadden TA, Berkowitz RI, Silvestry F, et al. The fen-phen finale: a study of weight loss and valvular heart disease. Obes Res 1998;6:278–284.
34. Buchwald H, Avidor Y, Braunwald E, et al. Bariatric surgery: a systematic review and meta-analysis. JAMA 2004;292:1724–1737.
35. Balsiger BM, Luque de Leon E, Sarr MG. Surgical treatment of obesity: who is an appropriate candidate? Mayo Clin Proc 1997;72:551–557; quiz 558.
36. Consensus Development Conference Panel. NIH conference. Gastrointestinal surgery for severe obesity. Ann Intern Med 1991;115:956–961.
37. Presutti RJ, Gorman RS, Swain JM. Primary care perspective on bariatric surgery. Mayo Clin Proc 2004;79:1158–1166; quiz 1166.
38. Monteforte MJ, Turkelson CM. Bariatric surgery for morbid obesity. Obes Surg 2000;10:391–401.
39. Buchwald H. A bariatric surgery algorithm. Obes Surg 2002;12:733–746; discussion 747–750.
40. Brolin RE. Bariatric surgery and long-term control of morbid obesity. JAMA 2002;288:2793–2796.
41. Balsiger BM, Murr MM, Poggio JL, Sarr MG. Bariatric surgery. Surgery for weight control in patients with morbid obesity. Med Clin North Am 2000;84:477–489.
42. Peltonen M, Lindroos AK, Torgerson JS. Musculoskeletal pain in the obese: a comparison with a general population and long-term changes after conventional and surgical obesity treatment. Pain 2003;104:549–557.

43. Henry R. Obesity and type II diabetes mellitus. In: Eckel RH, ed. Obesity: Mechanisms and Clinical Management. Lippincott Williams Wilkins, Philadelphia, PA, 2003, pp. 229–272.

44. Aronne LJ. Obesity as a disease: etiology, treatment, and management considerations for the obese patient. Obes Res 2002;10:95S–96S.

45. Lee A, Morley JE. Metformin decreases food consumption and induces weight loss in subjects with obesity with type II non-insulin-dependent diabetes. Obes Res 1998;6:47–53.

46. Ogden CL, Carroll MD, Flegal KM. Epidemiologic trends in overweight and obesity. Endocrinol Metab Clin North Am 2003;32:741–760, vii.

47. Ryan DH, Espeland MA, Foster GD, et al. Look AHEAD (Action for Health in Diabetes): design and methods for a clinical trial of weight loss for the prevention of cardiovascular disease in type 2 diabetes. Control Clin Trials 2003;24:610–628.

19 The Patient at Risk for Diabetes
Considering Prevention

Sarah E. Capes, MD, MSc, FRPC

CONTENTS

INTRODUCTION

More than 170 million people worldwide have diabetes, and the World Health Organization (WHO) projects that this number will more than double by the year 2030. Most of the increase is expected to occur in developing countries, where diabetes already affects people in their most productive years, the 45- to 64-yr age bracket *(1)*. In the United States, an estimated 17.7 million people have diabetes, and this number is expected to increase to 30.3 million by 2030 *(2)*. Thus, diabetes is poised to become one of the primary causes of disability and death worldwide within the next 25 yr. From these data, it is clear that there is an urgent need to develop and implement effective strategies to prevent diabetes. This chapter will review the evidence regarding predictors of diabetes and therapies to prevent diabetes, and will discuss how diabetes prevention strategies can be applied in the "real world."

WHO IS AT RISK FOR DIABETES?

Predisposition to diabetes is likely to be caused by a complex interaction among genetic, environmental/lifestyle factors, and possibly perinatal factors. Large cohort studies have identified several key predictors of diabetes.

Age

In most populations, type 2 diabetes is rare before age 30 but increases with age. In 6000 men enrolled in the Usual Care group of the Multiple Risk Factor Intervention

From: *Contemporary Endocrinology: Evidence-Based Endocrinology*
Edited by: V. M. Montori © Mayo Foundation for Medical Education and Research

Table 1
Risk Factors for Type 2 Diabetes

Definite risk factors
  Increasing age
  Obesity
  Central fat distribution
  Weight gain in adulthood
  Ethnicity
  Low birthweight
  Sedentary lifestyle
  Family history of diabetes
  Impaired glucose tolerance and impaired fasting glucose
  Hypertension
  Dyslipidemia (high triglyceride, low HDL cholesterol, high VLDL cholesterol levels)
  Polycystic ovary syndrome
Probable risk factors
  Gestational diabetes
  Diet: High-glycemic load
        Low-cereal fiber content
Possible risk factors
  Abstention from alcohol
  Cigarette smoking
  Schizophrenia

Trial (MRFIT), the incidence of diabetes over 5 yr follow-up increased by 30% for each 5-yr increment in age *(3)*. In NHANES III, the prevalence of diabetes (diagnosed and undiagnosed) in the United States rose from 1–2% at ages 20–39 to 18–20% at ages 60–74, with a plateau after age 75 *(4)*.

Obesity and Central Fat Distribution

Risk of type 2 diabetes also increases with increasing body mass index (BMI), defined as weight in kilograms per height in meters squared) (Table 2). In men in the MRFIT Usual Care cohort, the risk of diabetes almost doubled for each 5 kg/m^2 increase in BMI *(3)*. The risk may extend into the "normal" range of BMI (20–25 kg/m^2); for women in the Nurses' Health Study, the risk of self-reported diabetes doubled for BMI 22–22.9 kg/m^2, tripled for BMI 23–23.9 kg/m^2, and was five times higher for BMI 25–26.9 kg/m^2 compared to BMI under 22 kg/m^2 *(5)*. Central fat distribution further increases the risk of type 2 diabetes for a given BMI *(6–8)*. In American men, waist circumference >40 in. (101 cm) or waist-to-hip ratio >0.99 were associated with a significantly increased risk of self-reported diabetes *(7)*. In American women, waist circumference >29 in. (76 cm) or waist-to-hip ratio >0.75 indicated an increased risk *(8)*. Weight gain in adulthood of more than 10 kg after age 18 in women *(5)* or more than 8 kg after age 21 in men *(7)* was also associated with an increased risk of clinical diabetes independent of BMI in early adulthood.

Ethnicity

The prevalence of type 2 diabetes varies substantially among different ethnic groups. The most accurate estimates of prevalence come from large population-based surveys

Table 2
Clinical Trials of Diabetes Prevention

Reference (no.)	Study population	Intervention	Results
Finnish Diabetes Prevention Study (62)	522 middle-aged men and women with IGT. Mean BMI 31 kg/m².	Lifestyle modification (individualized counseling to reduce weight and fat intake, and increase fiber intake and physical activity)	Mean 3.2 yr incidence of DM 11% (95%; CI 6–15%) in intervention group vs 23% (95%; CI 17–29%) in control group. RRR = 58% (p < 0.001).
Diabetes Prevention Program Study (63)	3234 nondiabetic men and women, mean BMI 34.0 kg/m² + fasting hyperglycemia (5.3–6.9 mmol/L) and IGT.	Lifestyle modification (16-lesson curriculum and individualized support to achieve ≥7% weight loss through low-calorie and low-fat diet + physical activity ≥150 min/wk)	After mean follow-up 2.8 yr, incidence of DM 4.8/100 person-yr in the lifestyle group vs 11.0/100 person-yr in placebo group. RRR = 58% (95%; CI 48–66%) vs placebo.
		Metformin 850 mg bid	Incidence of DM 7.3/100 person-yr in metformin group. RRR = 31% (95%; CI 17–43%) vs placebo.
STOP-NIDDM Study (64)	1429 patients with fasting hyperglycemia (5.6–7.7 mmol/L) and IGT	Acarbose 100 mg tid	After mean follow-up 3.3 yr, incidence of DM 32% in acarbose group vs 42% in placebo group. RRR = 25% (95%; CI 10–37%).
XENDOS Study (65)	3305 obese men and women (BMI ≥ 30 kg/m²) with either normal or impaired glucose tolerance	Lifestyle modification + orlistat 120 mg tid	DM incidence over 4 yr = 6.2% in orlistat group vs 9.0% in placebo group. RRR = 37.3% (95%; CI 13.7–54.5%). Preventive effect of orlistat seen only in pts with IGT at baseline (RRR = 52%, p = 0.02).
TRIPOD Study (66)	236 Hispanic women with past GDM	Troglitazone	After 2.2 years follow-up, RRR = 55% (95% CI 17% –75% with troglitazone vs placebo.

Abbr: I GT, impaired glucose tolerance; DM, type 2 diabetes mellitus; GDM, gestational diabetes; RRR, relative risk reduction.

of randomly selected individuals in whom diabetes was diagnosed by plasma glucose levels 2 h after a 75 g oral glucose load. Using these standardized criteria, striking differences in the prevalence of diabetes mellitus (DM) are observed between countries and ethnic groups *(1)*. In many traditional communities in the least industrialized countries, such as sub-Saharan Africa, rural China, and rural India, the prevalence of diabetes is extremely low (<3%). A moderate prevalence of DM (5–10%) is observed among the people of Tunisia, Thailand, and among people of European origin who live in Europe and North America. A high prevalence (>20%) of DM is observed among migrant South Asians, Arab populations in the Middle East, and Chinese migrants living in Mauritius. Groups with extremely high rates of DM include aboriginal populations who have experienced marked changes in their energy consumption and physical activity patterns such as the Pima and Papago Indians of Arizona (50%), the Micronesian Naurans (41%), Oji-Cree Aboriginals of Northern Canada (26%), and the Australian Aborigines (24%). The effect that changes in lifestyle have on the prevalence of DM is also highlighted by intra-ethnic group comparisons. For example, among people of South Asian origin, the relative prevalence of DM compared with the rural dwelling South Asians (1.0), is 3- to 6-fold among urban South Asians in India, and increases to 6- to 12-fold among South Asians living in urban areas of Fiji. Similar increases in the relative prevalence of DM are observed among Chinese, Black African, and Japanese migrants. In general, the prevalence of diabetes in urban areas of developing countries is about two to four times higher than that of rural areas in the same country *(2,9)*.

The reasons why selected populations appear "protected" from developing diabetes while others are at "high risk" are difficult to discern, and are likely attributable to unique gene-environment interactions. Comparisons between and within certain ethnic groups reveal that populations who have replaced a traditional lifestyle with an urban lifestyle are at high risk. The common risk factors associated with urbanization are decreased physical activity, increased energy consumption, and increased body weight. Among migrants, the "thrifty genotype" theory is widely accepted and hypothesizes that populations who are exposed to periods of famine develop insulin resistance as a protective mechanism to use the least energy expending mechanism to store energy as fat *(10)*. However, when exposed to an abundance of energy (as is found in urban environments), this once protective gene action becomes deleterious, and results in increased abdominal obesity and DM.

Family History of Diabetes

First-degree relatives of people with type 2 diabetes have a twofold increased risk of diabetes *(11–13)*. In the United States, the prevalence of type 2 diabetes in adults with one diabetic parent is four times as high as in adults without a parental history of diabetes (6.0 vs 1.5%); the risk is almost doubled again if both parents have diabetes *(14)*.

Impaired Glucose Tolerance and Impaired Fasting Glucose

Impaired glucose tolerance (IGT) (i.e., plasma glucose level 2 h after a 75 g oral glucose load ≥7.8 mmol/L but <11.1 mmol/L *[15]*) and impaired fasting glucose (IFG) (i.e., fasting plasma glucose ≥5.6 but <7.0 mmol/L *[16]*) strongly predict the subsequent development of type 2 diabetes. In the Paris Prospective Study, subjects with IGT (defined as fasting glucose <7.8 m*M* and 2-h glucose after a 75 g glucose load ≥7.8 and <11.1 m*M*) had a 9.6-fold increased risk of diabetes, whereas subjects with IFG (defined as fasting glucose >6.1 and <7.8 mM, and 2-h glucose <7.8 mM) had a 5.6-fold increased risk of diabetes compared to subjects with normal glucose tolerance *(17)*. In an analysis of six prospective studies, the risk of conversion from IGT to type 2 diabetes ranged from 3.6–8.7% per year. Higher fasting plasma glucose (with a sharp increase in risk above 6.0 mM), higher 2-h post-challenge glucose, and increased BMI (>27), waist circumference and waist-to-hip ratio predicted conversion from IGT to diabetes *(18)*.

Gestational Diabetes

There is general consensus that a diagnosis of gestational diabetes also predicts the development of type 2 diabetes in women. Estimates of the rate at which women with previous gestational DM (GDM) develop type 2 diabetes vary greatly. A published systematic review of the literature found crude rates of conversion from GDM to type 2 DM ranging from 2.6 to 70% over follow-up periods ranging from 6 wk to 28 yr postpartum in 28 cohort studies *(19)*. Much of the variability among studies could be attributed to important differences in factors such as completeness of follow-up, duration of follow-up after the index GDM pregnancy, diagnostic criteria used to diagnose diabetes, and selection of the study cohort. Predictors of higher risk of conversion from GDM to type 2 diabetes included higher fasting glucose at the time of diagnosis of GDM *(20)*, higher maternal BMI before pregnancy *(20,21)* and at diagnosis of GDM *(21)*, preterm delivery *(20)*, abnormal glucose tolerance in the first 2 mo postpartum *(20)*, longer time since the index GDM pregnancy *(21)* and more weight gain during that time *(21)*, use of insulin in pregnancy *(21)*, and diabetes in a first degree relative *(21)*. Of course, some cases of GDM may represent new onset, or new recognition, of type 1 diabetes. For example, a study of 298 Danish women with a previous diagnosis of GDM found that more than 20% of those women who developed diabetes postpartum actually had type 1 diabetes; these women were leaner and younger than those who developed type 2 diabetes *(20)*.

Birthweight and Other Early Life Influences

Low birthweight (<2500 g) has been associated with the development of type 2 diabetes in adulthood in Pima Indians *(22)*, British men *(23)*, Swedish men *(24)*, and American men *(25)* and women *(26)*. This association is further supported by the observation that in monozygotic twins discordant for diabetes, birthweight was significantly lower in the diabetic twin than in the nondiabetic individual *(27)*. Although the mechanism of the association between diabetes and low birth weight is uncertain, a plausible hypothesis is that fetal under-nutrition impairs pancreatic development, leading to inadequate β-cell function in the face of dietary abundance later in life *(22)*. This theory, known as the "thrifty phenotype" hypothesis, also provides an alternative explanation for the high incidence of diabetes in migrants from underdeveloped countries to more affluent countries; however, it does not explain the low prevalence of diabetes in those populations who do not migrate and maintain a traditional lifestyle. Another explanation that has been proposed for the increased incidence of type 2 diabetes in people with low birthweight is that low-birthweight infants who survive to adulthood have some genetic feature (such as a predisposition to insulin resistance), which allows them to survive, but also predisposes to diabetes later in life *(10)*.

Among Pima Indians, high birthweight (>4500 g) is also associated with the subsequent development of diabetes. This association is no longer significant, however, after controlling for maternal diabetes in pregnancy *(10)*. Further observations that offspring of Pima Indian women who were diabetic during pregnancy have a higher risk of diabetes than offspring of nondiabetic mothers or mothers who developed diabetes after pregnancy suggest that the diabetic environment *in utero* may itself be a risk factor for the subsequent development of diabetes *(28)*.

Many other influences in infancy and childhood may affect an individual's diabetes risk. These include nutrition, childhood growth, and physical activity in childhood, all of which interact with an individual's genetic susceptibility to affect diabetes risk. For example, among Pima Indians, people who were breast-fed for at least 2 mo were half as likely to develop diabetes in adulthood as those who were exclusively bottle-fed *(29)*. In another study of 7086 Finnish adults aged 67–76, the highest risk of diabetes was seen in adults with birthweight less than 3000 g and accelerated growth between ages 7 and 15 *(30)*. Several cross-sectional studies have demonstrated a correlation between lack of physical activity and increased risk of obesity in children, but there are few data addressing how quantitative aspects of physical activity in children (such as frequency and intensity) affect body composition and health, including diabetes risk. Further, parent–child interactions and the home environment have been shown to affect behaviors related to obesity and diabetes risk. For example, children who eat dinner at home with their family watch less television, eat a better diet (less fried food, less trans and saturated fat, lower glycemic load carbohydrates, more fiber, fewer soft drinks, and more fruits and vegetables), and have increased social support, which positively correlates with participation in physical activity *(31)*. Behaviors established in early life are likely to persist into adulthood and are likely to influence the long-term risk of type 2 diabetes.

Diet

The hypothesis that poor diet might lead to type 2 diabetes was proposed centuries ago and remains an attractive hypothesis because diet is more easily modified than many other risk factors. Older studies of the association between diet and type 2 diabetes showed contradictory results, with no relationship reported in several prospective studies *(32–34)*. Recently, however, two large prospective studies in American men and women found that a diet containing both a high glycemic load (i.e., high in easily digestible carbohydrates, which produce a marked rise in blood glucose and insulin levels) and a low-cereal fiber content increased the risk of self-reported type 2 diabetes up to 2.5-fold *(35,36)*. Similarly, a prospective study of 31,641 Australian men and women showed that the risk of developing type 2 diabetes was positively associated with increasing glycemic index of the diet *(37)*. High-glycemic diets are thought to create a chronically high demand for insulin. Patients with a genetic predisposition to type 2 diabetes may initially be able to produce enough insulin to meet these demands and maintain a normal blood glucose level. Diabetes may develop, however, if the ability of the pancreatic β-cell to secrete these large amounts of insulin fails. Total energy intake was not related to the risk of type 2 diabetes in these studies after adjustment for age, BMI, physical activity, alcohol intake, smoking, and family history of diabetes. Interestingly, magnesium intake was inversely related to the risk of type 2 diabetes. This is consistent with the observation that magnesium increases insulin sensitivity in vitro *(38)*. In both of these studies, the risk of diabetes fell with increasing alcohol intake. Men with moderate alcohol intake (30–49.9 g/d) and women with alcohol intake of >15 g/d had about a 40% lower risk of diabetes than nondrinkers *(39,40)*. In contrast, alcohol intake of more than 176 g of alcohol per week (or more than 25 g/d) significantly increased the risk of diabetes in men but not in women in the Rancho Bernardo study *(41)*. Although the discrepancies between these studies remain to be resolved, increased insulin sensitivity has been demonstrated in moderate drinkers compared to abstainers *(42)* and might contribute to a protective effect of moderate alcohol intake.

Sedentary Lifestyle

A sedentary lifestyle (i.e., vigourous exercise less than once per week) increases the risk of type 2 diabetes in men and women by 20–40% in both obese and nonobese individuals, independent of BMI *(43,44)*. The amount of daily physical activity appears to have a continuous inverse relationship with the risk of type 2 diabetes, with a reduction in risk of 10% for each 500 kcal increase in leisure-time energy expenditure *(36,38,45,46)*. Exercise may be beneficial both by promoting weight loss and by increasing insulin sensitivity even in the absence of weight loss *(47)*.

Smoking

Cigarette smoking has been associated with an increased risk of diabetes in some cohort studies *(3,48,49)* but others have failed to show this association *(50–52)*.

Hypertension and Other Cardiovascular Risk Factors

A positive association between systolic blood pressure *(51,53,54)* or use of antihypertensive drugs *(55,56)* and the subsequent risk of diabetes has been noted in several prospective studies. On the other hand, treatment with certain antihypertensive drugs (e.g., angiotensin-converting enzyme inhibitors, angiotensin receptor blockers, and calcium antagonists) have been associated with lower risk of developing diabetes compared to β-blockers and diuretics *(57)*. High triglyceride *(47,48)*, low HDL cholesterol, and high VLDL cholesterol *(51)* levels have also been associated with an increased risk of diabetes in some studies.

Polycystic Ovary Syndrome

Women with polycystic ovary syndrome clearly are at increased risk of type 2 diabetes. In a cross-sectional study of 254 American women with polycystic ovary syndrome, aged 14–44, 39% had abnormal glucose tolerance on a 75-g oral glucose tolerance test. Three percent of these women had previously undiagnosed diabetes, 31% had impaired glucose tolerance, and 5% had impaired fasting glucose based on American Diabetes Association (ADA) criteria *(58)*. Furthermore, in the Nurses' Health Study (a prospective study of 116,671 mostly Caucasian female nurses aged 24–43 at study inception in 1989), women with highly irregular or long (≥40 d) menstrual cycles had twice the risk of developing diabetes compared to women with regular, 26–31 d cycles (RR 2.1 [95% CI 1.6–2.7] after adjustment for other risk factors) *(59)*.

Schizophrenia and Antipsychotic Drugs

The prevalence of type 2 diabetes in people with schizophrenia may be two- to four-fold higher than in the general population. Although the precise prevalence of diabetes in this population is difficult to determine from the existing literature, recent studies suggest that approx 15% of people with schizophrenia may have diabetes and an equal proportion may have impaired glucose tolerance *(60)*. Adverse metabolic effects of antipsychotic drugs may increase the risk, although more prospective studies are needed *(61)*.

Summary of Diabetes Risk Factors

Epidemiologic studies have identified a number of clinical risk factors for diabetes, including increasing age and BMI, weight gain in adulthood, central fat distribution, ethnicity, family history of diabetes, low birthweight, sedentary lifestyle, higher systolic blood pressure, impaired glucose tolerance and impaired fasting glucose, and polycystic ovary syndrome. Diets rich in easily digestible carbohydrates and low in cereal fiber may increase the risk of type 2 diabetes; moderate alcohol intake may be protective. Gestational diabetes and schizophrenia may also be risk factors for type 2 diabetes.

CAN DIABETES BE PREVENTED?

This question has been addressed by a number of recent, large clinical trials. All of these trials have focused on preventing diabetes in adults with strong risk factors.

Lifestyle Interventions

Two large, randomized controlled trials have shown unequivocally that a program of lifestyle modification, incorporating regular exercise and modest weight loss, can prevent or delay progression of impaired glucose tolerance to type 2 diabetes. The Finnish Diabetes Prevention Study enrolled 522 middle-aged men and women with mean BMI of 31 kg/m^2 and impaired glucose tolerance (IGT) according to WHO criteria (i.e., fasting glucose <7.8 mmol/L and 2-h glucose after a 75 g glucose challenge of 7.8–11.0 mmol/L). Patients were randomly assigned to either a lifestyle intervention group (consisting of individualized counseling to reduce weight and fat intake, and increase fiber intake and physical activity) or to a control group. After 2 yr, the lifestyle intervention group lost a mean of 3.5–5.5 kg compared to 0.8–4.4 kg in the control group ($p < 0.001$). After mean follow-up of 3.2 yr, the cumulative incidence of diabetes in the intervention group was 11% (95%; confidence interval [CI] 6–15%) compared to cumulative incidence of 23% (95%; CI 17–29%) in the control group. The risk of incident diabetes was reduced by 58% ($p < 0.001$) in the lifestyle intervention group *(62)*. The Diabetes Prevention Program (DPP) Study similarly showed that sustained healthy lifestyle changes reduce the incidence of diabetes in high-risk individuals. In the DPP Study, a group of 3234 ethnically diverse, nondiabetic men and women with mean BMI 34.0 kg/m^2 plus fasting hyperglycemia (5.3–6.9 mmol/L) and IGT (glucose level 7.8–11.0 mmol/L 2 h after a 75 g glucose load) were randomly assigned to one of three interventions: standard lifestyle recommendations plus metformin 850 mg twice daily; standard lifestyle recommendations plus placebo twice daily; or an intensive lifestyle intervention (consisting of a 16-lesson curriculum and individualized support to help patients achieve the goals of weight reduction of at least 7% of initial body weight through healthy, low-calorie, and low-fat diet, as well as physical activity for at least 150 min/wk). After mean follow-up of 2.8 yr, the incidence of diabetes was 4.8 cases per 100 person-years in the lifestyle group vs 11.0 cases per 100 person-years in the placebo group. The lifestyle intervention reduced the incidence of diabetes by 58% (95%; CI 48–66%) compared to placebo; results for the metformin group are described next *(63)*.

Pharmacotherapy

There is strong clinical trial evidence that pharmaceutical agents—including metformin, acarbose, and orlistat—may also prevent progression to type 2 diabetes in high-risk individuals. Patients with high fasting glucose and IGT who were treated with metformin in the DPP Study showed a diabetes incidence of 7.8 cases per 100 person-year, representing a risk reduction of 31% (95%; CI 17–43%) compared to placebo. Metformin was most effective in preventing diabetes in patients with higher BMI and higher fasting glucose levels. Nevertheless, in the entire study group, metformin was less effective than lifestyle modification at preventing diabetes: the lifestyle intervention resulted in a 39% lower incidence of diabetes (95%; CI 24–51%) than treatment with metformin. The advantage of lifestyle intervention over metformin was most pronounced in older people and in those with lower body-mass index *(63)*.

In the STOP-NIDDM Trial, 1429 patients with high fasting glucose (5.6–7.7 mmol/L) and IGT (2-h plasma glucose of 7.8–11.0 mmol/L after a 75 g glucose load) were randomized to treatment with acarbose 100 mg three times daily, or placebo. Patients treated with acarbose had a 25% lower risk of developing diabetes than those on placebo (32 vs 42%; relative risk 0.75 [95%; CI 0.63–0.90], $p = 0.0015$) over mean follow-up of 3.3 yr. However, mild to moderate gastrointestinal side effects (commonly flatulence and diarrhea) were significantly more common in patients treated with acarbose compared to placebo ($p < 0.0001$) and almost one-third of patients treated with acarbose discontinued treatment early *(64)*.

In the XENDOS Study, 3305 obese men and women (BMI ≥30 kg/m^2) with either normal or impaired glucose tolerance were randomized to lifestyle changes plus either orlistat 120 mg or placebo, three times per day. The cumulative incidence of diabetes over 4-yr follow-up was 6.2% in patients treated with orlistat, compared to 9.0% in patients on placebo. Treatment with orlistat reduced the incidence of diabetes by 37.3% (95%; CI 13.7–54.5%, $p = 0.0032$). Exploratory analyses showed that the preventive effect of orlistat was confined to subjects with IGT at baseline (21% of the group), within whom treatment with orlistat reduced the incidence of diabetes by 52% *(65)*. Thiazolidinedione drugs also may prevent diabetes in individuals at high risk. In the TRIPOD Study, 236 Hispanic women with previous history of gestational diabetes were randomized to treatment with troglitazone (a thiazolidinedione drug that was withdrawn from the market owing to liver toxicity) vs placebo. After treatment for 2.5 yr, the cumulative risk of developing diabetes was reduced by 55% (relative risk reduction 0.55 [95%; CI 0.17–0.75], $p = 0.009$) in patients treated with troglitazone compared to placebo *(66)*. Clinical trials are underway to assess whether other thiazolidinedione drugs may have similar effects in preventing diabetes *(67)*.

Analysis of secondary endpoints from cardiovascular trials have suggested that ACE inhibitors *(68)*, angiotensin receptor blockers *(69)*, and lipid-lowering agents *(70)* also may prove to lower the risk of incident diabetes. Further studies are underway to explore the possible role of these agents in diabetes prevention *(71)*.

Surgical Approaches

At least one observational study has suggested that surgical treatment for obesity (gastric banding, vertical banded gastroplasty, or gastric bypass) might reduce the incidence of diabetes in obese patients, compared to matched controls who were not treated surgically *(72)*. Liposuction does not appear to have beneficial effects on glucose metabolism *(73)*.

PREVENTING DIABETES

Research described above has clearly shown that intensive lifestyle modification and medications can prevent or delay onset of type 2 diabetes. Potential benefits of translating these research findings to the community include lower population rates of cardiovascular disease, renal failure, blindness, and premature mortality. For example, an epidemiologic analysis projected that if all diabetes could be avoided in white American males through effective primary prevention, the rate of all-cause and CVD mortality in the American population could be reduced by up to 6.2 and 9.0%, respectively *(74)*. The challenge for clinicians, and public health providers, will be in finding the most effective ways of implementing diabetes prevention strategies within a practice or community.

Diabetes prevention strategies can be implemented at a number of different levels. These include: (1) directing diabetes prevention initiatives at high-risk subgroups of a population (such as high-risk ethnic groups); (2) promoting healthy lifestyle changes in the general population to lower the population risk of diabetes; and (3) identifying and treating high-risk individuals (such as those with IGT or strong family history of diabetes) with interventions proven to lower diabetes risk. To date, there has been a paucity of research into the first two approaches. Indeed, a systematic review of community-based interventions to delay or prevent diabetes was able to identify only 16 relevant reports in peer-reviewed journals, most of which lacked a rigorous research design. Most of the studies examined the effect of community-based interventions on intermediate outcomes (such as healthy eating behaviors and physical activity) rather than plasma glucose levels or other diabetes risk factors. Results of the interventions were varied, with no study showing consistent positive effects on the outcomes of interest *(75)*.

The third approach to diabetes prevention, which involves identifying and treating high-risk individuals, is most familiar to clinicians in the context of everyday practice. Both the Canadian Diabetes Association (CDA) and the ADA have recommended routine screening and intervention for pre-diabetes in primary care. The ADA recommends routine screening for diabetes every 3 yr for individuals 45 yr old and above, particularly those with BMI ≥25 kg/m². Early or more frequent testing is suggested for overweight individuals who have one or more of the other risk factors for diabetes. The ADA recommends counseling to promote weight loss and increased physical activity in people with pre-diabetes, but does not recommend the routine use of drugs to prevent diabetes due to lack of information about their cost-effectiveness *(76)*. Similarly, the CDA recommends screening every 3 yr for people 40 yr old and older, with implementation of strategies to prevent diabetes and modify CVD risk factors in those with pre-diabetes *(77)*. However, a number of challenges are inherent in this "high-risk" approach. For example, the "high-risk" approach requires screening for risk factors or for pre-diabetes, which may take place either in a primary care office or in a community setting. If screening is done in a community setting, strategies must be put in place to provide adequate follow-up and treatment of people that are identified as high-risk. On the other hand, opportunistic screening in primary-care settings may miss individuals who lack access to health care. Once identified, people at high risk for diabetes must have access to adequate professional and nonprofessional resources to support lifestyle change, and to sustain the changes in the long term. Furthermore, the cost-effectiveness of these interventions in "real world" settings needs to be evaluated. The challenges surrounding the implementation of diabetes prevention research in the community have been highlighted in recent reviews *(78,79)*.

CONCLUSIONS

Predisposition to diabetes is likely to be caused by a complex interaction among genes, perinatal and early life influences, and environmental/lifestyle factors in adulthood. Recent research has focused on treatments to prevent diabetes in adults at high risk, in whom both lifestyle modification and pharmaceutical agents have been shown to prevent or delay the onset of diabetes. There has been less research into interventions in children and adolescents that might prevent the onset of diabetes later in life. More efforts need to be made to translate the research findings into effective, "real life" diabetes prevention strategies.

REFERENCES

1. From World Health Organization website http://www.who.int/diabetes/facts/world_figures/en/index. html.
2. Wild S, Roglic G, Green A, et al. Global prevalence of diabetes. Diabetes Care 2004;27:1047–1053.
3. Shaten BJ, Davey Smith G, Kuller LH, Neaton JD. Risk factors for the development of type II diabetes among men enrolled in the Usual Care group of the Multiple Risk Factor Intervention Trial. Diabetes Care 1993;16:1331–1339.
4. Harris MI, Flegal KM, Cowie CC, et al. Prevalence of diabetes, impaired fasting glucose, and impaired glucose tolerance in U.S. adults. Diabetes Care 1998;21:518–524.
5. Colditz GA, Willett WC, Stampfer MJ, et al. Weight as a risk factor for clinical diabetes in women. Am J Epidemiol 1990;132:501–513.
6. Cassano PA, Rosner B, Vokonas PS, Weiss ST. Obesity and body fat distribution in relation to the incidence of non-insulin-dependent diabetes mellitus. Am J Epidemiol 1992;136:1474–1486.
7. Chan JM, Rimm EB, Colditz GA, Stampfer MJ, Willett WC. Obesity, fat distribution, and weight gain as risk factors for clinical diabetes in men. Diabetes Care 1994;17:961-969.
8. Carey VJ, Walters EE, Colditz GA, et al. Body fat distribution and risk of non-insulin-dependent diabetes mellitus in women. Am J Epidemiol 1997;145:614–619.
9. Ramachandran A, Snehalatha C, Latha E et al. Impacts of urbanization on the lifestyle and on the prevalence of diabetes in native Asian Indian population. Diabetes Res Clin Pract 1999;44: 207–213.
10. Neel V. Diabetes mellitus: a thrifty genotype rendered detrimental by progress? Am J Hum Genetics 1962;14:353–362.
11. Ohlson L-O, Larsson B, Bjorntorp P, et al. Risk factors for Type 2 (non-insulin-dependent) diabetes mellitus. Thirteen and one-half years of follow-up of the participants in a study of Swedish men born in 1913. Diabetologia 1988;31:798–805.
12. Kawakami N, Takatsuka N, Shimizu H, Ishibashi H. Effects of smoking on the incidence of non-insulin-dependent diabetes mellitus. Am J Epidemiol 1997;145:103–109.
13. Anand S, Yusuf S. Ethnicity and vascular disease. In: Salim Yusuf ed. Evidence Based Cardiology. BMJ, London, 1998, pp. 329–352.
14. Rewers M, Hamman RF. Risk factors for non-insulin-dependent diabetes. In: National Diabetes Data Group, ed. Diabetes in America, 2nd ed. National Institutes of Health/NIDDK, Bethesda, MD, 1995, pp. 179–220.
15. Report of The Expert Committee on the Diagnosis and Classification of Diabetes Mellitus. Diab Care 1997;20:1183–1197.

16. Genuth S, Alberti KG, Bennett P et al. Follow-up report on the diagnosis of diabetes mellitus. Diabetes Care 2003;26:3160–3167.

17. Charles MA, Fontbonne A, Thibult N, Warnet J-M, Rosselin GE, Eschwege E. Risk factors for NIDDM in white population. Paris Prospective Study. Diabetes 1991;40:796–799.

18. Edelstein SL, Knowler WC, Bain RP, et al. Predictors of progression from impaired glucose tolerance to NIDDM. An analysis of six prospective studies. Diabetes 1997;46:701–710.

19. Kim C, Newton KM, Knopp RH. Gestational diabetes and the incidence of type 2 diabetes. Diabetes Care 2002;25:1862–1867

20. Damm P, Kuhl C, Bertelsen A, Molsted-Pedersen L. Predictive factors for the development of diabetes in women with previous gestational diabetes. Am J Obstet Gynecol 1992;167:607–616.

21. Coustan DR, Carpenter MW, O'Sullivan PS, Carr SR. Gestational diabetes: predictors of subsequent disordered glucose metabolism. Am J Obstet Gynecol 1993;168:1139–1145.

22. McCance DR, Pettitt DJ, Hanson RL, Jacobsson TH, Knowler WC, Bennett PH. Birth weight and non-insulin-dependent diabetes: thrifty genotype, thrifty phenotype, or surviving small baby genotype? BMJ 1994;308:942–945.

23. Hales CN, Barker DJP, Clark PMS, et al. Fetal growth and impaired glucose tolerance at age 64. BMJ 1991;303:1019–1022.

24. Carlsson S, Persson P-G, Alvarsson M, et al. Low birth weight, family history of diabetes, and glucose intolerance in Swedish middle-aged men. Diabetes Care 1999; 22:1043–1047.

25. Curhan GC, Willett WC, Rimm EB, Spiegelman D, Ascherio AL, Stampfer MJ. Birth weight and adult hypertension, diabetes mellitus, and obesity in US men. Circulation 1996;94:3246–3250.

26. Rich-Edwards JW, Colditz GA, Stampfer MJ, et al. Birthweight and the risk of type 2 diabetes mellitus in adult women. Ann Intern Med 1999;130:278–284.

27. Poulsen P, Vaag AA, Moller Jensen D, Beck-Nielsen H. Low birth weight is associated with NIDDM in discordant monozygotic and dizygotic twin pairs. Diabetologia 1997;40:439–446.

28. Pettitt DJ, Aleck KA, Baird HR, Carraher MJ, Bennett PH, Knowler WC. Congenital susceptibility to NIDDM: role of intrauterine environment. Diabetes 1988;37:622–628.

29. Pettitt DJ, Forman MR, Hanson RL, Knowler WC, Bennett PH. Breastfeeding and incidence of non-insulin-dependent diabetes mellitus in Pima Indians. Lancet 1997;350:166–168.

30. Forsen T, Eriksson J, Tuomilehto J, Reunanen A, Osmond C, Barker D. The fetal and childhood growth of persons who develop type 2 diabetes. Ann Intern Med 2000;133:176–182.

31. Ebbeling CB, Pawiak DB, Ludwig DS. Childhood obesity: public-health crisis, common sense cure. Lancet 2002;360:473–482.

32. Feskens EJM, Kromhout D. Cardiovascular risk factors and the 25-year incidence of diabetes mellitus in middle-aged men. Am J Epidemiol 1989;130:1101–1108.

33. Lundgren H, Bengtsson C, Blohme G, et al. Dietary habits and incidence of noninsulin-dependent diabetes mellitus in a population study of women in Gothenburg, Sweden. Am J Clin Nutr 1989;49:708–712.

34. Medalie JH, Papier CM, Goldbourt U, Herman JB. Major factors in the development of diabetes mellitus in 10 000 men. Arch Intern Med 1975;135:811–817.

35. Salmeron J, Manson JE, Stampfer MJ, Colditz GA, Wing AL, Willett WC. Dietary fiber, glycemic load, and risk of non-insulin-dependent diabetes mellitus in women. JAMA 1997;277:472–477.

36. Salmeron J, Ascherio A, Rimm EB, et al. Dietary fiber, glycemic load, and risk of NIDDM in men. Diabetes Care 1997;20(4):545–550.

37. Hodge AM, English DR, O'Dea K, Giles GG. Glycemic index and dietary fiber and the risk of type 2 diabetes. Diabetes Care 2004;27:2701–2706.

38. Resnick LM. Ionic basis of hypertension, insulin resistance, vascular disease, and related disorders: the mechanism of syndrome X. Am J Hypertens 1993;6:123s–134s.

39. Rimm EB, Chan J, Stampfer MJ, Colditz GA, Willett WC. Prospective study of cigarette smoking, alcohol use, and the risk of diabetes in men. BMJ 1995;310:555–559.

40. Stampfer MJ, Colditz GA, Willett WC, et al. A prospective study of moderate alcohol drinking and risk of diabetes in women. Am J Epidemiol 1988;128:549–558.

41. Holbrook TL, Barrett-Connor E, Wingard DL. A prospective population-based study of alcohol use and non-insulin-dependent diabetes mellitus. Am J Epidemiol 1990;132:902–909.

42. Facchini F, Chen Y-DI, Reaven GM. Light-to-moderate alcohol intake is associated with enhanced insulin sensitivity. Diabetes Care 1994;17:115–119.

43. Manson JE, Rimm EB, Stampfer MJ, et al. Physical activity and incidence of non-insulin-dependent diabetes mellitus in women. Lancet 1991;338:774–778.
44. Manson JE, Nathan DM, Krolewski AS, Stampfer MJ, Willett WC, Hennekens CH. A prospective study of exercise and incidence of diabetes among US male physicians. JAMA 1992;268: 63–67.
45. Perry IJ, Wannamethee SG, Walker MK, Thomson AG, Whincup PH, Shaper AG. Prospective study of risk factors for development of non-insulin dependent diabetes in middle aged British men. BMJ 1995;310:560–564.
46. Helmrich SP, Ragland DR, Leung RW, Paffenbarger RS. Physical activity and reduced occurrence of non-insulin-dependent diabetes mellitus. N Engl J Med 1991;325:147–152.
47. Ruderman N, Apelian AZ, Schneider SH. Exercise in therapy and prevention of type II diabetes: implications for blacks. Diabetes Care 1990;13: 1163–1168.
48. Rimm EB, Manson JE, Stampfer MJ, et al. Cigarette smoking and the risk of diabetes in women. Am J Public Health 1993;83:211–214.
49. Rimm EB, Chan J, Stampfer MJ, Colditz GA, Willett WC. Prospective study of cigarette smoking, alcohol use, and the risk of diabetes in men. BMJ 1995;310: 555–559.
50. Njolstad I, Arnesen E, Lund-Larsen PG. Sex differences in risk factors for clinical diabetes mellitus in a general population: a 12-year follow-up of the Finnmark Study. Am J Epidemiol 1998;147: 49–58.
51. Stolk RP, van Splunder IP, Schouten JSAG, Witteman JCM, Hofman A, Grobbee DE. High blood pressure and the incidence of non-insulin dependent diabetes mellitus: findings in a 11.5 year follw-up study in the Netherlands. Eur J Epidemiol 1993;9:134–139.
52. Perry IJ, Wannamethee SG, Walker MK, thomson AG, Whincup PH, Shaper AG. Prospective study of risk factors for development of non-insulin dependent diabetes in middle aged British men. BMJ 1995;310:560–564.
53. McPhillips JB, Barrett-Connor E, Wingard DL. Cardiovascular disease risk factors prior to the diagnosis of impaired glucose tolerance and non-insulin-dependent diabetes mellitus in a community of older adults. Am J Epidemiol 1990;131:443–453.
54. Balkau B, King H, Zimmet P, Raper LR. Factors associated with the development of diabetes in the Micronesian population of Nauru. Am J Epidemiol 1985;122:594–605.
55. Skarfors ET, Selinus KI, Lithell HO. Risk factors for developing non-insulin dependent diabetes: a 10 year follow up of men in Uppsala. BMJ 1991;303:755–760.
56. Wilson PWF, Anderson KM, Kannel WB. Epidemiology of diabetes mellitus in the elderly. The Framingham Study. Am J Med 1986;80:3–9.
57. Pepine CJ, Cooper-DeHoff RM. Cardiovascular therapies and risk for development of diabetes. J Am Coll Cardiol 2004;44:509–12.
58. Legro RS, Kunselman AR, Dodson WC, Dunaif A. Prevalence and predictors of risk for type 2 diabetes mellitus and impaired glucose tolerance in polycystic ovary syndrome: a prospective, controlled study in 254 affected women. J Clin Endocrinol Metab 1999;84:165–169.
59. Solomon CG, Hu FB, Dunaif A, et al. Long or highly irregular menstrual cycles as a marker for risk of type 2 diabetes mellitus. JAMA 2001;286:2421.
60. Bushe C, Holt R. Prevalence of diabetes and impaired glucose tolerance in patients with schizophrenia. Br J Psychiatry Suppl 2004;47:s67–s71.
61. "Schizophrenia and Diabetes 2003" Expert Consensus Meeting, Dublin, 2-3 October 2003: consensus summary. Br J Psychiatry Suppl 2004;184:s112–s114.
62. Tuomilehto J, Lindström J, Eriksson JG, et al. Prevention of type 2 diabetes by changes in lifestyle among subjects with impaired glucose tolerance. N Engl J Med 2001;344:1343–1350.
63. Diabetes Prevention Program Research Group. Reduction in the incidence of type 2 diabetes with lifestyle intervention or metformin. N Engl J Med 2002;346:393–403.
64. Chiasson J-L, Josse RG, Gomis R, et al. Acarbose for prevention of type 2 diabetes mellitus: the STOP-NIDDM randomised trial. Lancet 2002;359:2072–2077.
65. Torgerson JS, Hauptman J, Boldrin MN, Sjöström L. XENical in the prevention of diabetes in obese subjects (XENDOS) Study. Diab Care 2004;27:155–161.
66. Buchanan TA, Xiang AH, Peters RK et al. Preservation of pancreatic β-cell function and prevention of type 2 diabetes by pharmacological treatment of insulin resistance in high-risk Hispanic women. Diabetes 2002;51:2796–2803.

67. The DREAM Trial Investigators. Rationale, design and recruitment characteristics of a large, simple international trial of diabetes prevention: the DREAM trial. Diabetologia 2004;47:1519–1527.
68. Heart Outcome Protection Evaluation Study Investigators. Effects of ramipril on cardiovascular and microvascular outcomes in people with diabetes mellitus: results of the HOPE study and MICRO-HOPE substudy. Lancet 2000;355:253–9.
69. Lindholm LH, Ibsen H, Dahlof B et al. Cardiovascular morbidity and mortality in patients with diabetes in the Losartan Intervention For Endpoint reduction in hypertension study (LIFE): a randomised trial against atenolol. Lancet 2002;359:1004–1010.
70. Freeman DJ, Norrie J, Sattar N et al. Pravastatin and the development of diabetes mellitus: evidence for a protective treatment effect in the West of Scotland Coronary Prevention Study. Circulations 2001;103:357–362.
71. Simpson RW, Shaw JE, Zimmet PZ. The prevention of type 2 diabetes- lifestyle change or pharmacotherapy? A challenge for the 21st century. Diabetes Res Clin Pract 2003;59:165–180.
72. Torgerson JS, Sjöström L. The Swedish Obese Subjects (SOS) study- rationale and results. Int J Obesity 2001;25 Suppl 1:S2–S4.
73. Klein S, Fontana L, Young VL et al. Absence of an effect of liposuction on insulin action and risk factors for coronary heart disease. N Engl J Med 2004;350:2549–2457.
74. Narayan KM, Thompson TJ, Boyle JP et al. The use of population attributable risk to estimate the impact of prevention and early detection of type 2 diabetes on population-wide mortality risk in US males. Health Care Manag Sci 1999;2:223–227.
75. Satterfield DW, Volansky M, Caspersen CJ et al. Community-based lifestyle interventions to prevent type 2 diabetes. Diabetes Care 26:2643-2652, 2003.
76. American Diabetes Association. Standards of medical care in diabetes. Diabetes Care 2005;28:S4–S36.
77. Canadian Diabetes Association 2003 Clinical Practice Guidelines for the Prevention and Management of Diabetes in Canada. Can J Diab 2003;27:S10–S13.
78. Centers for Disease Control and Prevention Primary Prevention Working Group. Primary prevention of type 2 diabetes mellitus by lifestyle intervention: implications for health policy. Ann Int Med 2004;140:951–957.
79. Zimmet P, Shaw J, Alberti KGMM. Preventing type 2 diabetes and the dysmetabolic syndrome in the real world: a realistic view. Diabet Med 2003;20:693–702.

20

An Evidence-Based Approach to Type 2 Diabetes

Robert K. Semple, MA, MB, BChir
and Sean F. Dinneen, MD, MSC, FRCP(I), FACP

INTRODUCTION

The past century has been witness to a dramatic transformation in the health care challenges facing both the industrialized and developing world. Among the most striking of these has been a surge in the prevalence of obesity and type 2 diabetes. In developed countries this has been caused by the conjunction of the waning societal threat posed by communicable disease, a technology-driven rise in sedentary lifestyles, and the availability of aggressively marketed, mass produced, and calorically rich food. Some 150 million people worldwide are believed to presently have diabetes at present (90% of which is type 2), and this is projected to rise to 300 million by 2025 *(1)*.

This burgeoning pandemic not only poses prodigious challenges for those planning health care at the population level, but also means that the diabetes-related workload of physicians will dramatically increase over the coming years. Mindful of this, the research community has directed intense efforts toward understanding the molecular and physiological basis of type 2 diabetes, toward further refinement of our appreciation of its natural history, and toward improvement and innovation in its therapy. This has lead to a clinical literature that can seem bewilderingly large, spread across a range of specialist and general journals, often beyond the scope of full time clinicians. It is in this context that the approach of evidence-based medicine (EBM) becomes not just a convenience but a necessity, as a tool to distill clinically useful information for the patient in clinic.

From: *Contemporary Endocrinology: Evidence-Based Endocrinology*
Edited by: V. M. Montori © Mayo Foundation for Medical Education and Research

We shall attempt to illustrate the use and limitations of EBM, and to explore the evolving diabetes-related clinical evidence base by considering the therapeutic options for a single patient at three key points in his course through type 2 diabetes.

SCENARIO 1

A 54-yr-old Caucasian man is referred by his primary-care physician for further advice regarding treatment for diabetes. He was diagnosed some 2 yr before after investigation of fatigue, and successfully abrogated his initial symptoms through dietary observance, guided by a local dietician, and a program of aerobic exercise for 30 min, three to four times a week. As of late, demands at work have curtailed this, and his weight has increased slightly. His HbA1c has risen to 8.1%, though he remains asymptomatic. He takes no other medication, and is otherwise well, but smokes 10–15 cigarettes a day. He drinks alcohol in moderation. His mother died of a stroke in her early 70s.

On examination he has evidence of early background retinopathy, and an elevated albumin:creatinine ratio of 4:5. His blood pressure is 148/90, and his body mass index (BMI) 29 kg/m^2, with a centripetal pattern of adiposity.

A fasting lipid profile shows total cholesterol 4.8 mmol/L, low-density lipoprotein cholesterol (LDL) 3.4 mmol/L, high-density lipoprotein cholesterol (HDL) 0.9 mmol/L triglyceride 2.9 mmol/L.

The patient himself is, in general, reluctant to take medication, especially as he feels well, and would like to discuss whether there is a strong reason why he should.

Discussion

This man's presentation is typical, and it poses a large number of potential clinical questions. Central to answering the patient's initial enquiry, and in formulating therapeutic recommendations, are the following:

1. What is the prognosis in terms of morbidity and mortality of untreated type 2 diabetes?
2. Which interventions have been demonstrated to improve the prognosis?
3. Which interventions have the greatest impact on risk?
4. Where there are multiple possible interventions, are they equally or more effective when combined? If so, what is the hierarchy of importance of these interventions with respect to outcome?
5. What is the balance of benefit and harm which will best accommodate this man's preferences and values?

WHAT IS THE PROGNOSIS OF UNTREATED TYPE 2 DIABETES?

This is already answerable in its current form.

Acquisition of Evidence

The epidemiological evidence necessary to inform this man about his prognosis without treatment derives largely from historical studies, and has not been systematically reviewed according to the modern principles of EBM. However searching Medline and the bibliographies of intervention studies soon provides the appropriate data. The most informative study design for addressing the natural history of a disease is a prospective cohort study. Such a study in untreated type 2 diabetes has been unethical for many years based on the accrual of clinical evidence over the last century. However, evidence from such prospective studies from the 1960s and 1970s does give information of relevance to this man: the Whitehall prospective study of around 18,000 male English civil servants between 40 and 64 yr old *(2)*, and the Paris Prospective Study of 7000 French civil servants between 43 and 54 yr old *(3)* each analyzed the prognosis of those with undiagnosed diabetes mellitus, and found it to be modestly worse than those with diagnosed diabetes, presumably receiving the conventional treatment of the time. The large prospective studies of prognosis in those with diagnosed diabetes (Whitehall *[2]* , Paris *[3]*, NHANES I *[4]*, and Framingham *[5]*) show a pronounced increase in all cause, coronary heart disease-related and cardiovascular mortality in patients with diabetes. In general the relative risk of death is around twice that of the nondiabetic population, and the risk of cardiovascular death is around 2.5 times that of nondiabetics. Thus this man could be informed that simply because he has diabetes, he has double the risk of dying over the next decade as someone from the same population without diabetes. However in his case, he also has a constellation of other risk factors for atherosclerosis, including cigarette smoking, a family history of complications of atherosclerosis, borderline hypertension, and dyslipidaemia. On the basis of the Framingham data, these appear to confer the same risks in diabetes as in those without diabetes (although Framingham diabetes was not diagnosed according to modern diagnostic criteria). Rather than enumerating the relative risks conferred by each individual parameter or behavior, more meaningful to the patient would be an overall level of risk. Such an assessment is offered through the various risk engines generated from the available evidence. Many are based on Framingham data, such as the UK Joint Societies Charts *(6)*, which incorporate age, diabetes status, gender, smoking, total cholesterol, HDL cholesterol, and left ventricular hypertrophy by voltage criteria. Based on the largely Caucasian population of Framingham, these data are likely pertinent to this patient, although it has been demonstrated in various different ethnic groups that some recalibration of the risk calculation is required before it becomes accurate in those populations. Applying this man's profile to the risk calculator, his 10-yr risk of coronary events is estimated at between 15 and 30%. However this is likely to underestimate the risk, as it does not, critically, take into account his raised alb:Cr ratio, which may betoken incipient diabetic nephropathy. This should be repeated, and perhaps be corroborated by a formal determination of the albumin excretion rate. This is important because a systematic review of published trials has shown that microalbuminuria (i.e., 30–299 mg albumin excretion/24 h) confers an additional relative risk of around 2.5 for cardiovascular morbidity and mortality compared to diabetes alone *(7)*, possibly because it serves as a surrogate marker of endothelial dysfunction *(8)*. Thus the best estimate of this patient's 10-yr cardiovascular risk is in excess of 30%.

In considering his prognosis, attention must also be given to his chances of suffering morbidity from microvascular disease—the classical "diabetic complications" of retinopathy, nephropathy, and neuropathy—over the coming years. Unlike the case of cardiovascular disease, it is now well established that the level of glycemic control is the major factor influencing progression of microvascular damage, as evidenced by extensive observational data over the past 80 yr since the discovery of insulin. Indeed, the currently accepted, arbitrary thresholds for the diagnosis of diabetes are largely based on the levels of glycaemia at which the incidence of microvascular complications rapidly starts to increase. This appears to show a threshold at about an HbA1c of 6%. This is supported by cross-sectional data from the Wisconsin Epidemiological Study of Diabetic Retinopathy *(9)*, and by cross-sectional and longitudinal studies in the

Pima Indians *(10)*. Perhaps the most relevant data to this patient, however, comes from the United Kingdom Prospective Diabetes Study (UKPDS). Discussed in more detail below, this complex study demonstrated in type 2 diabetes that "tight" diabetic control, characterized by a mean HbA1c of 7.0%, resulted in an improvement in microvascular endpoints of 25% compared to the less-tight control group, which had mean HbA1c of 7.9% *(11)*. However, despite the risks of progressive microvascular disease, it is clear that the greater threat to this man lies in cardiovascular morbidity and mortality.

Appraisal/Application of the Evidence

Thus, synthesizing this disparate but fairly consistent historical evidence, this patient should be advised that, although the term "diabetic complications" is most commonly recognised as denoting eye, renal, and foot disease, by far the greatest threat to his well-being over the coming years is cardiovascular disease, and that this is where efforts should be directed at present. In terms of clarity of focus of the immediate management steps, cardiovascular risk reduction should be pre-eminent.

WHICH INTERVENTIONS HAVE BEEN SHOWN TO IMPROVE RISK?

This rather open question is not currently easily answerable using an evidence based approach. The first step is, thus, to articulate the question in a manner that will facilitate the acquisition of clinical evidence. Indeed, EBM does not substitute for theoretical, experimental, and observational knowledge of disease. Rather, it allows the specific testing of hypotheses, which derive from this base. Thus, as we have decided to concentrate on lowering this man's cardiovascular risk, we must ask specific questions about those factors and interventions, which we believe influence the progression of atherosclerosis. Such factors include:

Factor	Intervention
• Extent of established disease	Screening for existing atherosclerosis
• Lifestyle	Dietary advice/exercise training
• Glycemic control	Oral hypoglycemic agents
• Blood pressure	Antihypertensive agents
• Lipid profile	Lipid lowering agents
• Smoking	Support for smoking cessation
• Platelet aggregation	Aspirin

Thus, the specific question for each factor is "Does intervention X improve the cardiovascular prognosis in type 2 diabetes?"

Acquisition of Evidence

The best study design for assessing the effect of an intervention on a disease is a prospective, randomized controlled clinical trial (RCT), and the best possible confidence in the results comes from a systematic review of such studies with homogeneity among studies (i.e., consistent findings). Over the past 30 yr in the field of diabetes many RCTs have been undertaken, and a large number have been encompassed by systematic reviews carried out either *ad hoc*, or, increasingly, by one of the bodies interested either in promulgating good diabetes care specifically—notably the American Diabetes Association— or interested in facilitating the process of EBM, such as the Cochrane Collaboration, *Evidence-Based Medicine/ACP Journal Club*, or *Bandolier*. Thus, a reasonable first step for a busy clinician is to consult these sources of organized and appraised data, which effectively bypasses the acquisition and appraisal of individual pieces of evidence. This is particularly easy in this more-or-less treatment naïve man.

It is clear from the patient's initial question that he is loath to be over-burdened by medication. Equally, consideration of the number of potential medications used to control the above risks is very large. Thus, consideration of the evidence must be focused on providing a pragmatic and robust case for the recommended regimen, if any.

Consider each intervention in turn.

Screening for Existing Disease

On one hand, this man is currently asymptomatic. However conversely, he has potent risk factors for atherosclerosis, and the gradual and progressive pathogenesis of atheromata is such that he is likely already to be harboring disease. As there is clear and growing evidence that medical, percutaneous, and surgical interventions can improve prognosis in various degrees of clinical disease, there is a clear suggestion that in patients such as this, baseline screening for coronary disease with a suitable noninvasive test (e.g., treadmill testing or myocardial scintigraphy) may improve outcomes. However, data to this effect do not currently exist from prospective RCTs. Nevertheless, appraisal of the existing data at an ADA-sponsored conference in 1998 led to the recommendation in the United States that subjects with diabetes and one further (prespecified) risk factor should undergo screening *(12)*. Although informed and pragmatic, this recommendation, thus, has a low level of direct supporting evidence, and was recently subjected to direct testing in the Detection of Ischemia in Asymptomatic Diabetics (DIAD) study: over 1000 patients with type 2 diabetes, between 50 and 75 yr old, with no known coronary artery disease, were randomly assigned to either stress testing (with adenosine technetium-99m sestamibi SPECT myocardial perfusion imaging) and 5-yr clinical follow-up or to follow-up only. Twenty-two percent of subjects who underwent stress testing had silent ischemia, and 73% of those had regional myocardial perfusion abnormalities (moderate or large in 29%) The strongest predictors for abnormal tests were abnormal Valsalva, male sex, and diabetes duration. Traditional cardiac risk factors were not predictive, such that selecting only patients who met ADA guidelines would have failed to identify 41% of patients with silent ischemia. This study is testimony to the importance of direct testing of guidelines based largely on expert opinion alone, and deserves further work *(13)*.

Lifestyle Modification (Exercise/Diet)

Adoption of a healthy lifestyle involving aerobic exercise at least three to four times a week, and a healthy diet aimed at weight loss, optimizing glycaemic control, and lipid parameters, have long been the mainstay of the therapeutic approach in type 2 diabetes. They are believed, based on a wealth of experimental evidence, to promote weight loss and insulin sensitization. The detailed evidence pertinent to both diet and exercise has already been appraised and presented by the ADA with levels of recommendation indicated *(14–17)*, whereas dietary interventions have been examined by the Cochrane collaboration *(18)*. Both groups note that there is no significant direct evidence that such an approach impacts upon hard cardiovascular endpoints, instead examining only surrogate markers of metabolic control and cardiovascular risk, and were of variable design, comparing several different interventions, and making general conclusions difficult. There is an urgent need for formal studies to address this issue, and this may be met in part by the current NIH-sponsored Look AHEAD study, which plans to follow up 5000 subjects with obesity and type 2 diabetes for up to 11 yr, comparing diabetes education and support with intentional weight loss *(19)*. Despite the relative lack of evidence, extrapolation from three recent large diabetes prevention trials *(20–22)* strongly suggests that dietary and exercise interventions are likely to improve outcomes also in frank type 2 diabetes.

The case patient here has already been following dietary and exercise advice, although he remains overweight, so it seems doubtful that this alone will lead to the desired improvement on his risk profile. Nevertheless he should receive tailored dietary and exercise advice at the first appointment with support thereafter.

Smoking

Smoking is well established as the leading avoidable cause of death in the developed world, much of which is attributable to cardiovascular disease *(23,24)*. Although the epidemiological cohort and case–control studies, which have established this, have not generally reported patients with diabetes separately, and although no randomized controlled intervention trial of smoking cessation in diabetes has been undertaken, the available evidence suggests that the same smoking-related risks apply in diabetes as in the general population, and are likely to amplify the already high cardiovascular risk. Thus, although the formal level of evidence upon which the recommendation is based specifically in diabetes is low, the ADA and other organizations recommend focused intervention based on repeated counselling and support, with the use of nicotine replacement and newer adjunctive therapies such as buproprion *(23,24)*.

Drugs

In general, pharmaceutical agents have been subjected to more rigorous scrutiny than the less easily definable interventions above, not least because many of the pharmaceutical innovations have fallen in the era of the RCT. Furthermore, the case patient as at the most easily studied point in the natural history of diabetes—at the point of instigation of drug therapy. Thus, for the physician in clinic most of the work of evidence accrual and appraisal has already been undertaken by national diabetes associations, or by bodies such as the Cochrane collaboration. Thus, in line with the EBM ideal, good quality data can quickly be accessed to inform patient advice.

Oral Hypoglycemic Agents. The slow and progressive pathogenesis of atherosclerosis, and the heterogeneity of both type 2 diabetes and its therapies makes a formal examination of the impact on macrovascular endpoints of improving glycemic control a formidable undertaking. For this reason, only one study has had sufficient power to address this question. Long and complex in design, the UKPDS randomized nearly 4000 patients with newly diagnosed diabetes to either intensive or less intensive glycemic control, and permitted comparison of initial therapy with insulin, sulphonylureas, and metformin. Ultimately the intensive control group had a mean HbA1c of 7.0%, compared with 7.9% in the conventional control group. Despite this, the difference in myocardial infarction between the two groups failed to achieve conventional significance, although there was a trend toward improvement in the intensive group, but the stroke rate showed a trend toward an increase in the intensive group *(11)*. Only on subgroup analysis of obese subjects was a significant improvement in myocardial infarction rates discovered, in those patients initially treated with metformin, compared with diet alone. On this basis, most professional bodies have now adopted the recommendation that metformin be used in obese patients as first line oral treatment of type 2 diabetes. The case patient, although his BMI does not exceed the arbitrary threshold for obesity, is nevertheless close, with moreover a centripetal fat distribution.

Newer agents such as the short acting meglitinide insulin secretagoges, and the thiazolidinedione PPARγ agonists rosiglitazone and pioglitazone, are largely untested in terms of hard cardiovascular endpoints, although with pioglitazone in particular, its beneficial effect on lipid profile make it an agent of promise, and prospective studies are underway.

Anti-Hypertensives. The data relating to the use of anti-hypertensives in patients with diabetes is relatively abundant, and has been systematically reviewed by the American Diabetes Association (ADA) and others. Individual trials are well summarized in the systematic reviews, but all emphasize the importance of the UKPDS: some balm for the rather disappointing macrovascular outcome of the full UKPDS was provided by its smaller and shorter hypertension-focussed sub-study, which examined prospectively the effect of tight or less tight blood pressure control on diabetes-related endpoints and death *(25)*. The actual blood pressures achieved were 144/82 mmHg (tight) and 154/87 mmHg (less tight), with initial treatment either with captopril or atenolol. This 10/5 mmHg difference in mean blood pressure was associated with impressive reductions in both microvascular, and macrovascular event rates, indeed, rather more impressive than the reduction with improved glycemic control. Epidemiological analysis of the data suggested that for each 10 mmHg decrement in systolic blood pressure, there was a 15% decrease in deaths related to diabetes, and 11% for myocardial infarction, with no difference between the initial β-blocker and angiotensin-converting enzyme (ACE) inhibitor groups. The headline reduction in macrovascular events has been supported in other trials reporting subjects with diabetes, so that the importance of blood pressure reduction in subjects with type 2 diabetes is beyond doubt. Related questions are which target blood pressure to aim for, and which agent or combination of agents to use. A recurring feature has been the failure in RCTs to define a lower threshold of blood pressure where benefit is no longer seen *(26,27)*, and epidemiological analyses show that blood pressures above 120/70 mmHg are associated with increased cardiovascular event rates and mortality in persons with diabetes. Most authorities at present recommend a target of no higher than 135/80 in subjects with diabetes, and current trials may address specifically the effect of even lower targets. The question of which agent to use is rather more complex, yet several consistent patterns have emerged from the available RCTs. ACE inhibitors have proved superior in terms of mortality to calcium channel blockers *(28,29)*, although the direct comparisons with β-blockade have been less clear cut *(29,30)*. However, in view of the strong evidence of their beneficial effects on mortality *(61,62)* and renoprotection (SFD *27,63*), it is generally now recommended that ACE inhibitors or angiotensin II blockers be first-line pharmacological treatment for patients with diabetes and hypertension, with thiazide diuretics as additive agents, followed by β-blockers or calcium channel blockers (although these should be avoided in patients who have suffered a myocardial infarction).

Lipid-Lowering Therapy. Despite the well established literature relating to LDL cholesterol lowering for both primary and secondary prevention of macrovascular events in the general population, until fairly recently few studies existed dedicated to lipid lowering in diabetes. Instead, recommendations were largely based on a combination of epidemiological studies and subgroup analyses from the large general trials such as the

4S study *(31)*. The most important recent addition to the diabetes-specific data has been the large Heart Protection Study, which included 5963 patients with diabetes and compared the effects of simvastatin and placebo in patients over 40 yr with total cholesterol >3.5 m*M (32)*. Those assigned to simvastatin had a 22% reduction in the event rate for macrovascular events, and this risk reduction was similar across all LDL subcategories, including patients with pretreatment LDL cholesterol levels below 3.0 m*M* and those without pre-existing vascular disease. This finding has since been supported by the Collaborative Atorvastatin Diabetes Study (CARDS) study, which examined solely those with type 2 diabetes together with retinopathy, albuminuria, current smoking, or hypertension, but with mean baseline LDL cholesterol of only 3 mmol/L, and found atorvastatin to reduce macrovascular events by 37% and death by 27% *(33)*. In the case patient, who has a high 10-yr risk of vascular disease, treatment with a statin as well as reenforcement of dietary and lifestyle advice is clearly warranted. Later questions will be determined by the response of his LDL, HDL, and triglycerides to this initial therapy.

Aspirin. A final event in the occlusion of a coronary artery in atherosclerosis is the development of thrombus on the ruptured shoulder of a complicated atheroma. Thus, aspirin, with its capacity to inhibit platelet cyclooxygenase and hence aggregation, is an obvious therapeutic approach. The ADA have reviewed this, and, based principally on a subgroup analysis of the Physicians' Health Study *(34)*, a primary prevention trial comparing low-dose aspirin to placebo in male physicians, the Early Treatment Diabetic Retinopathy Study *(35)*, a mixed primary and secondary prevention trial involving both type 1 and type 2 diabetes, and the Hypertension Optimal Treatment study *(27)*, which examined the effects of 75 mg/d of aspirin vs placebo in 18,790 hypertensive patients who were also randomized to achieve diastolic blood pressure goals of 90, 85, or 80 mmHg, it recommends that low dose aspirin (between 75 and 162 mg/d) be used for primary prevention in those with type 2 diabetes at increased cardiovascular risk, which encompasses the case patient.

Synthesis/Application of Evidence

Thus, the process of acquisition and appraisal of evidence related to the initial care of this treatment-naïve man has been a straightforward process, mostly relying on published systematic reviews. Whereas the recommendations appended to these reviews may vary according to the health care climate in which they were formulated, consideration of the evidence alone means that the following possible interventions can reasonably be presented and discussed with the case patient. Note that extrapolations from studies not explicitly examining patients with diabetes are not incorporated in this scheme:

1. Evaluation and optimisation of his current medical nutritional therapy and exercise programs.
2. Screening for asymptomatic coronary disease by treadmill testing or scintigraphy.
3. Counselling and supportive intervention as required to promote smoking cessation.
4. Pharmacotherapy:
   a. Metformin.
   b. An ACE inhibitor.
   c. A statin such as atorvastatin.
   d. Low-dose aspirin.

The patient has already pre-empted the discussion by showing his reluctance to take any medication, and although each of these recommendations has proven or likely benefit, this suggested plan involves taking four tablets initially, with the likelihood of more in future if targets are to be adhered to. He may reasonably ask if it is proven that combining all these interventions still confers the benefit of each individually. Although this cannot be answered precisely, some evidence that intensive management of multiple risk factors is beneficial comes from the Steno 2 study *(36)*. This study was a randomized, open, parallel trial, looking at 160 patients with diabetes and microalbuminuria randomly assigned to receive either conventional treatment from their primary-care physician—according to the recommendations of the Danish Medical Association at the time—or intensive multifactorial intervention involving stricter treatment goals (on a par with those currently espoused by the ADA) to be achieved through behavioral modification and stepwise pharmacological therapy overseen by a specialist diabetes center. Behavioral modification included dietary and exercise programs and support for smoking cessation. On average, patients in the intensive-therapy group were offered consultations every 12 wk during the 8-yr follow-up. Taken together, the results showed that the long-term, targeted, intensive intervention reduced the risk of both cardiovascular and microvascular events by about 50%. This demonstrates that, whereas the burden both on the patient and the care delivery system required for a similarly focused level of management may be onerous, the ultimate benefits are likely to be significant. However the therapeutic decision must be taken entirely collaboratively with the patient, and be in accord with his own preferences and values, or poor compliance is a likely result.

SCENARIO 2

The same man, 5 yr later, has managed to stop smoking. Appropriate annual screening has shown bilateral background retinopathy and mild peripheral sensory neuropathy. His microalbuminuria was confirmed after initial presentation, and has remained stable. He is now taking aspirin, ramipril 10 mg od, and atorvastatin 10 mg od. His oral hypoglycemic therapy has been progressively increased such that he now takes metformin 850 mg tds and gliclazide 160 mg bid. Despite this, his HbA1c is now 9.1%. He undertakes around 20–30 min aerobic exercise daily and is generally adherent to an appropriate diet. His fasting lipid profile shows total chol 3.9 mmol/L, LDL chol 2.7 mmol/L, HDL chol 0.9 mmol/L, triglyceride 2.0 mmol/L. He is very reluctant to have any insulin injections.

Discussion

The principal problem is now deteriorating glycemic control despite maximal doses of two oral hypoglycaemic agents. It is clear that further intervention will be required to minimize the risk of progressive microvascular, and perhaps macrovascular, complications, as previously described. The central question is whether it is now necessary to recommend an insulin-containing regimen, whereas a subsidiary question is how best to formulate this regimen. The most obvious alternative to starting insulin would be to introduce one of the two currently available thiazolidinediones, relatively recently introduced agents that act via agonism of PPARγ to enhance insulin sensitivity. Framing this in an answerable format, three questions arise:

1. In patients who experience secondary failure of a sulphonylurea and metformin to maintain adequate glycaemic control (defined by consensus targets), will addition of a

thiazolidinedione result in sufficient improvement in glycemia to achieve those targets without undue side effects?

2. Which insulin or insulin-analog-based regimen is optimal in terms of both glycemic control and side effects?

3. Is triple oral therapy superior to the optimal insulin-based regime in terms of these clinical outcomes?

Is Triple Oral Therapy Effective?

Acquisition of Evidence

Being relatively recently introduced into clinical practice, data regarding the use of the currently available thiazoldinediones (TZDs)—rosiglitazone and pioglitazone—in triple oral therapy has only latterly begun to emerge, and has not been systematically reviewed. Searching PubMed for prospective trials reveals three recent studies incorporating oral triple therapy with the current agents *(37–39)*, as well as two older studies using troglitazone *(40,41)*, the prototypic clinical TZD, which was withdrawn as a result of idiosyncratic hepatotoxicity.

Appraisal of Evidence

Troglitazone, rosiglitazone, and pioglitazone, all TZDs, are believed to exert their beneficial influence through potent activation of the transcription factor PPARγ. One placebo-controlled RCT *(40)* and a second, longitudinal study *(41)*, which compared triple therapy with SUR, metformin, and troglitazone with SUR/metformin alone, established the efficacy of troglitazone in this setting, but this early promise was nullified by its occasional hepatotoxicity and withdrawal from use. Encouragingly, however, post-marketing surveillance of rosiglitazone and pioglitazone appears to support the belief that the liver damage with troglitazone was caused by a chemical moiety in troglitazone, that was not intrinsic to its pharmacological activity, and that is not found in the newer drugs, which have not experienced these problems. Prospective RCTs have now begun to emerge looking directly at the newer TZDs in triple therapy. One multicenter prospective placebo-controlled study examined the effect of adding rosiglitazone to optimized glyburide/metformin co-therapy in subjects with a mean HbA1c of 8.1% *(37)*. Three hundred and sixty-five patients were randomized, and over 24 wk there was a mean HbA1c improvement of 1.0% in the triple therapy group compared to placebo, with 43% achieving a level below 7% compared to 14% doing so in the placebo group. Eight percent of triple therapy patient experienced mild-moderate oedema, and 22% had symptoms of hypoglycaemia.

The study subjects in that trial were well matched demographically to the patient in this case, but the starting HbA1c was significantly better in the study. This suggests intuitively that the chance of this patient achieving the target HbA1c on this regimen would be significantly less than 43%. Two further studies compared oral triple therapy to insulin-based regimens *(38,39)*. The comparisons are discussed in more detail next. However in the triple therapy arm of each study, mean starting HbA1cs approached 10%, rather worse than the level in this patient. Despite this, both studies, including 98 *(38)* and 31 *(39)* patients in the triple therapy arms, found improvements in HbA1c of around 2% in this group over 24 and 16 wk, respectively. This led to 31% of patients in the first study, and 23% in the second study, achieving an HbA1c below 7%. In the larger study, which employed rosiglitazone in half the patients and pioglitazone in the others, 10.2% were deemed treatment failures, whereas three had therapy stopped because of intercurrent problems, not thought to be a result of treatment. There were no episodes of severe hypoglycaemia. In the smaller trial, 30% of triple therapy subjects experienced leg oedema, 9% nausea, and a single subject had a 1.4-fold increase in liver aminotransferase levels, but all were deemed mild. There was no hypoglycemia requiring assistance.

WHAT IS THE OPTIMAL INSULIN-CONTAINING REGIMEN?

Acquisition of Evidence

There are two components to this question. The first is whether both basal and prandial insulin replacement are required in some form and the second is whether insulin should be given alone or in combination with oral therapy. Numerous studies, often small and of duration less than 1 yr, have addressed different aspects of these questions. Because of the number of studies involved, practicing clinicians must rely on reviews of the literature to some extent in formulating recommendations. The problem is exemplified by published expert opinion, which, based on the same evidence, can be diametrically opposed on key issues *(42,43)*.

Appraisal of Evidence

Searching Medline reveals the first important and relevant study to have been reported in 1992 *(44)*. In this study, 153 patients failing on oral therapy were randomized to continued oral hypoglycaemic agents (OHA) with NPH insulin either in the morning or evening, to a twice daily 70/30 insulin mix, to a full basal bolus regimen combining basal and prandial components, or to continued OHA therapy (control group). The study was only of 3 mo duration and demonstrated significant improvements in HbA1c in all insulin treated groups (around –1.8%). The differences between the groups were not significant, but the bedtime NPH-containing regimen resulted in less weight gain and daytime hyperinsulinemia. This offered the possibility of simple insulin regimens for patients with type 2 diabetes at the point of OHA failure, which is appealing in terms of patient satisfaction and compliance. This is particularly relevant in this case as the patient has volunteered that he is very reluctant to have any insulin injections. On the other hand, the very short duration (3 mo) and surrogate endpoints of the study should be noted.

Although evidence from the UKPDS and elsewhere suggests that supplementary prandial insulin may be required with time in those patients on a basal-only regimen *(45)*, trial evidence for the use of a single basal insulin in patients failing on oral therapy has accumulated steadily. Indeed, the focus of several recent trials has not been a comparison of basal and mixed regimens, but rather the comparison of conventional basal NPH insulin and the newer, "peakless" insulin glargine: two of these studies involved adding insulin glargine to existing combination therapy with SUR and metformin, and so are very relevant to the patient in question here. The first study randomized 426 patients to NPH insulin or insulin glargine in addition to existing OHA therapy, and targeted a fasting plasma glucose of 6.7 mmol/L *(46)*. Starting HbA1cs were around 9.0%, as is the case here, and the population was well matched demographically to him. After 1 yr, both groups had similar drops in HbA1c to just above 8%, but with significantly less hypoglycaemia in the glargine group. The second study adopted a more aggressive approach to insulin dose titration, with a FPG target of less 5.6 mmol/L, and randomized 756 patients *(47)*. Again, study subjects were well matched demographically to this patient, and this time had mean baseline HbA1cs of around 8.6%. After 24 wk, the decreases in HbA1c were again similar, although rather more impressive than the previous study, with around 60% of subjects achieving target HbA1cs below 7%. Insulin glargine was superior in terms of episodes of hypoglycaemia, with 13.9 episodes per patients per year, compared to 17.7 for the NPH group.

Given this patient's professed desire to avoid insulin injections if possible, it seems highly desirable to be able to offer him a regimen of only one injection per day. It appears that this is efficacious in lowering HbA1c in the short term, and that insulin glargine may help to reduce episodes of hypoglycemia and thus potentially improve compliance in comparison to NPH insulin. However although this assumption of improved patient satisfaction seems reasonable, it has yet to be formally tested. The accumulated evidence suggests that he should be advised that further prandial injections may eventually be required as an inevitable consequence of the disease process, and the paucity of longer term studies of combined regimens and pure basal regimens should be noted.

Thus, it seems tenable to include a once daily regimen of insulin glargine in the evidence-based options presented to the patient, but a remaining question is whether to continue either or both OHAs. The protocols adopted by the studies of glargine attest that continuing both does work, but whether it is superior in terms of glycaemic endpoints or side effects to glargine alone, or glargine in combination with a single OHA has not been tested. There have, however, been a variety of studies that have addressed combination of other insulins with oral hypoglycemic therapy. The most directly relevant study to this patient was undertaken in Finland, and compared the effects of: (1) evening NPH plus SUR plus placebo, (2) evening NPH plus metformin plus placebo, (3) evening NPH plus SUR and metformin, and (4) twice daily NPH plus placebo *(48)*. The subjects studied had suboptimal glycemic control on SUR monotherapy with HbA1cs around 10% in each group, and the study ran for 12 mo. Ninety-six patients were randomized, and all groups had a marked fall in HbA1c of around 2–2.5%. The greatest improvement in HbA1c was seen in the metformin plus NPH group, and this achieved significance compared to the other groups. Strikingly, this group alone also failed to gain weight, and suffered significantly fewer episodes of hypoglycemia despite higher levels of NPH insulin being used. An important caveat in applying the results of this study to the case in hand is that the patients at enrolment were metformin-naïve, and thus not wholly representative of this case, or indeed routine clinical practice. Other studies making two-way comparisons between insulin alone and insulin with SUR or SUR and metformin (reviewed in ref. *49*) mostly demonstrate equivalent glycemic control between groups, although 2 meta-analyses of combination therapy with SUR and insulin have pointed to modest improvements in glycemia compared to insulin alone. However all studies do demonstrate a marked sparing effect of either SUR or SUR and metformin on exogenous insulin dose, with weighted mean decrements 62% for SUR and metformin, and 42% for SUR alone. There is also a suggestion from some studies that metformin use mitigates the weight gain seen with insulin therapy. Apart from the Finnish study, no other studies examine metformin combined with insulin in previously insulin-naïve patients, but studies of addition of metformin to insulin-based regimenns consistently show marked improvement in glycemic control with metformin as well as reduced weight gain.

Is Oral Triple Therapy Better Than or As Good As Insulin-Containing Regimens?

Acquisition of Evidence

This very specific question gets at the heart of the problem posed by this patient, yet evidence is only just beginning to emerge to address it. Medline searching reveals two prospective studies that are relevant *(38,39)*.

Appraisal of Evidence

Both studies address patient groups and a clinical problem highly relevant to the case at hand. The first, published in 2003, randomized 188 patients who had failed glycemic targets on combined SUR and metformin, with HbA1cs of around 9.6%, to a twice daily insulin 30/70 mix combined with metformin alone, or oral triple therapy including rosiglitazone or pioglitazone (50% each) *(38)*. Over 24 wk of follow up, no difference in glycemic improvement between groups was shown, with around 60% achieving HbA1c <8 and 30% an HbA1c <7% in both groups. However 10.2% of the oral triple therapy group were deemed therapeutic failures, and were changed to the insulin-based regimen, whereas only 2.4% in the twice daily 70/30 group failed and required switching to a basal bolus regimen. Furthermore, cost analysis suggested that the triple therapy approach was less cost effective than the metformin/insulin combination. A second study in 2004 used a nonblinded, open-label RCT to compare oral triple therapy with SUR/metformin plus bedtime NPH insulin in a similar group of patients *(39)*. Over 16 wk the mean HbA1c improved from approx 10% to approx 7.8% in both groups, but the oral triple therapy group also had significantly less hypoglycaemia and greater improvement in HDL cholesterol, at the expense of a 30% incidence of dependent oedema.

These studies together suggest that in the short term, oral triple therapy results in similar glycemic improvement to the insulin regimens studied, although only a minority achieved treatment goals in the periods studied.

Application to This Patient

The question of how to proceed once dual therapy with SUR and metformin has failed is a central issue in managing type 2 diabetes. It is important both for the physician and, crucially, the patient, who faces the possibility of crossing the rubicon of the initiation of insulin treatment. Despite this, the trial data summarized above almost universally addresses only short-term treatment, and measures surrogate endpoints such as HbA1c. This means that there is very little evidence that assesses the key endpoints of microvascular and macrovascular complications, and long-term quality of life. Furthermore, little is known about therapeutic factors that influence the decline in β cell function, and to what extent this is clinically important in improving outcomes. In the face of this uncertainty, the patient's preferences are important in navigating this part of the therapeutic course. In this case, oral triple therapy, dual therapy with insulin (twice daily or basal alone) and either metformin or metformin and SUR, and insulin alone should all be discussed. Uncertainty over their relative long-term outcomes, and also the liklelihood again of secondary failure should be presented before a decision is made.

SCENARIO 3

The same man, a further 8 yr later, is re-evaluated. He has now been taking subcutaneous insulin for 5 yr. Although he has now achieved some stability on a twice daily mixed insulin regimen, with an HbA1c of 8.1%, his course has been rather stormy, with poor and erratic glycemic control.

He has received retinal photocoagulation for diabetic maculopathy, now said to be stable by the ophthalmologist, and has albuminuria of 350 mg/24 h. His blood pressure, and lipids are well under control, he remains an exsmoker, and is established on a high dose of ACE inhibitor.

Unfortunately he now presents with a foot ulcer, which developed from a blister incurred during a weekend's hiking some 5 wk before. On examination there is a 2 × 2 cm ulcer on the plantar aspect of his right hallux, covered in slough but with no surrounding erythema or evidence of systemic infection. The ulcer appears superficial on probing. There is absent sensation in both feet on testing with a 10 g monofilament, but both feet are warm with normal pulses.

Discussion

The annual incidence of diabetic foot ulceration in patients with diabetic neuropathy is between 5 and 7.5% *(50)*, and the personal and economic burden of this ulceration in its own right is enormous. Furthermore, 85% of lower limb amputations in diabetes are preceded by foot ulceration *(51,52)*, leading to the concept that intervening effectively at the stage of ulceration may improve chances of limb preservation later, although this has yet to be formally demonstrated. Despite the enormous impact of this late complication of diabetes, the evidence base for its management is strikingly sparse. Most conventional approaches include debridement of necrotic tissue, good wound care, optimization of glycemic control and general care, pressure off-loading of the affected foot, treatment of infection, and sometimes adjunctive therapy. Adjunctive therapies that have been tested in small clinical trials are numerous, but in general are expensive of unproven benefit in larger scale studies. For this reason, they tend to be reserved for refractory ulcers. In this case, an evidence-based indication of likely prognosis would thus be of great use in guiding treatment.

Prognostic Indicators in Neuropathic Diabetic Foot Ulcers

Medline searching reveals a meta-analysis from 2000 which incorporates data from "standard care" groups from five RCTs, consisting of 586 subjects *(52)*. All patients in these groups received standard wound care, debridement, and pressure off-loading. Comparing the groups of patients whose ulcer healed within 20 wk with those who failed to heal within 20 wk, it was found that early healers statistically had smaller ulcers of shorter duration, and also were more likely to be nonwhite. Age, gender, and glycemic control as assessed by HbA1c were not significantly different between groups. Thus the case patient can be classified as having a reasonably good prognosis.

Preparation of the Ulcer Bed and Wound Dressing

Sharp debridement of necrotic tissue from ulcers has been universally adopted as the standard of care for patients with diabetic foot ulcers, based on the belief that it reduces the risk of infection, and exposes the full extent of the ulcer. Despite this well-established belief, there is little evidence to support this approach directly, although a *post hoc* analysis of a nonrandomized trial in 1996 correlated frequency of debridement with time to ulcer healing *(53)*. More recently there has been a Cochrane review of the debridement of diabetic ulcers *(54)*. This observed that trials were generally small and of poor methodological quality. Furthermore, classification of ulcers and their etiology varied, as did the agents investigated. Three of the studies compared formulations of hydrogel (a sodium carboxymethylcellulose-based gel) with other dressings and standard care. Despite methodological differences, there was a significant improvement in time to wound closure with each of the three hydrogel-based regimens compared to saline or dry gauze-based dressings. Although the review was described as addressing debridement, however, the hydrogel also has hydrating properties locally in the ulcer, clouding the issue. Thus sharp debridement should be undertaken regularly in this patient despite the formal lack of evidence, and additional hydrogel remains a possibility to promote wound healing.

PRESSURE OFF-LOADING OF THE ULCER

Abnormal pressure distribution on bony protruberances, and loss of pain sensation, which impairs the natural off-weight bearing response of limping, are believed to be central features of the route to ulceration in neuropathic diabetic feet, and removal of pressure on the affected area has long been a key plank of the therapeutic strategy. A Cochrane review (55) of the evidence behind this strategy identified only one relevant RCT which compared total contact casting (TCC) and limitation of weight bearing to accommodative footware and instruction to avoid weight bearing alone (56). Despite the small size of this study there was clear evidence of improved time to wound healing in the TCC group, with 19/21 ulcers healing in 42 ± 29 d compared with 6 of 19 ulcers healing in 65 ± 29 d. On the basis of this study and previous case series, the ADA consensus conference in 1999 adopted TCC as the standard of care (57). This early RCT was later followed up by a further study comparing TCC to a removable cast walker and a half shoe (58). The patients in the TCC group had significantly improved time to complete healing compared to the other groups, and were also significantly less active. As TCC was known to reduce foot pressure only to around the same degree as removable cast walkers, it was later tested whether the difference in ulcer outcome was attributable to differences in compliance—TCCs are not removable, unlike the cast walkers. Correlation of activity recorded by waist-worn and concealed cast-walker mounted accelerometers in 20 subjects showed that despite advice to wear the cast walker whenever walking, only 28% of daily activity in fact was taken while wearing it (59). This volitional factor might have significant implications for many of the trials of proposed new agents that have proved to have little benefit.

On the basis of this evidence, this patient should be advised of the crucial importance of off-weight bearing as much as possible, and TCC should be discussed. Use of TCC is time and labor-intensive, and requires sufficient skill to avoid the risks of further damage to neuropathic feet, but the limited available evidence suggests that it should be recommended in the first instance.

ADJUNCTIVE TREATMENTS

This man has an ulcer with good prognostic features, and diligent off-weight bearing and regular debridement with good wound care (perhaps in conjunction with hydrogel) is very likely to lead to ulcer healing in a few weeks. Thus, consideration of more innovative adjunctive therapies is probably not necessary. Many such approaches have been tested in small pilot studies, including topical growth factor-based treatments, hyperbaric oxygen, and negative pressure dressings, but at present there is insufficient evidence to recommend any of these strongly, as discussed in a recent comprehensive review (60).

SUMMARY AND PERSPECTIVE

Therapeutic issues facing this patient and his physician have been discussed at three key points in the natural history of his diabetes—at the point of failure of lifestyle measures alone, at the point of failure of dual oral therapy with sulphonylurea and metformin, and at the point of development of a major foot complication. Many of the recommendations at the first decision point have a good evidence base, but even for this patient, who in many ways is prototypic—male, Caucasian, mildly obese, aged 50–65, and representative of most large type 2 diabetes study populations—there are no hard data looking at important clinical outcomes to guide the transition to insulin therapy, whereas the evidence underpinning the management of diabetic foot ulcers is also limited. These weaknesses of the clinical evidence would be more pointed still were the case patient to have been a woman, or from a different ethnic group. The difficulty in accumulating evidence for many therapeutic decisions in type 2 diabetes reflects in part the long-term, progressive nature of the disease and its pathological heterogeneity, and the divergent appearance of complications between patients in the later stages. Nevertheless, huge strides have been made, particularly over the past 15 yr, and although informed decision making based on observational evidence will always have an important role to play in guiding patients, direct evidence of efficacy of particular interventions can increasingly be drawn upon.

REFERENCES

1. Zimmet P, Alberti KG, Shaw J. Global and societal implications of the diabetes epidemic. Nature 2001;414:782–787.
2. Jarrett RJ, Shipley MJ. Type 2 (non-insulin-dependent) diabetes mellitus and cardiovascular disease—putative association via common antecedents; further evidence from the Whitehall Study. Diabetologia 1988;31:737–740.
3. Eschwege E, Richard JL, Thibult N, et al. Coronary heart disease mortality in relation with diabetes, blood glucose and plasma insulin levels. The Paris Prospective Study, ten years later. Horm Metab Res Suppl 1985;15:41–46.
4. Kleinman JC, Donahue RP, Harris MI, Finucane FF, Madans JH, Brock DB. Mortality among diabetics in a national sample. Am J Epidemiol 1988;128:389–401.
5. Kannel WB, McGee DL. Diabetes and glucose tolerance as risk factors for cardiovascular disease: the Framingham study. Diabetes Care 1979;2:120–126.
6. Joint British recommendations on prevention of coronary heart disease in clinical practice: summary. British Cardiac Society, British Hyperlipidaemia Association, British Hypertension Society, British Diabetic Association. BMJ 2000;320:705–708.
7. Dinneen SF, Gerstein HC. The association of microalbuminuria and mortality in non-insulin-dependent diabetes mellitus. A systematic overview of the literature. Arch Intern Med 1977;157:1413–1418.
8. Deckert T, Feldt-Rasmussen B, Borch-Johnsen K, Jensen T, Kofoed-Enevoldsen A. Albuminuria reflects widespread vascular damage. The Steno hypothesis. Diabetologia 1989;32:219–226.
9. Klein R, Klein BE, Moss SE, Cruickshanks KJ. The Wisconsin Epidemiologic Study of Diabetic Retinopathy: XVII. The 14-year incidence and progression of diabetic retinopathy and associated risk factors in type 1 diabetes. Ophthalmology 1998;105:1801–1815.
10. McCance DR, Hanson RL, Charles MA, et al. Comparison of tests for glycated haemoglobin and fasting and two hour plasma glucose concentrations as diagnostic methods for diabetes. BMJ 1994; 308:1323–1328.
11. Intensive blood-glucose control with sulphonylureas or insulin compared with conventional treatment and risk of complications in patients with type 2 diabetes (UKPDS 33). UK Prospective Diabetes Study (UKPDS) Group. Lancet 1998;352:837–853.
12. Consensus development conference on the diagnosis of coronary heart disease in people with diabetes: 10-11 February 1998, Miami, Florida. American Diabetes Association. Diabetes Care 1998;21:1551–1559.

13. Wackers FJ, Young LH, Inzucchi SE, et al. Detection of silent myocardial ischemia in asymptomatic diabetic subjects: the DIAD study. Diabetes Care 2004;27:1954–1961.

14. Franz MJ, Bantle JP, Beebe CA, et al. Nutrition principles and recommendations in diabetes. Diabetes Care 2004;27:S36–S46.

15. Franz MJ, Bantle JP, Beebe CA, et al. Evidence-based nutrition principles and recommendations for the treatment and prevention of diabetes and related complications. Diabetes Care 2002;25: 148–198.

16. Zinman B, Ruderman N, Campaigne BN, Devlin JT, Schneider SH. Physical activity/exercise and diabetes. Diabetes Care 2004;27:S58–62.

17. Exercise and NIDDM. Diabetes Care 1990;13:785–789.

18. Moore H SC, Hooper L, Cruickshank K, et al. Dietary advice for treatment of type 2 diabetes mellitus in adults. The Cochrane Database of Systematic Reviews: Art. No.: CD004097.pub3. DOI: 10.1002/14651858.CD004097.pub3, 2004.

19. Ryan DH, Espeland MA, Foster GD, et al. Look AHEAD (Action for Health in Diabetes): design and methods for a clinical trial of weight loss for the prevention of cardiovascular disease in type 2 diabetes. Control Clin Trials 2003;24:610–628.

20. Tuomilehto J, Lindstrom J, Eriksson JG, et al. Prevention of type 2 diabetes mellitus by changes in lifestyle among subjects with impaired glucose tolerance. N Engl J Med 2001;344:1343–1350.

21. Knowler WC, Barrett-Connor E, Fowler SE, et al. Reduction in the incidence of type 2 diabetes with lifestyle intervention or metformin. N Engl J Med 2002;346:393–403.

22. Pan XR, Li GW, Hu YH, et al. Effects of diet and exercise in preventing NIDDM in people with impaired glucose tolerance. The Da Qing IGT and Diabetes Study. Diabetes Care 1997;20:537–544.

23. Haire-Joshu D, Glasgow RE, Tibbs TL. Smoking and diabetes. Diabetes Care 1999;22:1887–1898.

24. Haire-Joshu D, Glasgow RE, Tibbs TL. Smoking and diabetes. Diabetes Care 2004;27:S74–S75.

25. UK Prospective Diabetes Study Group. Tight blood pressure control and risk of macrovascular and microvascular complications in type 2 diabetes: UKPDS 38. BMJ 1998;317:703–713.

26. Adler AI, Stratton IM, Neil HA, et al. Association of systolic blood pressure with macrovascular and microvascular complications of type 2 diabetes (UKPDS 36): prospective observational study. BMJ 2000;321:412–419.

27. Hansson L, Zanchetti A, Carruthers SG, et al. Effects of intensive blood-pressure lowering and low-dose aspirin in patients with hypertension: principal results of the Hypertension Optimal Treatment (HOT) randomised trial. HOT Study Group. Lancet 1998;351:1755–1762.

28. Estacio RO, Jeffers BW, Gifford N, Schrier RW. Effect of blood pressure control on diabetic microvascular complications in patients with hypertension and type 2 diabetes. Diabetes Care 2000;23: B54–B64.

29. Lindholm LH, Hansson L, Ekbom T, et al. Comparison of antihypertensive treatments in preventing cardiovascular events in elderly diabetic patients: results from the Swedish Trial in Old Patients with Hypertension-2 Study Group. J Hypertens 2000;18:1671–1675.

30. Lindholm LH, Ibsen H, Dahlof B, et al. Cardiovascular morbidity and mortality in patients with diabetes in the Losartan Intervention For Endpoint reduction in hypertension study (LIFE): a randomised trial against atenolol. Lancet 2002;359:1004–1010.

31. Scandinavian Simvastatin Survival Study. Randomised trial of cholesterol lowering in 4444 patients with coronary heart disease: the Scandinavian Simvastatin Survival Study (4S). Lancet 1994;344: 1383–1389.

32. Collins R, Armitage J, Parish S, Sleigh P, Peto R. MRC/BHF Heart Protection Study of cholesterol-lowering with simvastatin in 5963 people with diabetes: a randomised placebo-controlled trial. Lancet 2003;361:2005–2016.

33. Colhoun HM, Betteridge DJ, Durrington PN, et al. Primary prevention of cardiovascular disease with atorvastatin in type 2 diabetes in the Collaborative Atorvastatin Diabetes Study (CARDS): multicentre randomised placebo-controlled trial. Lancet 2004;364:685–696.

34. Steering Committee of the Physicians' Health Study Research Group. Final report on the aspirin component of the ongoing Physicians' Health Study. N Engl J Med 1999;321:129–135.

35. Early Treatment Diabetic Retinopathy Study Investigators. Aspirin effects on mortality and morbidity in patients with diabetes mellitus. Early Treatment Diabetic Retinopathy Study report 14. ETDRS Investigators. JAMA 1992;268:1292–1300.

36. Gaede P, Vedel P, Larsen N, Jensen GV, Parving HH, Pedersen O. Multifactorial intervention and cardiovascular disease in patients with type 2 diabetes. N Engl J Med 2003;348:383–393.

37. Dailey GE, 3rd, Noor MA, Park JS, Bruce S, Fiedorek FT. Glycemic control with glyburide/ metformin tablets in combination with rosiglitazone in patients with type 2 diabetes: a randomized, double-blind trial. Am J Med 2004;116:223–229.

38. Schwartz S, Sievers R, Strange P, Lyness WH, Hollander P. Insulin 70/30 mix plus metformin versus triple oral therapy in the treatment of type 2 diabetes after failure of two oral drugs: efficacy, safety, and cost analysis. Diabetes Care 2003;26:2238–2243.

39. Aljabri K, Kozak SE, Thompson DM. Addition of pioglitazone or bedtime insulin to maximal doses of sulfonylurea and metformin in type 2 diabetes patients with poor glucose control: a prospective, randomized trial. Am J Med 2004;116:230–235.

40. Yale JF, Valiquett TR, Ghazzi MN, Owens-Grillo JK, Whitcomb RW, Foyt HL. The effect of a thiazolidinedione drug, troglitazone, on glycemia in patients with type 2 diabetes mellitus poorly controlled with sulfonylurea and metformin. A multicenter, randomized, double-blind, placebo-controlled trial. Ann Intern Med 2001;134:737–745.

41. Gavin LA, Barth J, Arnold D, Shaw R. Troglitazone add-on therapy to a combination of sulfonylureas plus metformin achieved and sustained effective diabetes control. Endocr Pract 2000;6:305–310.

42. Garber AJ . Benefits of combination therapy of insulin and oral hypoglycemic agents. Arch Intern Med 2003;163:1781–1782.

43. Westphal SA, Palumbo PJ. Insulin and oral hypoglycemic agents should not be used in combination in the treatment of type 2 diabetes. Arch Intern Med 2003;163:1783–1785; discussion 1785.

44. Yki-Jarvinen H, Kauppila M, Kujansuu E, et al. Comparison of insulin regimens in patients with non-insulin-dependent diabetes mellitus. N Engl J Med 1992;327:1426–1433.

45. Wolffenbuttel BH, Sels JP, Rondas-Colbers GJ, Menheere PP, Nieuwenhuijzen-Kruseman AC. Comparison of different insulin regimens in elderly patients with NIDDM. Diabetes Care 1996;19:1326–1332.

46. Yki-Jarvinen H, Dressler A, Ziemen M. Less nocturnal hypoglycemia and better post-dinner glucose control with bedtime insulin glargine compared with bedtime NPH insulin during insulin combination therapy in type 2 diabetes. HOE 901/3002 Study Group. Diabetes Care 2000;23:1130–1136.

47. Riddle MC, Rosenstock J, Gerich J. The treat-to-target trial: randomized addition of glargine or human NPH insulin to oral therapy of type 2 diabetic patients. Diabetes Care 2003;26:3080–3086.

48. Yki-Jarvinen H, Ryysy L, Nikkila K, Tulokas T, Vanamo R, Heikkila M. Comparison of bedtime insulin regimens in patients with type 2 diabetes mellitus. A randomized, controlled trial. Ann Intern Med 1999;130:389–396.

49. Yki-Jarvinen H. Combination therapies with insulin in type 2 diabetes. Diabetes Care 2001;24: 758–767.

50. Abbott CA, Vileikyte L, Williamson S, Carrington AL, Boulton AJ. Multicenter study of the incidence of and predictive risk factors for diabetic neuropathic foot ulceration. Diabetes Care 1998;21: 1071–1075.

51. Palumbo PJ MLI. Peripheral Vascular Disease and Diabetes. In: Diabetes in America: diabetes data compiled 1984. Government Printing Office, Washington DC, August 1985:XV-1-XV-21. (NIH publication no. 85-1468).

52. Margolis DJ, Kantor J, Santanna J, Strom BL, Berlin JA. Risk factors for delayed healing of neuropathic diabetic foot ulcers: a pooled analysis. Arch Dermatol 2000;136:1531–1535.

53. Steed DL, Donohoe D, Webster MW, Lindsley L. Effect of extensive debridement and treatment on the healing of diabetic foot ulcers. Diabetic Ulcer Study Group. J Am Coll Surg 1996;183:61–64.

54. Smith J. Debridement of diabetic foot ulcers. Cochrane Database Syst Rev. 2002;(4):CD003556.

55. Spencer S. Pressure relieving interventions for preventing and treating diabetic foot ulcers. Cochrane Database Syst Rev. 2000;(3):CD002302.

56. Mueller MJ, Diamond JE, Sinacore DR, et al. Total contact casting in treatment of diabetic plantar ulcers. Controlled clinical trial. Diabetes Care 1989;12:384–388.

57. Consensus Development Conference on Diabetic Foot Wound Care: 7-8 April 1999, Boston, Massachusetts. American Diabetes Association. Diabetes Care 1999;22:1354–1360.

58. Armstrong DG, Nguyen HC, Lavery LA, van Schie CH, Boulton AJ, Harkless LB. Off-loading the diabetic foot wound: a randomized clinical trial. Diabetes Care 2001;24:1019–1022.

59. Armstrong DG, Lavery LA, Kimbriel HR, Nixon BP, Boulton AJ. Activity patterns of patients with diabetic foot ulceration: patients with active ulceration may not adhere to a standard pressure off-loading regimen. Diabetes Care 2003;26:2595–2597.

60. Eldor R, Raz I, Ben Yehuda A, Boulton AJ. New and experimental approaches to treatment of diabetic foot ulcers: a comprehensive review of emerging treatment strategies. Diabet Med 2004;21:1161–1173.

61. Tuomilehto J, Rastenyte D, Birkenhager WH, et al. Effects of calcium-channel blockade in older patients with diabetes and systolic hypertension. Systolic Hypertension in Europe Trial Investigators. N Engl J Med 1999;340:677–684.

62. Yusuf S, Sleight P, Pogue J, Bosch J, Davies R, Dagenais G. Effects of an angiotensin-converting-enzyme inhibitor, ramipril, on cardiovascular events in high-risk patients. The Heart Outcomes Prevention Evaluation Study Investigators. N Engl J Med 2000;342:145–153.

63. Effects of ramipril on cardiovascular and microvascular outcomes in people with diabetes mellitus: results of the HOPE study and MICRO-HOPE substudy. Heart Outcomes Prevention Evaluation Study Investigators. Lancet 2000;355:253–259.

21

Patients With Diabetes Using Alternative Medicine

Dugald Seely, ND, Edward Mills, MSC and Beth Rachlis, BSc

CONTENTS

INTRODUCTION
CASE SCENARIO
REFERENCES

INTRODUCTION

Clinicians need for valid information on herbal medicinal products is considerable. In the United States, the popularity of complementary and alternative medicine is growing at a remarkable, and possibly concerning, rate *(1)*. In particular, herbal medicine has grown faster than any other complementary or alternative medicine (CAM) treatment method in the United States *(1,2)*. The top-selling herbal medicinal products in the United States include: *Ginkgo biloba* (total 1998 retail sales of $151 million), St. John's wort ($140 million), ginseng ($96 million), garlic ($84 million), echinacea ($70 million), saw palmetto ($32 million), and kava ($17 million) *(3)*.

Physicians will often see patients who self-prescribe herbal medicinal products but do not discuss this with their physicians *(4)*. Some herbal medicines have adverse effects, and many can interact with prescription drugs *(5)*. A complete medical history should, therefore, include specific questions about the use of herbal medicinal products *(4)*, and physicians must acquire sufficient knowledge in this area to advise their patients responsibly.

In 2001, the American Diabetes Association issued a Position Statement on "Unproven Therapies" that suggest health care providers ask their patients about alternative therapies and practices, evaluate each therapy's effectiveness, be cognizant of any potential harm to patients, and acknowledge when new and innovative diagnostic or therapeutic measures might have a role to play in patient care *(6)*. Two US national surveys have now examined CAM use among those with diabetes. One study, using 1996 data, reported that 8% of respondents with diabetes saw a CAM provider for care *(7)*. A US national representative survey conducted in 1997–1998 reported that about one-third of respondents with diabetes

From: *Contemporary Endocrinology: Evidence-Based Endocrinology*
Edited by: V. M. Montori © Mayo Foundation for Medical Education and Research

use CAM to treat their condition *(8)*. In other surveys of specific diabetic populations, 39% of Navajo *(9)*, two-thirds of Vietnamese *(10)*, and 49% of a largely Hispanic population in South Texas used CAM *(11)*. However, the evidence supporting CAM use in diabetes is not well established. This may be, in part, a result of the issue that CAM incorporates many different interventions, including, but not limited to: acupuncture and Asian medicine, chiropractic, counseling and mind–body medicine, herbal medicines, homeopathy, nutrition, spirituality, and other treatments that may seem odd, even to those involved in CAM.

Most of the literature, however, has focused on herbs or other dietary supplements. Plant medicines with alleged diabetic control properties have been used in folk medicine and traditional healing systems around the world for centuries if not millennia (e.g., Native American, Chinese, East Indian, Mexican, Tibetan). Many modern pharmaceuticals used in conventional medicine today also have natural plant origins. Indeed metformin, one of the most commonly used drugs in diabetes care, was derived from the flowering plant, *Galega officinalis* (Goat's Rue or French Lilac), which was traditionally a remedy for diabetes *(12)*.

To provide context and emphasize the need to be aware of herbal medicinal use in diabetes we present a typical case scenario. Following the case, we will examine the best evidence available on herbal medicines, some nonherbal natural products, and specific dietary recommendations that are used to treat diabetes. We will look at the role these therapies may have in treatment with a principal emphasis on glycemic control.

CASE SCENARIO

Presentation

Jess Tarnaruk is a 53-yr-old Native American woman who has been referred to you by her medical doctor for treatment of type 2 diabetes. Ms. Tarnaruk has raised seven children and has been divorced for 12 yr. She appears somewhat anxious, and claims that in order to follow her deeply held beliefs, she is not interested in taking "drugs" for her treatment. She's very concerned about the side effects of prescription drugs, and feels that herbs are what she needs, and she wants to know what you can suggest.

Her chief complaint is mild blurring of her vision, which started about 6 mo ago, and now she finds it difficult to read small type. She also experiences a tingling sensation in her fingers and toes that started to come on sporadically 2 yr ago. Other complaints include deep calf pain in her left leg when she walks for more than 15 min (gets better with rest) and fatigue for most of the day every day.

Physical examination shows a body mass index (BMI) of 32, blood pressure 135/90 mmHg and some microaneurysms in both retinae (visual acuity 20/60 in both eyes). She has decreased light touch and vibration perception in both legs. Posterior tibial pulses are diminished and pedal pulses are nonpalpable. Otherwise the examination was normal.

Her HbA1c was 8.4% (normal hemoglobin) with a fasting glucose of 142 mg/dL, total cholesterol of 235 mg/dL, low-density lipoprotein (LDL) 143 mg/dL, high-density lipoprotein (HDL) 55 mg/dL, and triglycerides 178 mg/dL.

Your assessment is of an uncontrolled type 2 diabetes patient with micro- and macrovascular complications. Apart from usual management approaches this patient would want serious consideration to herbal medications as the mainstay of her therapy. You note how uncomfortable you are about this route but decide to try to determine if evidence-based approaches exist that can effectively and safely help this patient while respecting her beliefs.

In order to practice evidence-based medicine, we need to have a focused clinical question, conduct a systematic search, appraise the evidence, and then determine how to apply it to our patient.

The Question

In order to develop a focused question, we must ask who is our patient population, what is our intervention, and what is the outcome that we are interested in examining. In this case, we develop a question that resembles: in Type 2 diabetics, do any herbal medicines assist in glycemic control?

Now it is necessary to determine what kind of evidence we would like to have in order to determine whether Ms. Tarnaruk's desire for herbal medicine can be justified for a clinical recommendation. Considering the hierarchy of evidence, we would ideally like a systematic review or meta-analysis of homogeneous and valid randomized trials assessing the effectiveness and safety of herbal products in patients with diabetes. However, as with many fields of health care, there is a paucity of systematic reviews of interventions. Consideration of individual randomized trials would follow.

Literature Review

To adequately search for evidence on the use of herbal medicines to control blood glucose, we will perform a systematic search of the peer-reviewed literature. In our search, we will only include studies that have assessed glycemic control as a primary outcome in a population of patients with diabetes mellitus (type 1 or 2) or impaired glucose tolerance using any herbal medicine as therapy.

For the purpose of "sensitive" searching, we will access the MeSH database section of PubMed (www.pubmed.com). We are aware that the indexing of abstracts in PubMed is not always ideal, so we will want to identify a MeSH term that will capture all of the relevant studies, and likely some that are irrelevant. For the purpose of searching for articles relevant to our patient, we will use the MeSH term "Diabetes Mellitus." For the purpose of herbal medicines, we will use the combined search terms, using boolean operators, "Complementary therapies OR Medicine, herbal OR Medicine, traditional). We may also choose to examine only our outcome of interest, using the MeSh term "blood glucose."

RESULTS

We limited the evidence gathered to randomized controlled trials (RCTs) and systematic reviews of orally ingested herbal medicines and to systematic reviews of non-herbal supplements and dietary modification. We identified 34 RCTs and two systematic reviews of herbal medicines and five systematic reviews assessing non-herbal supplements and dietary modification. Figure 1 depicts the flow chart detailing the selection process of the articles found in the literature. Table 1 summarizes the trials assessed for the use of single herbal medicines; Table 2 summarizes the trials assessed for the use of combination herbal medicines; and Table 3 summarizes the details of systematic reviews of non-herbal supplements and dietary recommendations. All these tables include the herb,

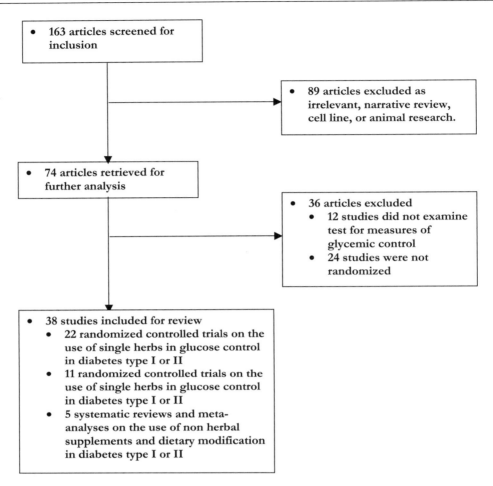

Fig. 1. Flow chart of studies selected for the systematic review.

supplement or diet, the reference, the number of participants, the intervention, the control, the outcomes measured, the results, and adverse events noted.

One of the systematic reviews of herbal medicines for glycemic control in type 1 or 2 diabetes included all clinical trials randomized or not *(13)*. The other systematic review specifically included only Chinese herbs in the treatment of type 2 diabetes *(14)*. Although there is some overlap between these reviews and ours, we specifically look at randomized controlled trials of herbs for glycemic control in both type 1 and 2 diabetes.

Single Herbs (Table 1)

A cursory assessment of whether or not there was a beneficial effect on blood sugar control using single herbs indicated that 78% of published trials showed benefit. Of the 22 RCTs assessed, 18 found a statistically significant and clinically beneficial effect comprising a total of 13 separate herbs. The herbs that were found to be beneficial included: *Cinnamomum cassia (15)*, *Coccinia indica (16)*, *Ficus carica (17,18)*, *Ganoderma lucidum (18)*, *Glycine max (19)*, Ginseng (unspecified species) *(20)*, *Ipomoea batatas (21,22)*, *Lagerstroemia speciosa (23)*, *Morus indica (24)*, *Ocimum sanctum*

(25), *Opuntia streptacantha (26)*, *Panax quinquefolius (27,28)*, *Pinus maritime (29)*, *Silybum marianum (30)*, and *Trigonella foenum graecum (31,32)*. The remaining four trials did not show any clinical efficacy of the following five herbs: *Allium sativum (33)*, *Bauhinia forficate (34)*, *Momordica charantia (35)*, *Myrcia uniflora (34)*, and *Tinospora crispa (36)*.

All of the trials examining these herbs were placebo controlled except for *Sylibum marianum*. Providing greater strength of evidence, there were two RCTs conducted of *Ipamoea batatas (21,22)*, *Trigonella foenum graecum (31,32)*, and at least two if not three of *Panax quinquefolius (20,27,28)*. It is proposed that these herbs are best suited for further research and if any single herbal medicine be suggested as a treatment to help control blood glucose, then it should be selected from one of these three herbs.

Given the small number of participants in most of the trials (mean *n* = 30; range: 9 to 71) and that for most of the herbs only one RCT has been conducted, even tentative conclusions on clinical efficacy would be premature. As an exercise, however, we will specifically examine the evidence on one of the herbs that has relatively more trials to support its use and also one that is commonly used.

Evidence-Based Appraisal of American Ginseng. *Panax quinquefolius* (American ginseng) is one of the most commonly used herbs available *(37)*. Because of the common use of American ginseng and the fact that it has at least two RCTs in support of its use to control blood sugar in type 2 diabetics, we decided to take a closer look at the evidence *(27,28)*. We have excluded from the analysis a third study by Sotaniemi et al. *(20)* because it is not entirely clear which species of ginseng was tested.

The first study, a crossover trial, conducted by Vuksan et al. *(27)* examined the effect of combining 3 g of encapsulated American ginseng together with a glucose challenge test, or 40 min prior to the glucose challenge in 10 healthy volunteers and 9 patients with type 2 diabetes. In the case of consumption together with the glucose challenge in the diabetic patients, ginseng significantly lowered incremental glycemia at 45 min (4.2 ± 1.3 mmol/L vs 5.4 ± 1.3 mmol/L, $p < .05$) and 60 min (3.6 ± 1.4 mmol/L vs 4.9 ± 1.5 mmol/L, $p < .05$) compared with placebo. When it was given 40 min before the glucose challenge, significant results were found at 30 min (3.8 ± 1.2 mmol/L vs 4.8 ± 0.9 mmol/L, $p < .05$) and 45 min (4.5 ± 1.1 mmol/L vs 5.3 ± 1.2 mmol/L, $p < .05$) compared to placebo. These findings translated to significant reductions in incremental area under the curve (AUC). There was a 22 ±17% reduction and 19 ± 22% reduction in the incremental 2 h postprandial glycemic AUC when given together and 40 min prior to the 25-g glucose challenge test, respectively.

In looking at the quality of the trial itself, we noted that selection of the treatments (two test, two control for each participant) was randomized with a placebo identical to the intervention given as control. Allocation concealment and intention to treat analysis were not relevant in this case owing to the crossover design. All patients were accounted for and follow up was complete. Washout periods of 1 wk were set so as to eliminate any carry over effect from prior doses of ginseng.

The second trial also by Vuksan et al. *(28)* was similar in design to the latter except that this time the sample population was confined to 10 patients with type 2 diabetes only. The other principal difference is that multiple doses of American ginseng were used at different time points (0, 40, 80, and 120 min) to assess its effect on postprandial glycemia. Results of the trial showed that regardless of the time the ginseng was administered (0 min to 2 h) prior to a 25-g glucose challenge; there was a similar and

Table 1
Randomized Controlled Trials Assessing Single Herbs Used in the Treatment of Diabetes

Herb	Reference	Participants	Intervention	Control	Outcomes measured	Results	Adverse effects
Allium sativum (Garlic)	Sitprija S et al. (1987) (33)	33 DM 2 on diet alone	Garlic; 700 mg/d for 4 wk	Placebo	FG, PPG, insulin	No change in any of the measures for treatment or placebo groups	No adverse effects; no effect on liver function
Bauhinia forficata (Brazillian orchid-tree)	Russo EMK et al. (1990) (34)	16 DM 2 on diet and/or OHA	Bauhinia forficata tea; 3 3 g/d for 8 wk	Placebo herb tea	FG, HbA1c, insulin	No change in any of the measures for treatment or placebo groups	No adverse effects; no effect on liver/kidney function
Cinnamomum cassia (Cinnamon)	Khan A et al. (2003) (15)	60 DM 2 on OHA	Cinnamon: 3 separate groups consumed 1, 3, 6 g/d for 40 d	Placebo (corresponding amounts)	FG, TG, LDL, TC, HDL	All three treatment groups: decrease in FG, TG, LDL, TC; no change in HDL Placebo: no change in all measures	None reported
Coccinia indica (Ivy gourd)	Azad Khan AK et al. (1979) (16)	32 DM 2 uncontrolled or untreated	Ivy gourd leaf; 1800 mg/d for 6 wk	Placebo	FBG, PPG	Treatment group: decrease in both FBG and PPG Placebo: no change in either measure	No adverse effects; no effect on liver/kidney function
Ficus carica (Fig leaf)	Serraclara A et al. (1998) (17)	10 DM I on diet and insulin	Fig leaf tea; 13 g/d leaf decoction; for 4 wk	Open-label; Bitter commercial tea blend	PPG, insulin requirements, FG, C-pep, HbA1c	Treatment group: decrease in PPG and insulin requirements; no change in FPG, C-peptide, and HgbA(1c) Control: no change in all measures	No adverse effects noted

328

Species	Author (year)	Participants	Treatment/Dose	Control	Measures	Results	Adverse events
Ganoderma lucidum (Ling Zhi or reishi mushroom)	Gao Y et al. (2004) (18)	71 DM 2 on dietary treatment	Ganopoly (600 mg extract of G.lucidum) 1800 mg/3 times a day for 12 wk	Placebo	FG, FI, C-pep, HbA1c, PPG, TG, TC, HDL, BMI, BP	Treatment group: decrease in HbA1c, FG, and PPG Placebo: no changes in all measures	Adverse events included mild gastrointestinal complaints in treatment group
Glycine max (Soybean)	Jayagopal V et al. (2002) (19) phytoestrogens	33 DM 2 postmenopausal women on dietary treatment	Soy protein (30 g/d; isoflavones 132 mg/d) for 12 wk	Placebo	FI, IR, HbA1c, TC, LDL, total/HDL, free thyroxine	Treatment group: lower mean values for all measures Placebo: no change in all measures	Mild gastrointestinal side effects. 1 had heart attack during soy phase and withdrew
Ginseng (Unspecified species)	Sotaniemi EA et al. (1995) (20)	36 DM 2 on diet alone	Ginseng; 100 mg/d and 200 mg/d for 8 wk	Placebo	FBG, HgbA1C, BG, insulin, C-pep during OGTT	Treatment groups: Decrease in FBG, HgbA1C (200 mg); no change in BG, insulin, C-peptide during OGTT Placebo: no changes in all measures	No adverse effects
Ipomoea batatas (Caiapo)	Ludvik B et al. (2003) (21)	18 DM 2 (males only) on diet alone	Caiapo; (2 g/d) and (4 g/d) 3×/d for 6 wk	placebo	FG, FI, TC, LDL, HDL, TG, HbA1c, BP, BMI, IS	Treatment groups: low dose: no changes noted except in improved IS High dose: reduction of fasting plasma glucose and LDL cholesterol Placebo: no changes in all measures	No adverse effects reported

(continued)

Table 1 (continued)

Herb	Reference	Participants	Intervention	Control	Outcomes measured	Results	Adverse effects
Ipomoea batatas (Caiapo)	Ludvik B et al. (2004) (22)	61 DM 2 on diet alone	Caiapo: 4 g/d for 12 wk	Placebo	FG, PPG HbA1c, TC, TG, BP	Treatment group: decreased HbA1c, FG, PPG,TC; no change in TG or BP Placebo: no changes in all measures	Mild gastrointestinal effects
Lagerstroe mia speciosa Glucosol™ (Crepe Myrtle)	Judy WV et al. (2003) (23)	10 DM 2 on diet alone	Glucosol soft gel formulation with 16, 32, and 48 mg for 15 d	Glucosol hard gel-dry powder formula 16, 32, 48 mg for 15 d	FG	Both groups showed drop in FG, sig only at 48 mg. Soft gel showed 30% drop in BG, hard gel: 20%. No placebo control	Not mentioned
Momordica Charantia (Bitter Gourd)	John AJ et al. (2003) (35)	50 DM 2 on diet or OHA	Dried bitter gourd tablets; 2 gm tid for 4 wk	Placebo	FG, PPG, fruct levels	No change in any of the measures for treatment or placebo groups	None observed
Morus indica (Mulberry leaves)	Andallu B et al. (2001) (24)	24 DM 2	Mulberry leaves 3 g/d for 30 d	Glibenclamide 5 mg/d	TC, TG, FFA, LDL, VLDL, PP, UP, HDL, HbA(1c,) FG	Mulberry: greater decreased TC, TG, PFFA, LDL, VLDL, PP, UP. FBG, and increased HDL in comparison to control No change for both groups in HbA1c	Not mentioned
Myrcia uniflora (Pedra hume)	Russo EMK et al. (1990) (34)	18 DM 2 on diet and/or OHA	Pedra hume tea; 3 g/d for 8 wk	Placebo herb tea (sape, Imperata brasiliensis)	FG, HgbA(1c), FI	No change in any of the measures for treatment or placebo groups	No adverse effects

Ocimum sanctum (Holy basil)	Agrawal P et al. (1996) (25)	40 DM 2 on diet and/or OHA	Holy basil leaf; 2.5 g powder for 4 wk	Placebo (Fresh spinach leaf powder)	FG, PPG, urine glucose	Treatment group: decreased FBG, PPG, urine glucose; Placebo: no change in all measures	No adverse effects
Opuntia streptacantha (Nopal)	Frati AC et al. (1990) (26)	14 DM 2 on diet alone single dose	Grilled nopal stems; 500 g;	Open label: 400 mL H2O	FG, FI	Treatment group: decrease FG and FI; Control: no change in all measures	Not reported
Panax quinquefolius (American Ginseng)	Vuksan V et al. (2000) (28)	9 DM 2 on diet and/or OHA	Ground root of American Ginseng 3 g capsules at varying times prior to OGTT	Placebo	PPG	Treatment group: decreased PPG (given at 0 to 40 min pre OGTT) Placebo: no change observed	Mild transient insomnia in 1 case taking ginseng
Panax quinquefolius (American Ginseng)	Vuksan V et al. (2000) (28)	10 DM 2 on diet and/or OHA	Ground root of American Ginseng; 3 g vs 6 g vs 9 g capsules—single experimental dose at varying times prior to GTT	Placebo	PPG	Treatment group: decreased PPG (all doses) Placebo: no change observed	No adverse effects noted

(continued)

Table 1 (*continued*)

Herb	Reference	Participants	Intervention	Control	Outcomes measured	Results	Adverse effects
Pinus Maritima Pycnogenol® (French maritime pine bark extract)	Liu X et al. (2004) (29)	77 DM 2 on OHA	Pycnogenol: 100 mg/d for 12 wk	Placebo	FG, HbA1c, endothelin-1, 6-ketoprostaglandin F(1a)	Treatment group: decreased FG, HbA1c (only in 1st mo), endothelin-1; 6-ketoprostaglandin increased Placebo: no change in all measures	Mild transient effects in both groups
Silybum marianum "Legalon" (Milk Thistle)	Velussi M et al. (1997) (30)	60 DM 2 with cirrhosis on diet and insulin	Silymarin; 600 mg/d for 12 mo	No treatment	FG, BG, UG, HgbA1c, FI, insulin requirement, C-pep	Treatment group: decreased FG, BG, UG, HgbA(1c), FI, insulin requirement, C-pep Control: no change in all measures	No adverse effects
Tinospora Crispa (Makabuhai)	Sangsuwan C et al. (2004) (36)	40 DM 2 on OHA	*Tinospora crispa:* 1 gm 3×/d for 6 mo	Placebo	FG, HbA1c, FI	No change in any of the measures for treatment or placebo groups	Two in treatment group showed elevation of liver enzymes; slight increase in TC in treatment group

Herb	Study	Subjects	Intervention	Control	Outcomes measured	Results	Adverse effects
Trigonella foenum graecum (Fenugreek)	Sharma RD et al. (1990) (32)	10 DM I on diet and insulin (dose decreased during study)	Defatted debitterized fenugreek seed powder; 100 g/d in unleavened bread; for 10 d	No treatment	FG, PPG, urine glucose, TC, HDL, LDL, VLDL, TG, body weight, insulin	Treatment group: decrease in FG, PPG, urine glucose; no change body weight, insulin control: no change in all measures	Not reported
Trigonella foenum graecum (Fenugreek)	Gupta A et al. (2001) (31)	25 DM 2 on dietary and exercise regimen	Extract of fenugreek seeds: 1 gm/day for 2 mo	Placebo	FG, PPG, FI, IR, IS, TG, HDL	Treatment group: decreased FI, IR (in % b-cell secretion); no change in FG, PPG; increase in IS, TG, HDL Placebo: no change in all measures	None reported

significant reduction in postprandial glycemia. At the diagnostically important 2-hr end point, doses of 3, 6, and 9 g of American ginseng reduced glycemia by 59.1, 40.9, and 45.5% compared with placebo respectively. No side effects were noted for any of the doses given.

The methodology and analysis of the trial just described was thorough and lends credibility to the results. The trial was a crossover study in which each of the 10 participants received all three doses at each of the four different initial time point for a total of 12 separate glucose challenge tests. As in the first trial, the crossover design eliminated issues regarding allocation concealment, baseline differences, and intention to treat analysis. Follow up was complete and no one dropped out of the study. The placebo was adequately described and participant blinding appeared intact. One potential criticism is that the trial was single blind. However, because of the biological tests used, it is unlikely that this could have significantly affected the results.

The principal limitation to the two studies on American ginseng is in clinical application. The fact that long-term exposure was not measured and we have no real sense of what effect ginseng might have on long-term glycemic control is clearly a problem. Ideally a large parallel group RCT would be conducted on long-term ginseng use (i.e., at least 3 mo duration) with a validated outcome measure like HbA1c being assessed. This would provide much more relevant information on which to base any clinical decisions for our patient or any other seeking herbal treatment to help control their blood sugar. A final concern is long-term safety for the dosages used in these studies. There is a clear history of use for this herb, however, we do not have any confirmed evidence as to long-term safety with this herb. For that matter, we also do not have any evidence to show that ginseng will not interact with proven therapy for managing blood sugar in diabetics. At this point in time it would seem premature and unethical to suggest American ginseng as a safe and effective treatment for blood sugar control in a type 2 diabetic.

Combination Herbs (Table 2)

In assessment of the combination herbal formulas; of the 11 trials that examined 11 distinct herbal formulas, 9 showed a positive effect and 2 did not achieve statistically significant results. The trials involving the combination herbs were generally larger than those exploring single herbs with the average number of participants being 3 times that of the single trials (mean $n = 94$; range: 12 to 216). The herbal combinations that demonstrated clinical efficacy included: "Inolter" (38), "Pancreas tonic" (39), a Tibetan medicine formula (40), and six traditional Chinese medicine formulas (41–46). The two combinations that did not show any evidence of blood sugar control were the Xiaoke tea (47), and the Native American tea (48).

The herbal combinations that appeared to have the strongest evidence, based on number of participants ($n \geq 100$) included the Tibetan medicine combination ($n = 200$) (40), and three of the traditional Chinese formulas: Jiangtangkang Chrysanthemum product ($n = 188$) (41), the three herb combination (Astragalus, Coptis, and Lonicera) ($n = 216$) (45), and Qidan tongmai ($n = 128$) (46). Clearly further research needs to be conducted in this realm but there is support that efficacy in the control of blood sugar can be achieved through the use of combination herbal formulations. Whether this is a result of individual constituents found in one or more of the plants or, as is often claimed, whether there is some degree of synergy between the herbs is an issue worth

Table 2
Randomized Controlled Trials Assessing Herbal Combinations Used in the Treatment of Diabetes

Herb	Reference	Participants	Intervention	Control	Outcomes measured	Results	Comments/adverse events
"Inolter"—herbal product consisting of *Momordica charantia*, *Trigonella foenum-graecum*, Asphalt, *Gymnema sylvestre* and *Eugenia jambolena*	Agrawal RP et al. (2002) *(38)*	60 DM 2 on diet or OHA	Inolter: unspecified daily amount for 3 mo	Placebo	HbA1c, FG, TC, LDL, VLDL, HDL, TG	Treatment group: decreased FG, TC, TG, VLDL, LDL; increased HDL Placebo: no change in all measures	None reported
Jiangtangkang (JTK) Chrysanthemum product	Chen SH et al. (1997) *(41)*	188 DM 2 (71 new cases + 117 poorly controlled cases)	JTK 8 g/3×/d	Glibenclamide (only in new cases)	FG, PPG, HbA1c, PI, BV, TG	Treatment group: decrease in FG, PPG, HbA1c; PI unchanged and BV, TG decreased Control: FG, PPG lowered in control group (non significant difference with treatment)	No adverse effects
Jiangtang Bushen Recipe: Combination of 11 traditional Chinese herbs for kidney supplementation	Fan G et al. (2004) *(42)*	51 IGT with educational course, diet therapy, and kinetotherapy	Combination herbal recipe 2–3×/wk for 12 mo	No placebo	FG, FI, TC, TG, BMI, diabetes conversion rate	Treatment group: no change in FG; decrease in FI, TC, TG, BMI Control: no change in all measures	Six drop outs reasons not reported

(continued)

Table 2 (continued)

Herb	Reference	Participants	Intervention	Control	Outcomes measured	Results	Comments/adverse events
Xiaoke tea (uncharacterized herb preparation)	Hale PJ et al. (1989) (41)	12 DM 2 on diet and/or OHA	Xiaoke tea 2.72 g infusion/4x/d for 4 wk	Ordinary tea (2.72 g/4 ×/d)	HbA1c, FG, PI, TG, TC	No change in any of the measures for treatment or placebo groups	No adverse effects
"Pancreas Tonic"—mixture of 10 Ayurvedic herbs	Hsia SH et al. (2004) (39)	36 DM 2 on OHA divided into 2 strata of HbA1c levels (stratum 1: 8.0% to 9.9%; stratum 2: 10.0% to 12.0%)	Two capsules of "Pancreas Tonic"/3×/d for 3 mo	Placebo	HbA1c, FG, TC, HDL, LDL	Treatment group: reduction of HbA1c in higher HbA1c stratum alone Placebo: no change in all measures	Treatment well tolerated by participants
Traditional Chinese formula for Qi-supplementation and blood activation comprising 10 herbs	Lu W et al. (2003) (43)	63 DM 2 with foot ulcers using conventional "Western" treatment	Herbal formula	No placebo qd for 6 wk	FG, PPG,TC, TG, efficacy in ulcer healing	Treatment group: decrease in both FG, and PPG (same as in placebo); no change in TC and TG; improved ulcer healing Control: no significant difference in all measures except ulcers	Not mentioned
Tibetan Medicine including at least 2 of the following 4 herbs (Kyura-6, Aru-18, Yungwa-4, or Sugmel-9)	Namdul T et al. (2001) (40)	200 DM 2 with dietary treatment	Tibetan Medicine + lifestyle modification for 24 wk	Lifestyle modification only	TC, TG, HDL, HbA1c, FG, PPG, BMI, BP	Treatment group: decrease FG, PPG, HbA1c compared to control group. No change in BMI, BP, TC, HDL, TG	Not reported

Intervention description	Study	Patients	Regimen	Control/placebo	Measures	Results	Adverse effects
Traditional Chinese formula for kidney-supplementation and releasing fire comprising 13 herbs	Rao ZF et al. (2002) (44)	76 DM 2 on conventional medicine	Herbal formula tid for 3 mo	No placebo	FG, FI	Treatment group: decrease in FG,FI Control: no change in two measures	Not mentioned
Native American herbal tea composed of Populus tremuloides and Heracleum lanatum	Ryan EA et al. (2000) (42)	40 DM 2 on diet or OHA	250 mL of herbal tea for 10 d	Placebo tea	MBG, HbA1c, fruct and response to an "Ensure" meal challenge	Treatment group: No change in MBG; fruct decrease (similar to placebo); no change in HbA1c from "Ensure" challenge. Placebo: fruct decreased	One mild case of gastrointestinal discomfort in treatment group
Combination of three Chinese herbs (Astragalus membranaceus, Coptis chinensis, Lonicera japonica)	Vray M et al. (1995) (45)	216 DM 2	Group 1 (herbal formula: 7 caps tid + glibenclamide placebo); Group 2 (herbal formula 7 caps tid + glibenclamide) for 3 mo	A (herbal placebo + glibenclamide placebo); B (glibenclamide + herbal placebo)	HbA1c, FG, FI, PPG	Treatment groups: FG decreased only after OGTT with herbal formula, synergistic decrease in FG when both glibenclamide and herbal formula taken concurrently	Hypoglycemia occurred in 19 patients taking herbal formula and glibenclamide together
Qidan tongmai: Traditional Chinese formula for blood activation comprising 10 herbs	Zhang M et al. (2001) (46)	128 DM 2 on OHA	Herbal formula tid for 2 mo: 2 groups, 1 with no hyperlipidemia, 1 with hyperlipidemia	No placebo: 2 groups, 1 with no hyperlipidemia, 1 with hyperlipidemia	FG, PPG, HbA1c, TC, TG, HDL	Treatment group: decrease in FG, PPG, HbA1c, TC, TG; increase in HDL Control: no change in all measures	No adverse effects

Table 3
Systematic Reviews of Nonherbal Supplements Used in the Treatment of Diabetes

Supplement or dietary recommendation	Reference	Studies reviewed	Participants	Intervention	Control	Outcomes assessed	Results/conclusions	Adverse events
Chromium supplement	Althuis MD et al. (2002) (49)	15 RCTs (11 double-blind, 1 single, 3 not clear)	618 (193 DM 2, 425 good health or with IGT)	Chromium	12 used placebo	FG, PI, HbA1c	In DM 2 patients: 155 subjects (1 study): Chromium reduced FG, PI, HbA1c other 38 subjects (combined studies) showed no change	No evidence of any toxicity
Low-glycemic foods	Brand-Miller J et al. (2003) (53)	14 RCTs (3 parallel, 11 crossover)	356 (203 DM I + 153 DM 2)	Low-GI diet	High-GI diet or conventional diets	HbA1c, fruct	Low-GI diets reduced HbA1c and fruct more than high-GI diets. Small but clinically significant effect found	None reported
Fish oil: eicosapentaenoic acid (EPA) and docosahexaenoic acid (DHA)	Friedberg CE et al. (1998) (51)	26 trials (varying quality; 13 RCTs)	425 (240 DM 2; 185 DM I)	Fish oil (mean dose: 1.8 g EPA and 1.2 g DHA)	11 used placebo (9 olive oil, 2 safflower oil)	TG, TC, LDL, HDL, FG, HbA1c	Fish oil supplementation in: DM 2: decreased TG; increased FG (borderline); small increase in LDL DM I: decreased TG; FG decreased	None reported
High-monounsaturated fat diets	Garg A. (1998) (52)	10 RCTs	133 DM 2	High-monounsaturated fat diet (MSF)	High-carbohydrate diet	TG,TC, VLDL, LDL, HDL, FG, PI, PPG, HbA1c, fruct, UG	High MSF diet: decreased TG, VLDL, and TC; increase HDL; no change in LDL; lowered FG; no change in PI, HbA1c, fruct; PPG and UG changes varied within studies	None reported
Fish oil supplementation	Montori VM et al. (2000) (50)	18 RCTs (7 parallel and 11 crossover)	823 DM 2	3-18 g/d mean of 12 wk	Placebo	TG, LDL, FG, HbA1c, HDL, TC	Fish oil supplementation: TG decreased, LDL increased; no change in FG, HbA1c, TC, HDL	None reported

exploring. As with single herbs, however, the data gathered in our review is insufficient to make any real conclusions as to the clinical efficacy of the herbal combinations.

As mentioned above, the literature search also uncovered a systematic review by the Cochrane Collaboration that assessed all Chinese herbal medicines for type 2 diabetes *(14)*. Similar to our findings, the reviewer's conclusions were that some herbal medicines show hypoglycemic activity. However, low methodological quality, small sample size, and limited number of trials preclude any definite conclusions and that further research is warranted *(14)*.

Nonherbal Complementary and Alternative Medicine

The literature search for systematic reviews of nonherbal supplements and dietary modifications turned up a total of five systematic reviews. These reviews provide varying levels of evidence on the effectiveness of each of the treatments in question. In the systematic review and metaanalysis of chromium supplementation by Athuis et al. *(49)*, 15 RCTs were assessed. Only in one study, albeit the largest, was there a demonstrable reduction of fasting glucose, plasma insulin, and HbA1c through the use of chromium supplementation. Combining the results showed that changes to blood glucose control were not statistically significant at any of the dosages used. The overall conclusion of Althuis et al. is that there is currently insufficient evidence to recommend chromium supplementation for controlling blood glucose levels. There were two meta-analyses that specifically looked at fish oil supplementation and its effect on blood glucose control and blood lipid profiles. In both reviews it was found that triglyceride levels decreased with a slight concomitant rise in LDL *(50,51)*. In terms of blood sugar control, the earlier review of 26 trials (with 13 RCTs) by Friedberg et al. *(51)* found that in diabetes mellitus type 1 there was a slight decrease in fasting glucose whereas in type 2 there was a slight clinically insignificant increase. The more recent analysis by Montori et al. *(50)*, which included 18 RCTs examining only type 2 diabetes, found that there was no effect on blood sugar control through either of the indices fasting glucose or HbA1c. The conclusion drawn from both of these reviews concerning fish oil in diabetes is that supplementation can be an effective tool to reduce triglycerides without having an adverse effect on glycemic control.

There were two diet related systematic reviews found. One concerned the use of low glycemic index foods and the other was of the use of high levels of monounsaturated fats. The latter, a meta-analysis of ten RCTs found that a higher relative level of monounsaturated fat in comparison to a high carbohydrate consumption diet resulted in beneficial changes to the lipid profile with a slight concomitant reduction in fasting glucose *(52)*. The analysis of 14 RCTs by Brand-Miller et al. *(53)*, looking at the glycemic index of foods, found that patients with type 1 and type 2 diabetes consumed found that low-glycemic index foods (compared to high-glycemic index foods) caused a small but clinically significant reduction in HbA1c and fructosamine measures.

CASE RESOLUTION

Many approaches are probably adequate in managing Ms. Tarnaruk. An initial approach could be to point out the herbal origin of currently available prescription drugs, such as metformin or the natural origin of insulin. In addition, one could emphasize lifestyle changes in diet and exercise, perhaps suggesting low-glycemic index foods that are traditional to the Native American diet.

Directly addressing the patient's request requires acknowledgement of the uncertainty about the safety and efficacy of all herbal products that could be recommended for use. The clinician may decide to share with the patient the scant data available to support some of the single and combination herb products that could be helpful. In any event, it is crucial that Ms. Tarnaruk be aware of the gravity of the situation and the paramount importance of achieving control of her blood glucose levels.

REFERENCES

1. Kessler RC, Davis RB, Foster DF, et al. Long-term trends in the use of complementary and alternative medical therapies in the United States. Ann Intern Med 2001;135:262–268.
2. Eisenberg DM, Davis RB, Ettner SL, et al. Trends in alternative medicine use in the United States, 1990-1997: results of a follow-up national survey. JAMA 1998;280:1569–1575.
3. Blumenthal M. Herbal market levels off after five years of boom. HerbalGram 1999;47:64–65.
4. Busse JW, Heaton G, Wu P, Wilson KR, Mills EJ. Disclosure of natural product use to primary care physicians: a cross-sectional survey of naturopathic clinic attendees. Mayo Clin Proc 2005;80: 616–623.
5. Mills E, Montori VM, Wu P, Gallicano K, Clarke M, Guyatt G. Interaction of St John's wort with conventional drugs: systematic review of clinical trials. BMJ 2004;329:27–30.
6. American Diabetes Association. Unproven therapies. Diabetes Care 1994;17:1551.
7. Egede LE, Ye X, Zheng D, Silverstein MD. The prevalence and pattern of complementary and alternative medicine use in individuals with diabetes. Diabetes Care 2002;25:324–329.
8. Yeh GY, Eisenberg DM, Davis RB, Phillips RS. Use of complementary and alternative medicine among persons with diabetes mellitus: results of a national survey. Am J Public Health 2002;92: 1648–1652.
9. Kim C, Kwok YS. Navajo use of native healers. Arch Intern Med 1998;158:2245–2249.
10. Mull DS, Nguyen N, Mull JD. Vietnamese diabetic patients and their physicians: what ethnography can teach us. West J Med 2001;175:307–311.
11. Noel PH, Larme AC, Meyer J, Marsh G, Correa A, Pugh JA. Patient choice in diabetes education curriculum. Nutritional versus standard content for type 2 diabetes. Diabetes Care 1998;21:896–901.
12. Witters LA. The blooming of the French lilac. J Clin Invest 2001;108:1105–1107.
13. Yeh GY, Eisenberg DM, Kaptchuk TJ, Phillips RS. Systematic review of herbs and dietary supplements for glycemic control in diabetes. Diabetes Care 2003;26:1277–1294.
14. Liu JP, Zhang M, Wang WY, Grimsgaard S. Chinese herbal medicines for type 2 diabetes mellitus. Cochrane Database Syst Rev 2004(3):CD003642.
15. Khan A, Safdar M, Ali Khan MM, Khattak KN, Anderson RA. Cinnamon improves glucose and lipids of people with type 2 diabetes. Diabetes Care 2003;26:3215–3218.
16. Azad Khan AK, Akhtar S, Mahtab H. Coccinia indica in the treatment of patients with diabetes mellitus. Bangladesh Med Res Counc Bull 1979;5:60–66.
17. Serraclara A, Hawkins F, Perez C, Dominguez E, Campillo JE, Torres MD. Hypoglycemic action of an oral fig-leaf decoction in type-I diabetic patients. Diabetes Res Clin Pract 1998;39:19–22.
18. Gao Y, Lan J, Dai X, Ye J, Zhou S. A phase I/II study of Ling Zhi mushroom Ganoderma lucidum (W. Curt.:Fr.) Lloyd (Aphyllophoromycetideae) Extract in patients with type II diabetes mellitus. Intern J Med Mushrooms 2004;6:33–9.
19. Jayagopal V, Albertazzi P, Kilpatrick ES, et al. Beneficial effects of soy phytoestrogen intake in postmenopausal women with type 2 diabetes. Diabetes Care 2002;25:1709–1714.
20. Sotaniemi EA, Haapakoski E, Rautio A. Ginseng therapy in non-insulin-dependent diabetic patients. Diabetes Care 1995;18:1373–1375.
21. Ludvik B, Waldhausl W, Prager R, Kautzky-Willer A, Pacini G. Mode of action of ipomoea batatas (Caiapo) in type 2 diabetic patients. Metabolism 2003;52:875–880.
22. Ludvik B, Neuffer B, Pacini G. Efficacy of Ipomoea batatas (Caiapo) on diabetes control in type 2 diabetic subjects treated with diet. Diabetes Care 2004;27:436–440.
23. Judy WV, Hari SP, Stogsdill WW, Judy JS, Naguib YM, Passwater R. Antidiabetic activity of a standardized extract (Glucosol) from Lagerstroemia speciosa leaves in Type II diabetics. A dose-dependence study. J Ethnopharmacol 2003;87:115–117.

24. Andallu B, Suryakantham V, Lakshmi Srikanthi B, Reddy GK. Effect of mulberry (Morus indica L.) therapy on plasma and erythrocyte membrane lipids in patients with type 2 diabetes. Clin Chim Acta 2001;314:47–53.

25. Agrawal P, Rai V, Singh RB. Randomized placebo-controlled, single blind trial of holy basil leaves in patients with noninsulin-dependent diabetes mellitus. Int J Clin Pharmacol Ther 1996;34:406–409.

26. Frati AC, Gordillo BE, Altamirano P, Ariza CR, Cortes-Franco R, Chavez-Negrete A. Acute hypo-glycemic effect of Opuntia streptacantha Lemaire in NIDDM. Diabetes Care 1990;13:455–456.

27. Vuksan V, Sievenpiper JL, Koo VY, et al. American ginseng (Panax quinquefolius L) reduces post-prandial glycemia in nondiabetic subjects and subjects with type 2 diabetes mellitus. Arch Intern Med 2000;160:1009–1013.

28. Vuksan V, Stavro MP, Sievenpiper JL, , et al. Similar postprandial glycemic reductions with escala-tion of dose and administration time of American ginseng in type 2 diabetes. Diabetes Care 2000;23: 1221–1226.

29. Liu X, Wei J, Tan F, Zhou S, Wurthwein G, Rohdewald P. Antidiabetic effect of Pycnogenol French maritime pine bark extract in patients with diabetes type II. Life Sci 2004;75:2505–2513.

30. Velussi M, Cernigoi AM, De Monte A, Dapas F, Caffau C, Zilli M. Long-term (12 months) treatment with an anti-oxidant drug (silymarin) is effective on hyperinsulinemia, exogenous insulin need and malondialdehyde levels in cirrhotic diabetic patients. J Hepatol 1997;26:871–879.

31. Gupta A, Gupta R, Lal B. Effect of Trigonella foenum-graecum (fenugreek) seeds on glycaemic con-trol and insulin resistance in type 2 diabetes mellitus: a double blind placebo controlled study. J Assoc Physicians India 2001;49:1057–1061.

32. Sharma RD, Raghuram TC, Rao NS. Effect of fenugreek seeds on blood glucose and serum lipids in type I diabetes. Eur J Clin Nutr 1990;44:301–306.

33. Sitprija S, Plengvidhya C, Kangkaya V, Bhuvapanich S, Tunkayoon M. Garlic and diabetes mellitus phase II clinical trial. J Med Assoc Thai 1987;70:223–227.

34. Russo EM, Reichelt AA, De-Sa JR, et al. Clinical trial of Myrcia uniflora and Bauhinia forficata leaf extracts in normal and diabetic patients. Braz J Med Biol Res 1990;23:11–20.

35. John AJ, Cherian R, Subhash HS, Cherian AM. Evaluation of the efficacy of bitter gourd (momordica charantia) as an oral hypoglycemic agent—a randomized controlled clinical trial. Indian J Physiol Pharmacol 2003;47:363–365.

36. Sangsuwan C, Udompanthurak S, Vannasaeng S, Thamlikitkul V. Randomized controlled trial of Tinospora crispa for additional therapy in patients with type 2 diabetes mellitus. J Med Assoc Thai 2004;87:543–546.

37. Vogler BK, Pittler MH, Ernst E. The efficacy of ginseng. A systematic review of randomised clinical trials. Eur J Clin Pharmacol 1999;55:567–575.

38. Agrawal RP, Sharma A, Dua AS, Chandershekhar, Kochar DK, Kothari RP. A randomized placebo controlled trial of Inolter (herbal product) in the treatment of type 2 diabetes. J Assoc Physicians India 2002;50:391–393.

39. Hsia SH, Bazargan M, Davidson MB. Effect of Pancreas Tonic (an ayurvedic herbal supplement) in type 2 diabetes mellitus. Metabolism 2004;53:1166–1173.

40. Namdul T, Sood A, Ramakrishnan L, Pandey RM, Moorthy D. Efficacy of Tibetan medicine as an adjunct in the treatment of type 2 diabetes. Diabetes Care 2001;24:175–176.

41. Chen SH, Sun YP, Chen XS. [Effect of jiangtangkang on blood glucose, sensitivity of insulin and blood viscosity in non-insulin dependent diabetes mellitus]. Zhongguo Zhong Xi Yi Jie He Za Zhi 1997;17:666–668.

42. Fan GJ, Luo GB, Qin ML. [Effect of jiangtang bushen recipe in intervention treatment of patients with impaired glucose tolerance]. Zhongguo Zhong Xi Yi Jie He Za Zhi 2004;24:317–320.

43. Lu W, Zhong GL. [Clinical observation on treatment of diabetic foot by integrative Chinese and West-ern Medicine]. Zhongguo Zhong Xi Yi Jie He Za Zhi 2003;23:911–913.

44. Rao ZF. [Clinical observation on treatment of diabetes mellitus type 2 by medication with both Chi-nese and Western drugs]. Zhongguo Zhong Xi Yi Jie He Za Zhi 2002;22:140–141.

45. Vray M, Attali JR. Randomized study of glibenclamide versus traditional Chinese treatment in type 2 diabetic patients. Chinese-French Scientific Committee for the Study of Diabetes. Diabete Metab 1995;21:433–439.

46. Zhang M, Ma SP, Wang ZR. [Effect of qidan tongmai tablet on glucose and lipid metabolism in patients with diabetes mellitus type 2]. Zhongguo Zhong Xi Yi Jie He Za Zhi 2001;21:825–827.

47. Hale PJ, Horrocks PM, Wright AD, Fitzgerald MG, Nattrass M, Bailey CJ. Xiaoke tea, a Chinese herbal treatment for diabetes mellitus. Diabet Med 1989;6:675–676.
48. Ryan EA, Imes S, Wallace C, Jones S. Herbal tea in the treatment of diabetes mellitus. Clin Invest Med 2000;23:311-7.
49. Althuis MD, Jordan NE, Ludington EA, Wittes JT. Glucose and insulin responses to dietary chromium supplements: a meta-analysis. Am J Clin Nutr 2002;76:148–155.
50. Montori VM, Farmer A, Wollan PC, Dinneen SF. Fish oil supplementation in type 2 diabetes: a quantitative systematic review. Diabetes Care 2000;23:1407–1415.
51. Friedberg CE, Janssen MJ, Heine RJ, Grobbee DE. Fish oil and glycemic control in diabetes. A meta-analysis. Diabetes Care 1998;21:494–500.
52. Garg A. High-monounsaturated-fat diets for patients with diabetes mellitus: a meta-analysis. Am J Clin Nutr 1998;67:577S–582S.
53. Brand-Miller J, Hayne S, Petocz P, Colagiuri S. Low-glycemic index diets in the management of diabetes: a meta-analysis of randomized controlled trials. Diabetes Care 2003;26:2261–2267.

22

Evidence-Based Case Studies in Osteoporosis

Clifford J. Rosen, MD and Sue A. Brown, MD

CONTENTS

INTRODUCTION

Significant advances have been made in the care of the patient with osteoporosis in the last decade. Anti-fracture regimens have been tested in rigorous randomized-controlled trials (RCTs) and evidence supports several therapeutic options. The burden of fractures in the United States is high and accounts for over $14 billion in annual

From: *Contemporary Endocrinology: Evidence-Based Endocrinology*
Edited by: V. M. Montori © Mayo Foundation for Medical Education and Research

direct medical costs *(1)*. It is estimated that a white woman at age 50 in the United States has a 17% chance of sustaining a hip fracture and 32% chance of a vertebral fracture in her lifetime *(2,3)*. In the year following a hip fracture, mortality rates have been reported as high as 20–24% *(4,5)*, whereas up to 50% of patients are unable to walk without assistance and 33% are totally dependent or in a nursing home *(4,6,7)*. Despite the evidence for anti-fracture efficacy of multiple therapeutic regimens, it is alarming that reports find the majority of women and men with a recent hip or wrist fracture were not getting appropriate therapy *(8–10)*. The challenge is to ensure that those most in need of diagnosis or therapy are obtaining adequate care.

Most evidence guiding the management of osteoporosis has been developed for the postmenopausal female and it is, thus, reflected in our choice of case presentation. We will consider the case of a postmenopausal woman with low-bone density and follow the evolution of her management to discuss the evidence underlying the options for her care. There is accumulating evidence regarding appropriate care for men with osteoporosis as well as glucocorticoid-induced and post-transplantation osteoporosis. Evidence is emerging to address bone-related complications from diseases such as anorexia nervosa, Crohn's disease, and cystic fibrosis. However, there is comparatively less evidence to guide management in the healthy premenopausal woman or younger man with low bone mass or osteoporosis. We will discuss these clinical caveats as we consider the management of the following case.

CASE

A 62-yr-old white female is referred to her primary-care physician for osteopenia. At a local health fair, she had a screening bone density of the heel done by peripheral dual X-ray absorptometry (DXA) that showed a T-score of −1.4. She is an otherwise healthy nonsmoker and has had no loss in height or known fractures. She is 62 in. tall (155 cm) and 126 pounds (57.2 kg) with a body mass index (BMI) of 24. She underwent natural menopause 10 yr ago and took conjugated estrogens for 7 yr before electing to discontinue after learning of the results of the Women's Health Initiative. Her mother had a hip fracture in her 70s.

SCREENING RECOMMENDATIONS

The first question to consider is whether she was an appropriate candidate for a screening bone density test. A screening test must be able to identify individuals at risk for fracture or osteoporosis at a time in which reasonable interventions may be offered for altering the course of the disease. Fractures are the primary outcome of clinical relevance in osteoporosis rather than low-bone mass itself. Therefore, diagnostic testing and therapeutic interventions should be evaluated by their ability to predict or prevent fractures. Surrogate markers for fracture risk include bone density tests and bone turnover markers among others.

There is no adequate evidence that bone density measures should be used for mass or population screening for osteoporosis. However, there is evidence for a case-finding strategy to identify high-risk groups after an appropriate assessment of clinical risk factors. The US Preventative Task Force (USPTF) evaluated the evidence for appropriate screening for bone mineral density and fracture risk determination. Based on that evidence, the USPTF recommends screening should be routinely provided in women over age 65 and in those women ages 60–64 who are at increased risk *(11)*. There was good evidence that the benefits of screening and treatment are of at least moderate magnitude for women at increased risk. Low-body weight (<70 kg) was found to be the best single predictor of low bone density. Age and no current use of estrogen therapy have been consistently validated *(12)* but there is less evidence to support screening risk factors such as smoking, family history, weight loss, decreased physical activity, and lifelong calcium and vitamin D use. Additionally, the USPTF noted that African American women may be at lower risk than white women because of higher bone mineral densities and, therefore, are less likely to benefit from routine screening. The USPTF could make no recommendation for or against routine screening in women younger than 60 yr of age or women 60–64 who are not at increased risk. There was fair evidence that screening individuals at lower risk (younger age) can identify women eligible for treatment for osteoporosis but that the number of fractures prevented was small such that it is not clear that the benefits outweigh the risks. The National Osteoporosis Foundation recommendations also concur that women over age 65 should be screened as well as younger postmenopausal women who have had a fracture or who have one or more risk factors for osteoporosis (other than white, postmenopausal, female) *(13)*.

PERIPHERAL BONE MINERAL DENSITY MEASURES

Is there evidence to support the use of peripheral devices in bone density screening? Bone density can be measured at peripheral sites using a variety of techniques such as peripheral DXA and ultrasonography to assess individuals at risk for osteoporosis. However, fracture risk prediction is not as well studied for peripheral measures (e.g., calcaneus, phalanges, radius, tibia) as it is for the central skeletal sites of the hip and spine.

Different devices and sites may yield varying estimates of low bone mineral density (BMD) when used for population screening. The largest US clinical trial to utilize peripheral devices for population screening was the National Osteoporosis Risk Assessment (NORA). The study enrolled 200,160 postmenopausal, ambulatory women at least 50 yr old recruited from primary care practices throughout the US with no prior diagnosis of osteoporosis *(14)*. Each subject had a single BMD measurement at one of three peripheral sites using one of four devices: 54% had calcaneal single X-ray absorptiometry, 34% had radial peripheral DXA, 7% had phalangeal pDXA, and 5% had calcaneal ultrasound measures. Osteoporosis risk factors and fracture history were obtained from questionnaires at baseline and 12-mo follow-up.

The NORA results demonstrated that classification of individuals by osteoporosis or osteopenia using T-scores were different by device. A T-score is derived by comparing the BMD to a gender- and ethnically matched peak BMD and is expressed in standard deviations. A T-score that is 2.5 standard deviations or more below mean peak BMD ($\leq$ –2.5) is considered osteoporosis by the World Health Organization (WHO) categorization. The NORA study found that T-scores were lowest for calcaneal SXA (mean T = –0.97) and highest on calcaneal ultrasound (T = –0.56). A smaller proportion of women were identified by ultrasound as having very low BMD (T score $\leq$ –2.5) compared with phalangeal pDXA measures, which yielded the highest. Regardless of individual technology differences, the study concluded that low-peripheral BMD by any method was able to identify women at risk of fracture and when receiver operator curves were analyzed did not show significant differences by technology (15).

Ultrasound is appealing because of the low cost, portability, and lack of radiation exposure, as well as the theoretical benefits of evaluating an aspect of bone quality. Ultrasound has been correlated with fracture risk but is not standardized and varies across machines (16). Therefore, it is not certain that bone density of the hip or spine can be reliably predicted from measurements at peripheral sites (17). Fracture risk estimates derived from theoretical models and in vivo data vary almost threefold for the same group of patients undergoing BMD using DXA vs speed of sound measurements from ultrasound at multiple peripheral sites (18).

Peripheral DXA has been correlated with table-top DXA in an effort to determine an appropriate T-score threshold to identify patients at risk for osteoporosis. A study of 443 women (mean age 60 yr) with spine and femoral neck DXA as well as pDXA of calcaneus found that average T-scores from the femoral neck was –1.4 compared with –0.9 at the calcaneus and reported an optimal T-score of ≤1.4 with a sensitivity of 69.9% and specificity of 82.6% (19). Using pDXA, a study of 119 women (age 33–76) compared calcaneal BMD by pDXA with central DXA measures and concluded that a T-score ≤0 by pDXA was highly sensitive in predicting osteopenia or osteoporosis at the femoral neck of lumbar spine (20). A study of 100 patients referred for osteoporosis evaluation assessed by pDXA of calcaneus compared to central DXA of spine and hip found that T-scores of –1.6 and below by pDXA could be used to identify many high risk subjects (21). The population-based NORA study found only 82% of women with a self-reported incident fractures had a T-score greater than –2.5 on a peripheral device (22). Thus, the optimal T-score is not clear but consistently higher scores on peripheral devices are needed as a threshold when considering referral for central bone densitometry and the WHO diagnostic criteria do not apply to all types of peripheral devices. As these devices are often used for screening, it has been recommended that device-specific thresholds and higher T- or Z-score thresholds (e.g., T-score <–1) be used to refer for central (hip, spine, and/or radius) measures prior to diagnosing osteoporosis (23). Unfortunately, there are many site and manufacturer-specific differences in peripheral bone density assessment that limits the development of optimal, comprehensive strategies for utilization of peripheral bone density measurements in osteoporosis screening or diagnosis.

In this patient's scenario, it is appropriate that she obtained a screening test because she is between the ages of 60–64 and has one or more risk factors including estrogen deficiency, family history, and relatively thin build. It is also reasonable that her T-score of –1.4 by peripheral DXA prompted a referral for consideration of further work-up and diagnosis.

She is referred for bone mineral density of the hip and spine by dual-energy X-ray absorptiometry (DXA) and is found to have a T score of –1.8 and –2.6, respectively. Does she have osteoporosis? Is there evidence to define her risk of fracture?

BONE MINERAL DENSITY OF CENTRAL SKELETON

BMD testing by DXA has been the surrogate outcome of choice that is consistently and closely related to fracture risk. DXA is a noninvasive assessment generally requiring less than 5 min with minimal radiation exposure. Fracture risk is related to bone strength; however, there are no clinically available methods to assess bone strength directly. Fortunately, a strong relationship exists between bone density measurements and fracture risk, particularly in postmenopausal women. For every 10% decrease in BMD (1 SD below the mean) at any site (spine, hip, radius, calcaneus), the relative risk of hip fracture is estimated to be 1.6–2.6 and the relative risk of vertebral fracture is about 1.7–2.3 (24). BMD measured at the hip or spine are most predictive for hip or vertebral fractures respectively (24). Therefore, the most widely used and validated sites for the diagnosis and monitoring of therapy for osteoporosis is the central skeleton (spine and hip) using DXA scans.

The WHO developed diagnostic definitions based on BMD measures to standardize entry criteria into clinical trials in osteoporosis. As noted previously, the criteria are based on T-scores or the standard deviation from peak bone mass using a gender-matched and ethnically matched reference database. Osteopenia is defined by a T-score from –1 to –2.5 and osteoporosis by a T-score of –2.5 or below (25). The categorization of osteopenia encompasses individuals with greater variations in fracture risk and, therefore, often has limited clinical value (24). WHO criteria were developed as diagnostic categories rather than treatment thresholds. The reference databases are developed primarily in nonhispanic Caucasian women and more recent evidence is accumulating to establish databases for men, other ethnicities as well as children. The measurement of BMD should serve to estimate fracture risk over a defined future interval (e.g., 5- or 10-yr horizon) and new strategies to refine clinical reporting of fracture risk are being developed (26).

Our patient has a BMD of the hip that is 1.8 standard deviations below peak bone mass for a white woman and a BMD of the spine that is 2.6 standard deviations below. This patient would be considered to have osteoporosis by WHO criteria because the T-score in at least one site in the central skeleton is below –2.5. However, this patient would be at low to moderate risk for sustaining an osteoporotic fracture over the next 5 yr. Using data from population-based studies in Sweden, this patient's 10-yr risk of osteoporotic fractures is approx 5–10% with a hip T-score of –1.8 (26). Population-based studies in Minnesota suggest that her risk of fracture is approx 5% (27).

Is it expected that her hip and spine have different T-scores? T-scores derived from BMD as well as Z-scores (age-matched reference) can be discordant at different anatomic sites. Although BMD of the spine can be falsely elevated by the presence of osteophytes, discrepancies in T-scores usually result from differences in bone composition (trabecular vs cortical) at those sites. Trabecular or cancellous bone has high metabolic activity rates and includes sites such as the vertebral bodies, proximal femur, calcaneus, and ultradistal radius. Cortical bone in contrast has lower rates of activation frequencies of bone remodeling units and includes sites such as the distal one-third radius. Many sites, such as the femoral neck, have a mixture of both trabecular and cortical bone. Postmenopausal women often have rapid loss of bone at trabecular sites whereas other clinical conditions such as primary hyperparathyroidism are more likely to affect cortical bone. In addition to the differences in metabolic turnover between cortical and trabecular bone, genetic regulation of peak acquisition may also differ by skeletal site. Indeed, studies in mice and humans have recently recognized that there may be very distinct genetic determinants of peak bone mass that are compartment specific. Therefore it should not be surprising that acquisition of bone density, loss of bone mass, or differences in response to pharmacological therapy may differ by site of measurement.

Table 1
Selected Risk Factors for Low Bone Density

Genetic
    Personal history of fractures
    Family history of osteoporosis
    Low body weight
Reproductive
    Amenorrhea or history of amenorrhea (>1 yr)
    Estrogen deficiency or hypogonadism
Secondary diseases
    Hyperparathyroidism
    Renal failure
    Eating disorders
    Hyperthyroidism
    Multiple myeloma
    Type 1 diabetes mellitus
    Celiac sprue
    Cystic fibrosis
    Crohn's disease
    Osteogenesis imperfecta
    Homocystinuria
Nutrition
    Avoidance of calcium/dairy products
    Vitamin D deficiency
    Gastrectomy
Medications
    Glucocorticoids
    Anticonvulsants
Lifestyle
    Smoking
    Excess alcohol

Note: Adapted with permission from ref. *28*.

CLINICAL EVALUATION OF SECONDARY CAUSES

Can the BMD results be related to age- or menopause-related bone loss, or should secondary causes of osteoporosis be considered?

Common secondary causes of osteoporosis include glucocorticoid use, hyperparathyroidism, vitamin D deficiency, among others (Table 1) *(28)*. The true prevalence of secondary causes in individuals with osteoporosis is not known as most studies are done using clinical populations from bone-center referral bases. A cross-sectional study of 173 healthy postmenopausal women with osteoporosis at a University-based bone disease clinic without a known history of pre-existing conditions or treatments that affect bone metabolism were evaluated to assess the yield of routine laboratory testing *(29)*. In this study, 32% of women had an undiagnosed condition that was found by laboratory testing which included a complete blood count, chemistry profile, 24-h urinary calcium, 25 hydroxyvitamin D, and PTH assessment at an estimated cost of $75 per person screened. The most frequent predisposing conditions identified were hypercalciuria

(9.8%), malabsorption (8.1%), hyperparathyroidism (6.9%), and vitamin D deficiency (4.1%). The prevalence of primary hyperparathyroidism increases in postmenopausal women and, therefore, measuring the serum calcium and phosphorus should be included. Abnormal serum calcium or phosphorus values should prompt an appropriate workup including a PTH level and serum 25 hydroxyvitamin D; but it is unclear that PTH levels need to be included in the setting of normocalcemia. Vitamin D deficiency is increasing in prevalence and selected risk factors include advanced age, living at higher latitudes with less sun exposure, malabsorption, and African American race. Given this evidence, we advocate a low threshold for measuring 25 hydroxyvitamin D levels with a reliable assay in an established reference laboratory. With those caveats, the measurement of serum 25 hydroxyvitamin D provides an accurate measure of vitamin D stores, and can be used to guide therapeutic replacement. Vitamin D3 has been show to reduce fractures in selected populations (*see* Nutritional Interventions) but results are conflicting. Notably PTH and Vitamin D assays are among the more expensive initial laboratory testing options. Although it has been advocated that a 24-h urinary calcium be included in the initial work-up of a patient with osteoporosis, there are no outcome studies supporting routine measures in the initial workup. A thyroid stimulating hormone (TSH) is reasonable given the association of a suppressed TSH and decreased bone density although the evidence is not robust that endogenous hyperthyroidism contributes greatly to the burden of osteoporosis *(30)*. Multiple myeloma is often considered because most of these individuals have low bone mass. However, most individuals with osteoporosis do not have multiple myeloma. Therefore, it is reasonable to measure a complete blood count or serum creatinine as an indicator for multiple myeloma followed by a serum protein electrophoresis (SPEP) or urine protein electrophoresis (UPEP) if clinical suspicion warrants. Another indicator that would raise concern about the diagnosis of multiple myeloma would be a very suppressed PTH in an individual with significant osteoporosis but normocalcemia.

For men with osteoporosis, an assessment of testosterone levels is reasonable. There is accumulating evidence that estrogen levels in men may be a more important determinant of bone density and fracture risk than testosterone; however, the evidence for intervention options or thresholds is not yet sufficient to routinely measure estrogen levels *(31)*.

Less frequent causes of osteoporosis are often readily apparent during a complete clinical assessment and include hypercortisolism, Crohn's disease, and Celiac sprue, among others. The latter is one of the most common heritable disorders associated with low bone mass and its clinical presentation is quite variable. Because of widespread utilization of DXA, low bone mass can be the first clinically apparent manifestation of this disorder. Hence, the combination of low 25 dihydroxyvitamin D, high PTH and reduced BMD should raise suspicion about the diagnosis of Celiac sprue. Measurement of serum antibodies (e.g., tissue transglutaminase and/or endomysial antibodies) as indicators of disease activity would then be appropriate. Because aggressive vitamin D supplementation and a gluten-free diet can, in some studies, result in improvement in BMD, this cause of low bone mass should never be overlooked.

Secondary causes may be more likely with an unexplained accelerated bone loss. A low BMD measure could result from on-going accelerated bone loss and/or an inadequate accrual of peak bone mass. A single bone density reading may not be very helpful in a low-risk population, particularly younger women as it may simply represent a low peak bone mass. Bone turnover markers, therefore, may have a limited role in distinguishing high turnover and accelerated loss from low peak BMD, although there is not enough evidence to support the use of markers beyond identification of fracture risk in older postmenopausal women (*see* Bone Turnover Markers). This is particularly true in situations such as chronic renal failure where low bone density is associated with low bone turnover. A similar scenario has been noted in some men with idiopathic osteoporosis. Certainly an investigation is appropriate for determining the reasons for an inability to attain an adequate peak bone mass (e.g., family history, prolonged amenorrhea).

BONE TURNOVER MARKERS

Bone turnover markers have been shown to be independent predictors of fracture risk in older women *(32,33)* but have not yet been found to predict fractures in young perimenopausal women. These markers include bone resorption markers such as C-telopeptides and N-telopeptides in serum or urine among others and bone formation markers such as bone-specific alkaline phosphatase and osteocalcin. Overall, there is sparse evidence to support the routine use of bone turnover markers in the diagnosis or workup of an individual patient. At this point in time, most bone turnover markers are associated with high inter-individual and intra-individual variability. For example, urinary N-telopeptides has been reported to vary by 30–50% in an individual *(34)*. As noted above, bone turnover markers may have a role in understanding whether accelerated bone loss is occurring in a younger individuals to distinguish it from the inability to achieve an adequate peak bone mass but there is little evidence to support fracture risk prediction in that setting. These biochemical markers are sometimes used to assess early clinical response to bisphosphonate therapy prior to repeating a bone density since the markers are consistently decreased within 3 mo of starting therapy.

PHARMACOLOGICAL OPTIONS

Given the patient's low to moderate risk for fracture in the near term, it would be reasonable to consider therapeutic options. Following evidence-based guidelines, we focus on the data derived from meta-analyses and randomized controlled trials with fracture outcomes and appropriate validity *(35,36)*. BMD endpoints are discussed when fracture outcomes were not available.

NUTRITIONAL INTERVENTIONS

Calcium is an accepted component of osteoporosis treatment and prevention but its anti-fracture efficacy as a sole agent is not clear. Calcium administration results in modest increases in bone density at multiple sites (1.7% increase in spine; 95% confidence interval [CI] 0.9–2.4) in a meta-analysis of 15 trials. A trend toward vertebral fracture reduction was reported without evidence for nonvertebral fracture reduction *(37)*. Similarly, vitamin D is important for calcium absorption but fracture efficacy is limited and conflicting in postmenopausal women with effectiveness demonstrated in elderly women when combined with calcium *(38–41)*. A meta-analysis of all forms of vitamin D therapy found a reduction in vertebral fractures (RR 0.63; 95% CI 0.45–0.88) *(42)*. It is important to note that subjects participating in most RCTs of anti-osteoporosis therapies receive adequate calcium and vitamin D. The National Academy of Science and National Institutes of Health recommend calcium intakes of 1000–1500 mg/d and vitamin D of at least 400–800 IU for postmenopausal women (43,44). Vitamin D administration may be particularly important in individuals with little sun exposure such as the elderly. There is little evidence to guide nutritional interventions such as vitamin K and protein intake, but have been reported to be important frail elderly individuals (45,46).

LIFESTYLE INTERVENTIONS

According to a recent Cochrane Review, fall prevention interventions likely to be beneficial in the elderly include muscle strengthening and balance retraining, home hazard assessment, withdrawal of psychotropic medications and use of multidisciplinary risk factor assessment programs (47). Vitamin D supplementation in a meta analysis has also been shown to reduce falls by at least 20%, probably as a result of enhanced muscle strength (48,49). Hip protectors have been shown to reduce fracture risk in frail elderly adults (RH 0.4; 95% CI 0.2–0.8) but long term compliance is poor (50,51).

There is evidence from randomized trials that exercise intervention can increase BMD particularly in the femoral neck (52,53); however the BMD gains are often lost once the exercise regimen is stopped (54). There is little evidence to support fracture risk reduction although follow-up of a randomized controlled clinical trial in a small number of postmenopausal women found stronger back muscles owing to an exercise regimen resulted in fewer vertebral fractures (55).

Smoking cessation and decreased alcohol intake should be considered as they have been related to fracture risk although the effect of cessation on long-term outcomes is not clear (56,57).

MEDICATIONS

There are several pharmacological therapies available with demonstrated anti-fracture efficacy at vertebral and/or nonvertebral sites. Fracture efficacy results from major randomized placebo-controlled clinical trials are summarized in Table 2. The decision to choose one of these options depends highly on the short-term fracture risk assessment, particularly by site of fracture (e.g., spine vs hip) and acceptability of risks associated with each therapy. When considering the evidence for fracture prevention of these agents, a few points should be made regarding study design and reporting of fracture efficacy trials. Fracture efficacy is typically demonstrated in high-risk populations, such as elderly individuals with pre-existing vertebral fractures. The trials results are often difficult to generalize to individuals with similar T-scores and no prior fracture. The number needed to treat to prevent one fracture varies widely based on the underlying risk of the population studied. For example, treating a 50-yr-old recently menopausal women who has a low near-term risk of fractures requires over 1700 women be treated for 2 yr in order to prevent one vertebral fracture with most available pharmacological therapies (58). In contrast, an older postmenopausal woman at high risk of fracture requires only 90 women to be treated for 2 yr in order to prevent one vertebral fracture (58). The method of fracture ascertainment is relevant because trials that use radiographic surveillance of fractures as endpoints will report many more vertebral fractures than those that use clinical

Table 2
Vertebral and Hip Fracture Outcomes in Selected Randomized Placebo-Controlled Clinical Trials in Postmenopausal Women

Agent Dose	Ref. No.	Years	Sample size (PBO/drug)	Vertebral fractures			Hip fractures		
				% Placebo (n)	% Treatment (n)	RR Reduction (95% CI)	% Placebo (n)	% Treatment (n)	RR Reduction (95% CI)
Estrogen/Progesterone[a] 0.625 mg/2.5 mg	61	5.2	8102/8506	0.15 (60) annualized	0.09 (41) annualized	0.66 (0.44–0.98)	0.15 (62) annualized	0.1 (44) annualized	0.66 (0.45–0.98)
Estrogen[a] 0.625 mg	63	6.8	5429/5310	0.17 (64) annualized	0.11 (39) annualized	0.62 (0.42–0.93)	0.17 (64) annualized	0.11 (38) annualized	0.62 (0.41–0.91)
Raloxifene[b] 60 mg or 60 mg/120 mg pooled	68	3	I: 1522/3002 II: 770/1534	I: 4.5 (68) II: 21.2 (163)	I: 2.3 (35) II: 14.7 (113)	I: 0.5 (0.4–0.8) II: 0.7 (0.6–0.9)	0.7 (18)	0.8 (40)	1.1 (0.6–1.9)
Alendronate[c] 5 mg/10 mg[d]	76	3	1005/1022	15 (145)	8 (78)	0.53 (0.41–0.68)	2.2 (22)	1.1 (11)	0.49 (0.23–0.99)
Alendronate[d] 5 mg/10 mg[d]	77	4.2	2218/2214	3.8 (78)	2.1 (43)	0.56 (0.39–0.80)	1.1 (24)	0.9 (19)	0.79 (0.43–1.44)
Risedronate 5 mg	82	3	820/821	16.3 (93)	11.3 (61)	0.59 (0.43–0.82)	1.8 (15)	1.5 (12)	NR
Risedronate 5 mg	83	3	408/408	29 (89)	18.1 (53)	0.51 (0.36–0.73)	2.7 (11)	2.2 (9)	NR
Risedronate[e] 2.5 mg/5 mg pooled	85	3	I: 1821/3624 II: 1313/2573	NA	NA	NA	I: 3.2 (46) II: 5.1 (49)	I: 1.9 (55) II: 4.2 (82)	I: 0.6 (0.4–0.9) II: 0.8 (0.6–1.2)
Ibandronate[f] 2.5 mg daily	94	3	975/977	5.3 (41)	2.8 (22)	0.49 (NR)	8.2 (NR)	9.1 (NR)	NR, non-significant
PTH[g] 20 µg	101	1.5	544/541	14 (64)	5 (22)	0.35 (0.22–0.55)	0.7 (4)	0.2 (1)	NR
Calcitonin 200 IU	96	5	311/316	26 (70)	18 (51)	0.67 (0.47–0.97)	3 (9)	2 (5)	0.5 (0.2–1.6)

Abbr: PBO, placebo; RR, relative risk; CI, confidence interval; PTH, parathyroid hormone; NR, not reported.

[a]Nominal 95% CI reported.

[b]Hip fracture data reported as pooled estimate of both groups for 60 mg and 120 mg doses combined. Vertebral fracture data for 60 mg dose. Subgroup I had osteoporosis by T-scores of lumbar spine or femoral neck. Subgroup II included women with ≥2 prevalent vertebral fractures or low BMD and ≥1 prevalent vertebral fractures.

[c]Vertebral fracture data from morphometric (radiographic) analysis.

[d]5 mg for 2 yr followed by 10 mg for remainder of trial.

[e]Subgroup I enrolled women age 70–79 with a very low BMD at femoral neck (mean –3.7). Subgroup II enrolled women at least 80 yr old with nonskeletal risk factor for osteoporosis (e.g., prior-related fall injury) with or without osteoporosis.

[f] Clinical vertebral fractures. Hip fracture results shown are for nonvertebral fractures.

[g]Fragility hip fracture data presented. Median duration of observation was 21 mo. Approximate mean treatment duration was 18 mo.

Note: Table adapted and reprinted with permission from ref. 28.

vertebral fractures. Finally, BMD change does not always have a linear relationship to fracture risk reduction as several agents with similar fracture risk reductions may have smaller changes in BMD.

HORMONE THERAPY

Estrogen therapy increases BMD in both younger perimenopausal women and older postmenopausal women (59). In a meta-analysis, postmenopausal women treated with estrogen for 2 yr increased bone mineral density by 6.8% (95% CI 5.8–7.9; 21 trials) at the spine and 4.1% (95% CI 3.5–4.8; 9 trials) at the femoral neck (60). The Women's Health Initiative (WHI) represents one of the few RCTs to evaluate fracture efficacy. One arm of the WHI evaluated the effects of estrogen–progesterone combination therapy in 16,608 postmenopausal women (age 50–79, mean age 63) with an intact uterus and was halted early, after 5.2 yr, because of adverse events in primary outcomes of coronary heart disease and breast cancer (61). Women were not specifically recruited based on increased fracture risk and women with very low femoral neck BMD (Z-score <–3) were excluded (62). Hip and vertebral fractures were reduced by an estimated hazard ratio of 0.66 (nominal 95% CI 0.45–0.98 hip; 0.44–0.98 spine) and resulted in 5 fewer hip fractures per 10,000 person-years of use. The WHI arm in over 10,000 women without an intact uterus on conjugated-equine estrogens alone for a mean of 6.8 yr also demonstrated a reduction in hip fractures (six fewer hip fractures per 10,000 person-years) (63). These results are relevant because only one other class of agents, the bisphosphonates, alendronate, and risedronate, has convincingly resulted in hip fracture reduction. Determining the balance of risk and benefits regarding estrogen therapy in an individual is often difficult. If the goal is to decrease fracture risk, other options are available for the management of osteoporosis for most individuals.

Small RCTs using low-dose, or ultra-low-dose estrogen preparations have demonstrated increases in spine and hip BMD in postmenopausal women, although there are no data on fracture risk reduction (64–66). Currently, the evidence is not compelling to advocate low-dose estrogen therapy as an effective anti-osteoporosis therapy and long-term adverse effects have not been evaluated.

SELECTIVE ESTROGEN RECEPTOR MODULATORS

Selective estrogen receptor modulators (SERMs), such as raloxifene and tamoxifen, are potential alternatives to hormone therapy. These compounds interact with the estrogen receptor to selectively induce an agonist (bone, cholesterol) or antagonist (breast) action in estrogen-responsive target tissues (67).

Raloxifene improved BMD in postmenopausal women and has been shown to reduce vertebral fractures (68–70). The largest trial randomized 7705 postmenopausal women (mean age 67) to 60 mg or 120 mg of raloxifene per day or placebo for 3 yr. Two groups were studied: one group with T-score <–2.5 at spine or femoral neck and a second group with vertebral fractures. Both study groups taking 60 mg had decreased radiographic vertebral fractures with a relative risk of 0.7 (95% CI 0.5–0.8) but no significant decrease in nonvertebral fractures (RR 0.9, 95% CI 0.8–1.1). BMD increases were modest (2.1% at the femoral neck and 2.6% in the spine in the 60 mg group). The reduction in vertebral fractures was maintained in a 1-yr extension trial allowing the use of other bone-active agents (70). A meta-analysis reported pooled estimates for several adverse events including a significant increase in hot flashes (RR 1.46; 95% CI 1.23–1.74), deep venous thrombosis (RR 3.51; 95% CI 1.44–8.56) and slightly increased influenza-like syndrome (RR 1.18; 95% CI 1.04–1.34). No significant increased risks were found for leg cramps (RR 1.64; 95% CI 0.84–3.20), breast pain, and endometrial cancer (RR 0.8; 95% CI 0.2–2.7) *(68,71)*. *Post-hoc* analysis of secondary endpoints found decreased breast cancer risk (RR 0.24; 95% CI 0.13–0.44) and no overall change in cardiovascular or cerebrovascular risk but a potential benefit in women at increased baseline cardiovascular risk *(71,72)*. Studies are on-going with breast cancer, cardiovascular, and cerebrovascular endpoints as primary outcomes that will clarify the relationship between raloxifene and these outcomes *(73)*.

The raloxifene data demonstrate that significant absolute reduction in vertebral fractures can occur with only modest BMD increases. Raloxifene has not been shown to reduce nonvertebral fractures. This relegates the use of raloxifene to clinical scenarios when the short-term risk of vertebral fracture is higher than that of hip fracture, such as during early menopausal bone loss.

BISPHOSPHONATES

The oral bisphoshonates, alendronate and risedronate, have been shown to reduce vertebral and nonvertebral fractures. Bisphosphonates are potent inhibitors of bone resorption that act primarily through reducing the recruitment and action of bone-resorbing osteoclasts. The oral bioavailability is low and reports of pill-induced esophagitis require that patients remain upright, drink fluids and take on an empty stomach *(74)*. Despite a long half-life in bone, no detrimental effects have been reported in bone-biopsy studies in clinical trial subjects treated for up to 10 yr *(75)*.

Alendronate was the first oral bisphosphonate to be approved for the prevention and treatment of osteoporosis *(76,77)*. A meta-analysis found vertebral fractures reductions in subjects given 5 mg or more (RR = 0.52; 95% CI 0.43–0.65; 11 trials) as well as nonvertebral fracture reductions in subjects given 10 mg or more (RR 0.51; 95% CI 0.38–0.69) *(78)*. In pooled analysis of two RCTs, hip fractures were reduced in both women with existing vertebral fractures and women without vertebral fracture but a femoral neck T-score <–2.5 (RH 0.47; 95% CI 0.26–0.79) *(79)*. Alendronate has also been shown to increase BMD in recently menopausal women (<3 yr) without osteoporosis (spine T-score >–2) after 3-yr follow-up *(80,81)*.

Risedronate also has demonstrated anti-fracture efficacy *(82,83)*. A meta-analysis reported reductions in vertebral (RR 0.64; 95% CI 0.54–0.77) and nonvertebral fractures (RR 0.73; 95% CI 0.61–0.87) at doses of 2.5 mg or more *(84)*. The risedronate trials had significant loss to follow-up of 20 to greater than 35% compared to the alendronate trials reporting <10%; but the effect on the reported results is not clear *(84)*. Hip fracture reduction has been demonstrated in pooled analysis of 2.5 and 5 mg dose in an RCT of elderly women age 70–79 with very low femoral neck T-scores (mean –3.7) (RR 0.6; 95% CI 0.4–0.9) but not in women older than 80 years selected primarily based on non-skeletal risk factors (e.g., prior fall-related injury) with or without osteoporosis *(85)*. In a *post-hoc* subgroup analysis, the fracture benefits were only found in women with a prior vertebral fracture in the age 70–79 group (RR 0.4; 95% CI: 0.2–0.8) and not in those without a vertebral fracture. Risedronate has been reported to decrease nonvertebral fracture risk within 6 mo *(86)*. Taken together, these data suggest that patients at highest risk for fracture such as a prior history of fracture are the ones that are most likely to benefit from a bisphosphonate therapy for vertebral or hip fracture reduction.

Both alendronate and risedronate can increase BMD when given in once weekly doses but have not been studied for fracture outcomes. Alendronate given once weekly (70 mg) or once daily (10 mg) increases BMD by a similar degree in postmenopausal women treated for 1 yr (87). Similarly, once-weekly risedronate (35 mg) was comparable to the 5 mg daily dose in efficacy for BMD changes in 1146 postmenopausal women treated for 2 yr (88). Once-weekly alendronate resulted in higher BMD at several sites than once-weekly risedronate in a 12 mo RCT in postmenopausal women; however, it is not yet proved whether these changes result in greater fracture reduction efficacy (89,90). There does not appear to be a difference in upper gastrointestinal (GI) tract tolerability in short-term RCTs of once-weekly alendronate compared to placebo or once-weekly risedronate (89,91,92). Fracture efficacy data for all doses in ethnic/racial groups other than Caucasian women are limited (93).

Ibandronate, 2.5 mg daily is a third generation bisphosphonate recently approved by the US Food and Drug Administration (FDA) for the treatment of postmenopausal osteoporosis. Like risedronate and alendronate, it increases BMD in the spine and hip and reduces bone turnover markers. Daily ibandronate (2.5 mg) has been shown to reduce clinical vertebral fracture risk by 49% although nonvertebral fractures were not significantly reduced compared to placebo in a large 3-yr randomized placebo-controlled trial in postmenopausal women with prevalent vertebral fractures (94). Once monthly ibandronate, 100 mg orally, is currently being studied in phase III trials and may be the only marketed formulation of this drug, pending FDA approval.

CALCITONIN

Calcitonin is an endogenous peptide that decreases bone resorption by inhibiting osteoclast activity. It is available in nasal and subcutaneous forms and may be an alternative for patients who do not tolerate oral agents. However, no effect on nonvertebral fracture has been established and methodological flaws in the calcitonin trials limit the ability to conclude that vertebral fractures are decreased (95). In a meta-analysis, calcitonin decreased vertebral fractures with a pooled RR of 0.46 (95% CI 0.25–0.87; four trials; $n = 1404$) (95). The majority of those subjects were in one RCT which has been criticized because of the lack of dose-response effect because the vertebral fracture efficacy was only evident for the 200 IU dose and up to 59% of participants were lost to follow-up by the end of 5 yr (96). Calcitonin may have mild analgesic properties although it is not FDA-approved for this indication (97).

Our patient should be started on calcium (1200 mg in divided doses/d), vitamin D (800 IU daily if not deficient), encouraged to maintain an exercise regimen 3×/wk (e.g., walking or strength training) and given information on falls prevention. There are several reasonable first-line drug therapy alternatives for this individual including raloxifene, hormone therapy, and an oral bisphosphonate. Although data exists for PTH effectiveness as first-line therapy in individuals without a fracture (see Parathyroid Hormone), few would argue that the costs of PTH and its limited duration of use outweigh its antifracture benefits as first line therapy in a subject without a fracture.

She elects to begin oral bisphosphonate therapy. A repeat bone mineral density after two years of therapy demonstrates a T-score of –1.7 at the hip and –2.4 at the spine. She sustains a wrist fracture after falling on ice. Should you change your management?

This clinical scenario is common and several reasonable options face the clinician and patient including: (1) discontinue the bisphosphonate and switch to a different pharmacological therapy or lifestyle intervention, (2) continue the bisphosphonate and add another agent or lifestyle interventions, or (3) continue current management. First, wrist fractures can be considered an osteoporotic fracture and notably occur earlier in postmenopausal women followed by spine and hip fractures respectively as age increases. Individuals with osteoporosis are at increased risk of fracture given a loading force such as occurs during a fall and the majority of osteoporotic fractures occur in association with a fall. Therefore, it is a misconception that fractures owing to trauma are not attributable to the underlying osteoporosis. Falls prevention strategies should be reviewed with this patient.

What are the implications of her follow-up BMD results? First consider whether the interval is long enough to assess a change. In most scenarios, BMD should be repeated in 2 yr after beginning therapy. The evidence for these recommendations are often based on calculations of the least significant change that is clinically relevant and measurable based on the performance characteristics of DXA testing. This rate of changes varies by anatomic site and testing center and is often 2–3% at the spine and 4–6% at the hip for an individual (98). In select high-risk subjects, such as those on glucocorticoids who have sustained a fracture, more frequent follow-up may be considered. Again, it must be emphasized that fracture efficacy has been demonstrated in treatment trials despite small changes in BMD. Additionally, the concept of "regression to the mean" has been well-described in clinical trials and supports "watchful waiting" as those individuals who lose or fail to gain bone on repeated BMD measures tend to have a repeat measure that is higher (99).

In our patient, the most critical determinant of her therapeutic choice is the fact that she sustained an osteoporotic fracture rather than the lack of a robust BMD change. Consideration should be given as to whether the patient is effectively taking the bisphosphonate. This should prompt a review of adherence to therapy, taking on an empty stomach and consideration of bone turnover markers to assess evidence of bone turnover suppression. A note of caution however is that there may be high intraindividual variation such that a normal value of bone turnover marker may not be helpful whereas an elevated value may suggest an inadequate response to therapy or nonadherence. In the setting of an osteoporotic fracture in a patient on a bisphosphonate, combination therapies and parathyroid hormone may be considered.

PARATHYROID HORMONE

PTH is an anabolic agent that stimulates bone turnover and favors bone formation in contrast to most available agents which are primarily anti-resorptives. PTH is an 84 amino acid endogenous peptide with the human PTH 1-34 fragment (teriparatide) FDA-approved for clinical use and the PTH 1-84 fragment currently in clinical trials. Teriparatide requires daily subcutaneous injections and is among the most expensive anti-osteoporosis therapies. Elevated sustained levels of PTH have been known to contribute to cortical bone loss, but intermittent subcutaneous administration increases BMD, restores bone microarchitecture and increases bone size (100). The reason for this apparent paradox is not fully explained but may be due to intermittent exposure. Spine BMD increases have been reported up to 7–13% and are greater than at the femoral neck where no change or increases of 3% have been reported *(100)*. Several RCTs have demonstrated anti-fracture efficacy *(101–106)*. The largest trial studied 1637 postmenopausal women with prior vertebral fractures and found the 20 μg (marketed) dose reduced vertebral fractures (RR 0.35; 95% CI 0.22–0.55) and nonvertebral fragility fractures (RR 0.47; 95% CI 0.25–0.88) when compared to placebo for a median of 21 mo *(101)*. These vertebral fracture effects were greater in women with more than one fracture or more severe fractures. Recombinant hPTH (40 μg) compared to alendronate had significantly higher increases in spine BMD after 1 yr (12.2% vs 5.6%, respectively, $p < 0.001$) *(107)*. BMD gains with PTH can be preserved when followed by alendronate *(108)* or estrogen therapy *(103)*. Adverse events may include mild asymptomatic hypercalcemia (<11.2 mg/dL) but has not been observed in all trials *(101)*. Absolute and relative contraindications include renal stones, renal failure, open epiphyses, hyperparathyroidism, and a history of bone cancer. Pre-clinical studies in rats given long-term PTH at high doses found an increased risk of osteosarcoma *(109)*. This has not been observed in any human studies but had led the FDA to limit therapy duration to 2 yr. Additionally, the effect of prior anti-resorptive therapy on PTH efficacy is still being determined and preliminary evidence suggests the BMD response to teriparatide may differ by anti-resorptive agent *(110)*.

COMBINATION THERAPIES

What is the evidence for combination therapy or for direct comparison trials? Few data exist for direct comparison of fracture efficacy for different agents or for combination therapy. Estrogen and alendronate used in combination result in greater BMD increases than either agent alone *(111–113)*. Risedronate (5 mg) combined with CEE (0.625 mg) for 1 yr compared with CEE alone resulted in only slightly higher BMD at the femoral neck and radius with similar rates at the spine *(114)*. In postmenopausal women, it has been noted that BMD decreases after withdrawal of estrogen therapy are greater than that observed after withdrawal of alendronate *(115)*.

Raloxifene has been studied in combination with bisphosphonates for BMD outcomes. Combination therapy (raloxifene 60 mg and alendronate 10 mg) for 1 yr in 331 postmenopausal women was more effective at increasing BMD at the femoral neck than alendronate alone (3.7% combination vs 2.7% alendronate alone, $p = 0.02$) and the increases at other hip sites and the spine were similar for combination therapy and alendronate alone. Combination therapy increased BMD to a greater extent at all sites compared to raloxifene alone *(116)*. Alendronate (70 mg weekly) produced greater changes in BMD than raloxifene when directly compared in a 1-yr RCT in postmenopausal women *(117)*; however there was no fracture efficacy data limiting the clinical relevance of those results because it has been previously demonstrated that raloxifene effects on vertebral fracture reduction occur with smaller changes in BMD.

Calcitonin has not been studied in combination but the marketed dose of 200 IU had smaller BMD increases when compared to alendronate (10 mg) over 1 yr in older women with osteoporosis *(118)*.

Parathyroid hormone has been studied in combination with alendronate in both men and postmenopausal women and has not been shown to be more effective than either agent alone in respect to changes in BMD *(119,120)*.

In this patient, it is important to review adherence to therapy. Measurement of a bone resorption marker could be considered to determine whether she had an expected decrease in bone turnover markers in response to therapy; although as mentioned earlier these markers are difficult to interpret in an individual patient. These therapies greatly reduce the risk of fracture but certainly do not reduce the risk entirely. Now that she has sustained a wrist fracture, her chance of another osteoporotic fracture is increased significantly *(121)*. Adding raloxifene could be considered but there is no clear data to suggest that fracture risk reduction is greater in combination. Raloxifene use is probably most reasonable with a recently menopausal woman with low bone density who does not have contraindications to its use. Even though it does not have proven efficacy for hip fracture reduction *per se*, a perimenopausal woman with low-BMD has a relatively low short-term risk for hip fracture as the risk for Colle's or vertebral fractures is greater. We would consider continuing current bisphosphonate therapy and repeat BMD in 1–2 yr. We would maintain a high clinical suspicion for additional fractures. Vertebral fractures are often asymptomatic and undetected. Evidence from the placebo arm of an RCT with radiographic surveillance for vertebral fractures suggested that height loss of ≤2 cm over a 1–3 yr period is effective at ruling out a vertebral fracture whereas an upper limit for effectively ruling in a vertebral fracture was not clear *(122)*.

SURGICAL MANAGEMENT

What if she had sustained a painful vertebral fracture? Surgical management of hip fractures is usually indicated but there is little evidence guiding the surgical management of vertebral fractures. The techniques of vertebroplasty and kyphoplasty have been used in the management of painful vertebral body fractures in osteoporosis *(123)*. Vertebroplasty involves the percutaneous injection of polymetalmetacrylate cement into the vertebral body under fluoroscopic guidance. Kyphoplasty is a technique involving insertion of a balloon-like catheter (bone tamp) to expand the vertebral body prior to the injection of cement. A notable complication is extravasation of the cement that is usually asymptomatic but has been described in a case report to cause reversible paraplegia requiring surgical decompression *(124)*. Despite reports of decreased acute pain *(125)*, no RCTs have been performed and long-term complications are unclear. Studies suggest there may be an increased risk of new fracture in the vertebrae adjacent to fracture undergoing vertebroplasty *(125,126)*. For these reasons, these procedures should be used with caution and referral should be made to individuals with expertise in the area.

OSTEOPOROSIS MANAGEMENT IN MEN

How would the management options change if this patient had been a man? Current evidence is not as robust for guiding clinical management of osteoporosis in men. Epidemiological studies show that men account for a reasonable proportion of fractures and it has been estimated that 20–25% of hip fractures occur in men *(127)*. It is often advocated that an extensive search for secondary causes be done in men with osteoporosis but it is not well established that men have higher rates of secondary causes than women *(128,129)*. No clear evidence for BMD screening regimens have been validated. It is often suggested that older men (e.g., over age 70) should be considered for BMD testing. This is a result of the observation that men may suffer fractures at high rates at a later age later than women. Given the available evidence that the presence of a fracture connotes a greater risk for subsequent fracture, any man who has sustained a fracture should be considered for BMD testing. Special considerations for more frequent BMD testing and/or interventions include men undergoing androgen-deprivation therapy for prostate cancer treatment.

Compelling evidence for anti-fracture efficacy of therapeutic regimens except alendronate are lacking in men. Calcium, vitamin D, exercise recommendations, and lifestyle modifications to decrease falls risks are the same as women although there are no clear evidence for fracture reduction. One RCT in 41 men with idiopathic osteoporosis treated with calcium or calcitriol for 2 yr showed no changes in BMD or fracture risk (130). Testosterone therapy has not been proven to reduce fracture risk but has been shown to have modest improvements in BMD in hypogonadal older men (131). Therefore, testosterone therapy should be considered in the treatment of the hypogonadism but not in eugonadal men or for purposes of decreasing their fracture risk. Alendronate (10 mg/d) has been shown to increase BMD in small studies (132,133) and reduce vertebral fractures in 241 men with idiopathic osteoporosis treated for 2 yr (133). Intranasal calcitonin increases BMD at the spine but not the hip in a 1 yr RCT in 21 men (134). Teriparatide (134) has been shown to increase BMD in men in several treatment trials; none of which were powered to test fracture outcomes (135,136). Vertebral fracture incidence was evaluated in a follow-up study of 279 men with low BMD who originally participated in a treatment trial using two doses of teriparatide (20 mcg vs 40 mcg vs placebo). The trial was halted after 11 mo because of rat toxicity data and subjects were followed in a discontinuation study for an additional 30 mo of observation. Subjects initially assigned to the treatment arms (20 and 40 mcg combined) had a decrease in moderate or severe vertebral fractures by radiographs 18 mo after discontinuing teriparatide when compared to the placebo group. Confidence in these results is limited because it was an observational study in which up to 29% of subjects had other anti-osteoporosis therapy with bisphosphonates being most frequent (137). The ability of PTH to increase BMD is no better when used in combination with alendronate, than PTH alone, similar to the findings in women (119). Other agents have been studied for BMD responses in specific settings such as prostate cancer (e.g., raloxifene [138], intravenous pamidronate [139], zoledronate [140]). On-going studies should help clarify the benefits of these agents.

OSTEOPOROSIS MANAGEMENT IN GLUCOCORTICOID-INDUCED OSTEOPOROSIS

A common secondary cause of osteoporosis is long-term glucocorticoid therapy as a result of the multi-faceted detrimental effects that steroids have on normal bone physiology (141). Evidence from placebo arms of RCTs suggest that patients on oral glucocorticoids lose almost 3%/yr at the spine (142). Several bisphosphonates including alendronate, risedronate, etidronate, and intravenous pamidronate have been shown to increase BMD with more consistent effects at the lumbar spine than the femoral neck (143–145). The evidence for fracture reduction is limited. An RCT of alendronate in 477 men and women receiving ≥7.5 mg prednisone-equivalents daily initially reported a non-significant vertebral fracture reduction after 1 yr (145) and later found a decrease in new vertebral fractures in 208 of those subjects participating in 1-yr extension *(146)*. Risedronate therapy for 1-yr decreased new vertebral fracture in pooled estimates from two RCTs in 187 men taking glucocorticoids *(147)*. Teriparatide and hormone therapy have been shown to increase BMD at the spine whereas effects of calcitonin on BMD have been conflicting *(148)*. It has been suggested that BMD testing should be considered in patients receiving glucocorticoids for more than 3 mo and a lower threshold of BMD T-scores should be used when considering interventions because patients with glucocorticoid exposure may have a higher fracture risk than patients without glucocorticoid exposures at comparable BMD levels. Guidelines have suggested that therapy be considered in individuals receiving greater than 5–7.5 mg of prednisone-equivalents daily for 3–6 mo *(148)*.

SUMMARY

Several therapeutic regimens have demonstrated anti-fracture efficacy such that most individuals who have sustained an osteoporotic fracture can be offered beneficial therapy. Research is needed to clarify optimal clinical evaluation and management of patients with osteoporosis including recently menopausal women, men, and subjects with osteopenia. Current evidence strongly supports case-finding strategies in high-risk patients and use of agents with demonstrated anti-fracture efficacy in those who have already sustained a fracture.

REFERENCES

1. Ray N, Chan JK, Thamer M, and Melton J, 3rd. Medical expenditures for the treatment of osteoporotic fractures in the United States in 1995: report from the National Osteoporosis Foundation. J Bone Miner Res 1997;12:24–35.
2. Melton LJ, 3rd. Who has osteoporosis? A conflict between clinical and public health perspectives. J Bone Miner Metab 2000;15:2309–2314.
3. Cummings S, Black DM, Rubin S. Lifetime risks of hip, Colles', or vertebral fracture and coronary heart disease among white postmenopausal women. Arch Intern Med 1989;149:2445–2448.
4. Leibson C, Tosteson A, Gabriel, S, Ransom J, Melton LJI. Mortality, disability, and nursing home use for persons with and without hip fracture: a population–based study. J Am Geriatr Soc 2002;50: 1644–1650.
5. Cooper C, Atkinson EJ, Jacobsen S, O'Fallon WM, Melton LJ, 3rd. Population based study of survival after osteoporosis fracture. Am J Epidemiol 1993;137:1001–1005.
6. Riggs BL, Melton LJ, 3rd. The worldwide problem of osteoporosis: insights afforded by epidemiology. Bone 1995;17:505S–511S.
7. Kannus P, Parkkari J, Sievanen H, Heinonen A, Vuori I, Jarvinen M. Epidemiology of hip fractures. Bone 1996;18:57S–63S.
8. Torgerson DJ, Dolan P. Prescribing by general practitioners after an osteoporotic fracture. Ann Rheum Dis 1998;57:378–379.
9. Cuddihy M, Gabriel S, Crowson C, Atkinson EJ, C T, O'Fallon WM, Melton LJ, 3rd. Osteoporosis intervention following distal forearm fractures: a missed opportunity? Arch Intern Med 2002; 162:421–426.
10. Feldstein A, Elmer PJ, Orwoll E, Herson M, Hillier T. Bone mineral density measurement and treatment for osteoporosis in older individuals with fractures. Arch Intern Med 2003;163:2165–2172.
11. USPSTF. Screening for osteoporosis in postmenopausal women: recommendations and rationale. Ann Intern Med 2002;137:526–528.
12. Cadarette SM, Jaglal SB, Kreiger N, McIsaac WJ, Darlington GA, Tu JV. Development and validation of the osteoporosis risk assessment instrument to facilitate selection of women for bone densitometry. CMAJ 2000;162:1289–1294.

13. National Osteoporosis Foundation. Physician's Guide to Prevention and Treatment of Osteoporosis. 2003.
14. Siris ES, Miller PD, Barrett-Connor E, et al. Identification of fracture outcomes of undiagnosed low bone mineral density in postmenopausal women: results from the National Osteoporosis Risk Assessment. JAMA 2001;286:2815–2822.
15. Miller PD, Siris ES, Barrett-Connor E., et al. Prediction of fracture risk in postmenopausal white women with peripheral bone densitometry: evidence from the National Osteoporosis Risk Assessment. J Bone Miner Res 2002;17:2222–2230.
16. Miller PD, Siris ES, Barrett-Connor E., et al. Prediction of fracture risk in postmenopausal white women with peripheral bone densitometry:evidence from the national osteoporosis risk assessment. J Bone Miner Res 2002;17:2222–2230.
17. Bates DW, Black,DM, Cummings SR. Clinical use of bone densitometry: clinical applications. JAMA 2002;288:1898–1900.
18. Blake GM, Knapp KM, Fogelman I. Absolute fracture risk varies with bone densitometry technique used. J Clin Densitom 2002;5:109–116.
19. Fordham JN, Chinn DJ, Kumar N. Identification of women with reduced bone density at the lumbar spine and femoral neck using BMD at the oscalcis. Osteoporos Int 2000;11:797–802.
20. Sweeney AT, Malabana AO, Blake MA, et al. Bone mineral density assessment: comparison of dual-energy x-ray absorptiometry measurements of the calcaneus, spine and hip. J Clin Densitom 2002;5:57–62.
21. Williams ED, Daymond TJ. Evaluation of calcaneus bone densitometry against hip and spine for diagnosis of osteoporosis. Br J Radiol 2003;76:123–126.
22. Siris ES, Chen YT, Abbott TA, et al. Bone mineral density thresholds for pharmacological intervention to prevent fractures. Arch Intern Med 2004;164:1108–1112.
23. Miller P, Njeh C, Jankowski L, Lenchik L. What are the standards by which bone mass measurement at peripheral skeletal sites should be used in the diagnosis of osteoporosis? J Clin Densitom 2002;5:S39–S45.
24. Marshall D, Johnell O, Wedel H. Meta-analysis of how well measures of bone mineral density predict occurrence of osteoporotic fractures. BMJ 1996;312:1254–1259.
25. World Health Organization. Guidelines for preclinical evaluation and clinical trials in osteoporosis. Geneva, Switzerland, World Health Organization, 1998.
26. Kanis J, Black D, Cooper C, et al. A new approach to the development of assessment guidelines for osteoporosis. Osteoporos Int 2002;13:527–536.
27. Cooper C, Atkinson EJ, O'Fallon WM, Melton LJr. Incidence of clinically diagnosed vertebral fractures: a population-based study in Rochester, Minnesota, 1985–1989. J Bone Miner Res 1992;7:221–227.
28. Brown SA, Rosen CJ. Osteoporosis. Med Clin North Am 2003;87:1039–1063.
29. Tannenbaum C, Clark J, Schwartzman K, et al. Yield of laboratory testing to identify secondary contributors to osteoporosis in otherwise healthy women. J Clin Endocrinol Metab 2002;87:4431–4437.
30. Jamal SA, Leiter RE, Bayoumi AM, Bauer DC, Cummings SR. Clinical utility of laboratory testing in women with osteoporosis. Osteoporos Int 2004;16:534–540.
31. Barrett-Connor E, Mueller JE, von Muhlen DG, et al. Low levels of estradiol are associated with vertebral fractures in older men, but not women: the Rancho Bernardo Study. J Clin Endocrinol Metab 2000;85:219–223.
32. Garnero P, Hausherr E, Chapuy M, et al. Markers of bone resorption predict hip fracture in elderly women: the EPIDOS prospective study. J Bone Miner Res 1996;11:1531–1538.
33. Garnero P, Sornay-Rendu E, Claustrat B, Delmas PD. Biochemical markers of bone turnover, endogenous hormones and the risk of fractures in postmenopausal women: the OFELY study. J Bone Miner Res 2000;15:1526–1536.
34. Delmas P, Eastell R, Garnero P, Seibel M, Stepan J. The use of biochemical markers of bone turnover in osteoporosis. Osteoporos Int 2000;6:S2–S17.
35. Guyatt G, Sackett D, Cook D. Users' guides to the medical literature. II. How to use an article about therapy or prevention. A. Are the results of the study valid? Evidence-Based Medicine Working Group. JAMA 1993;270:2598–2601.
36. Moher D, Schulz K, Altman D. The CONSORT statement: Revised recommendations for improving the quality of reports of parallel-group randomised trials. Lancet 2001;357:1191–1194.

37. Shea B, Wells G, Cranney A, et al. Meta-analyses of therapies for postmenopausal osteoporosis. VII: Meta-analysis of calcium supplementation for the prevention of postmenopausal osteoporosis. Endocr Rev 2002;23:552–559.
38. Tilyard M, Spears G, Thomson J, Dovey S. Treatment of postmenopausal osteoporosis with calcitriol or calcium. N Engl J Med 1992;326:357–362.
39. Ott SM, Chestnut III C. Calcitriol treatment is not effective in postmenopausal osteoporosis. Ann Intern Med 1989;110:267–274.
40. Hayashi Y, Fujita T, Inoue T. Decrease of vertebral fracture in osteoporotics by administration of 1-alpha-hydroxy-vitamin D3. J Bone Miner Metab 1992;10:50–54.
41. Chapuy M, Arlot ME, DuBoeuf F, et al. Vitamin D3 and calcium to prevent hip fractures in elderly women. N Engl J Med 1992;327:1637–1642.
42. Papadimitropoulos E, Wells G, Shea B, et al. Meta-analyses of therapies for postmenopausal osteoporosis. VIII: Meta-analyses of the efficacy of vitamin D treatment in preventing osteoporosis in postmenopausal women. Endocr Rev 2002;23:560–569.
43. Institute of Medicine. DRI: Dietary Reference Intakes for Calcium, Phosphorus, Magnesium, Vitamin D and Fluoride. National Academy Press, Washington, DC, 1999.
44. Optimal calcium intake. National Institutes of Health. Conn Med 1994;58:613–623.
45. Hannan M, Tucker K, Dawson-Hughes B, Cupples L, Felson D, Kiel D. Effect of dietary protein on bone loss in elderly men and women: the Framingham osteoporosis study. J Bone Miner Res 2000; 15:2504–2512.
46. Booth S, Tucker K, Chen H, et al. Dietary vitamin K intakes are associated with hip fracture but not with bone mineral density in elderly men and women. Am J Clin Nutr 2000;71:1201–1208.
47. Gillespie L, Gillespie W, Robertson M, Lamb S, Cumming R, Rowe B. Interventions for preventing falls in elderly people. In: The Cochrane Library Issue 4:Oxford: Update software, 2002.
48. Bischoff-Ferrari HA, Dawson-Hughes B, Willett WC. et al. Effect of vitamin D on falls: a meta-analysis. JAMA 2004;291:1999–2006.
49. Bischoff-Ferrari HA, Dietrich T, Orav EJ, et al. Higher 25-hydroxyvitamin D concentrations are associated with better lower-extremity function in both active and inactive persons aged > or = 60 y. Am J Clin Nutr 2004;80:752–758.
50. Kannus P, Parkkari J, Niemi S, et al. Prevention of hip fracture in ambulatory elderly. N Engl J Med 2000;343:1506–1513.
51. Birks YF, Porthouse J, Addie C, et al. Randomized controlled trial of hip protectors among women living in the community. Osteoporos Int 2004;15:701–706. Epub 2004 Mar 2003.
52. Asikainen TM, Kukkonen-Harjula K, Miilunpalo S. Exercise for health for early postmenopausal women: a systematic review of randomised controlled trials. Sports Med 2004;34:753–778.
53. Kemmler W, Lauber D, Weineck J, et al. Benefits of 2 years of intense exercise on bone density, physical fitness and blood lipids in early postmenopausal osteopenic women: results of the Erlangen Fitness Osteoporosis Prevention Study (EFOPS). Arch Intern Med 2004;164:1084–1091.
54. Uusi-Rasi K, Sievanen H, Heinonen A, Kannus P, Vuori I. Effect of discontinuation of alendronate treatment and exercise on bone mass and physical fitness: 15-month follow-up of a randomized, controlled trial. Bone 2004;35:799–805.
55. Sinaki M, Itoi E, Wahner HW, et al. Stronger back muscles reduce the incidence of vertebral fractures: a prospective 10 year follow-up of postmenopausal women. Bone 2002;30:836–841.
56. Kanis JA, Johnell O, Oden A, et al. Smoking and fracture risk: a meta-analysis. Osteoporos Int 2005; 16:155–162.
57. Kanis JA, Johansson H, Johnell O, et al. Alcohol intake as a risk factor for fracture. Osteoporos Int 2005;16:737–742.
58. Cranney A, Guyatt G, Griffith L, Wells G, Tugwell P, Rosen C. Meta-analyses of therapies for postmenopausal osteoporosis. IX: Summary of meta-analyses of therapies for postmenopausal osteoporosis. Endocr Rev 2002;23:570–578.
59. Writing Group for the PEPI. Effects of hormone therapy on bone mineral density: results from the Postmenopausal Estrogen/Progestin Interventions (PEPI) Trial. JAMA 1996;276:1389–1396.
60. Wells G, Tugwell P, Shea B, et al. Meta-analyses of therapies for postmenopausal osteoporosis. V: Meta-analysis of the efficacy of hormone replacement therapy in treating and preventing osteoporosis in postmenopausal women. Endocr Rev 2002;23:529–539.
61. Writing group for the Women's Health Initiative investigators. Risks and benefits of estrogen plus progestin in healthy postmenopausal women. Principal results from the Women's Health Initiative randomized controlled trial. JAMA 2002;288:321–333.

62. The Women's Health Initiative Study Group. Design of the Women's Health Initiative clinical trial and observational study. Controlled Clin Trials 1998;19:61–109.
63. Anderson GL, Limacher M, Assaf AR, et al. Effects of conjugated equine estrogen in postmenopausal women with hysterectomy: the Women's Health Initiative randomized controlled trial. JAMA 2004;291:1701–1712.
64. Prestwood KM, Kenny AM, Kleppinger A, Kulldorff M. Ultralow-dose micronized 17 beta-estradiol and bone density and bone metabolism in older women: a randomized controlled trial. JAMA 2003; 290:1042–1048.
65. Gambacciani M, Ciaponi M, Cappagli B., et al. Postmenopausal femur bone loss: effects of a low dose hormone replacement therapy. Maturitas 2003;45:175–183.
66. Ettinger B, Ensrud KE, Wallace R, et al. Effects of ultralow-dose transdermal estradiol on bone mineral density: a randomized clinical trial. Obstet Gynecol 2004;104:443–451.
67. Riggs BL, Hartmann L. Selective estrogen-receptor modulators-mechanisms of action and application to clinical practice. N Engl J Med 2003;348:618–629.
68. Ettinger B, Black D, Mitlak B, et al. Reduction of vertebral fracture risk in postmenopausal women with osteoporosis treated with raloxifene. JAMA 1999;282:637–645.
69. Lufkin E, Whitaker M, Nickelsen T, et al. Treatment of established postmenopausal osteoporosis with raloxifene: a randomized trial. J Bone Miner Res 1998;13:1747–1754.
70. Delmas PD, Ensrud K, Adachi J, et al. Efficacy of raloxifene on vertebral fracture risk reduction in postmenopausal women with osteoporosis: four-year results from a randomized clinical trial. J Clin Endocrinol Metab 2002;87:3609–3617.
71. Cummings S, Eckert S, Krueger K, et al. The effect of raloxifene on risk of breast cancer in postmenopausal women: results from the MORE randomized trial. JAMA 1999;281:2189–2197.
72. Barrett-Connor E, Grady D, Sashegyi A, et al. Raloxifene and cardiovascular events in osteoporotic postmenopausal women: four-year results from the MORE (multiple outcomes of raloxifene evaluation) randomized trial. JAMA 2002;287:847–857.
73. Wenger N, Barrett-Connor E, Collins P, et al. Baseline characteristics of participants in the raloxifene use for the heart (RUTH) trial. Am J Cardiol 2002;90:1204–1210.
74. de Groen P, Lubbe D, Hirsch L, et al. Esophagitis associated with the use of alendronate. N Engl J Med 1996;335:1016–1021.
75. Bone HG, Hosking D, Devogelaer JP, et al. Ten years' experiences with alendronate for osteoporosis in postmenopausal women. N Engl J Med 2004;350:1189–1199.
76. Black D, Cummings S, Karpf D, et al.. Randomised trial of effect of alendronate on risk of fracture in women with existing vertebral fractures. Fracture Intervention Trial Research Group. Lancet 1996; 348:1535–1541.
77. Cummings S, Black D, Thompson D, et al.. Effect of alendronate on risk of fracture in women with low bone density but without vertebral fractures: results from the Fracture Intervention Trial. JAMA 1998;280:2077–2082.
78. Cranney A, Wells G, Willan A, et al.. Meta-analyses of therapies for postmenopausal osteoporosis. II: Meta-analysis of alendronate for the treatment of postmenopausal osteoporosis. Endocr Rev 2002; 23:508–516.
79. Black DM, Thompson DE, Bauer DC, et al. Fracture risk reduction with alendronate in women with osteoporosis: the Fracture Intervention Trial. J Clin Endocrinol Metab 2000;85:4118–4124.
80. McClung M, Clemmesen B, Daifotis A, et al. Alendronate prevents postmenopausal bone loss in women without osteoporosis. A double-blind, randomized, controlled trial. Alendronate Ostoeporosis Prevention Study Group. Ann Intern Med 1998;128:253–261.
81. Hosking D, Chilvers C, Christiansen C, et al. Prevention of bone loss with alendronate in postmenopausal women under 60 years of age. N Engl J Med 1998;338:485–492.
82. Harris S, Watts N, Genant H, et al. Effects of risedronate treatment on vertebral and nonvertebral fractures in women with postmenopausal osteoporosis: a randomized controlled trial. JAMA 1999; 282:1344–1352.
83. Reginster J, Minne H, Sorensen O, et al. Randomized trial of the effects of risedronate on vertebral fractures in women with established postmenopausal osteoporosis. Osteoporos Int 2000;11:83–91.
84. Cranney A, Tugwell P, Adachi J, et al. Meta-analyses of therapies for postmenopausal osteoporosis. III: Meta-analysis of risedronate for the treatment of postmenopausal osteoporosis. Endocr Rev 2002; 23:517–523.
85. McClung M, Geusens P, Miller P, et al.. Effect of risedronate on the risk of hip fracture in elderly women. N Engl J Med 2001;344:333–340.

86. Harrington JT, Ste-Marie LG, Brandi M, et al. Risedronate rapidly reduced the risk for nonvertebral fractures in women with postmenopausal osteoporosis. Calcif Tissue Int 2004;74:129-135. Epub 2003 Dec 2005.

87. Schnitzer T, Bone H, Crepaldi G, et al. Therapeutic equivalence of alendronate 70mg once-weekly and alendronate 10mg daily in the treatment of osteoporosis. Alendronate once-weekly study group. Aging (Milano) 2000;12:1–12.

88. Harris ST, Watts NB, Li Z, Chines AA, Hanley DA, Brown JP. Two-year efficacy and tolerability of risedronate once a week for the treatment of women with postmenopausal osteoporosis. Curr Med Res Opin 2004;20:757–764.

89. Rosen CJ, Hochberg MC, Bonnick SL, et al. Treatment with once-weekly alendronate 70 mg compared to once-weekly risedronate 35mg in women with postmenopausal osteoporosis: a randomized, double-blind study. J Bone Miner Res 2005;20:141–151.

90. Watts NB, Cooper C, Lindsay R, et al. Relationship between changes in bone mineral density and vertebral fracture risk associated with risedronate: greater increases in bone mineral density do not relate to greater decreases in fracture risk. J Clin Densitom 2004;7:255–261.

91. Greenspan S, Field-Munves E, Tonino R, et al. Tolerability of once-weekly alendronate in patients with osteoporosis: a randomized, double-blind, placebo-controlled study. Mayo Clin Proc 2002; 77:1044–1052.

92. Lanza F, Sahba B, Schwartz H, et al. The upper GI safety and tolerability of oral alendronate at a dose of 70 milligrams once weekly: a placebo-controlled endoscopy study. Am J Gastroenterol 2002; 97:58–64.

93. Bell NH, Bilezikian JP, Bone H, Kaur A, Maragoto A, Santora A. Alendronate increases bone mass and reduced bone markers in postmenopausal African-American women. J Clin Endocrinol Metab 2002;87:2792–2797.

94. Chesnut III CH, Skag A, Christiansen C, et al. Effects of oral ibandronate administered daily or intermittently on fracture risk in postmenopausal osteoporosis. J Bone Miner Res 2004;19:1241–1249.

95. Cranney A, Tugwell P, Zytaruk N, et al. Meta-analyses of therapies for postmenopausal osteoporosis. VI: Meta-analysis of calcitonin for the treatment of postmenopausal osteoporosis. Endocr Rev 2002;23:529–539.

96. Chesnut III C, Silverman S, Andriano K, et al. A randomized trial of nasal spray salmon calcitonin in postmenopausal women with established osteoporosis: the prevent recurrence of osteoporotic fractures study. Am J Med 2000;109:267–276.

97. Silverman S, Azria M. The analgesic role of calcitonin following osteoporotic fracture. Osteoporos Int 2002;13:858–867.

98. Gluer C. Sense and sensitivity: monitoring skeletal changes by radiological techniques. J Bone Miner Res 1999;14:1952–1962.

99. Cummings S, Palermo L, Browner W, et al. Monitoring osteoporosis therapy with bone densitometry. Misleading changes and regression to the mean. JAMA 2000;283:1318–1321.

100. Rosen,CJ, Bilezikian JP. Clinical review 123: Hot topic. Anabolic therapy for osteoporosis. J Clin Endocrinol Metab 2001;86:957–964.

101. Neer RM, Arnaud C, Zanchetta J, et al. Effect of parathyroid hormone (1–34) on fractures and bone mineral density in postmenopausal women with osteoporosis. N Engl J Med 2001;344:1434–1441.

102. Hodsman A, Fraher L, Watson P, et al. A randomized controlled tiral to compare the efficacy of cyclical parathyroid hormone versus cyclical parathyroid hormone and sequential calcitonin to improve bone mass in postmenopausal women with osteoporsosis. J Clin Endocrinol Metab 1997; 82:620–628.

103. Cosman F, Nieves J, Woelfert L, et al. Parathyroid hormone added to established hormone therapy: effects on vertebral fracture and maintenance of bone mass after parathyroid hormone withdrawal. J Bone Miner Res 2001;16:925–931.

104. Lindsay R, Nieves J, Formica C, et al. Randomised controlled study of effect of parathyroid hormone on vertebral-bone mass and fracture incidence among postmenopausal womenon oestrogen with osteoporosis. Lancet 1997;350:550–555.

105. Fujita T, Inoue T, Morii H, et al. Effect of an intermittent weekly dose of human parathyroid hormone (1–34) on osteoporosis: a randomized double-masked prospective study using three dose levels. Osteoporos Int 1999;9:296–306.

106. Reeve J, Mitchell A, Tellez M, et al. Treatment with parathyroid peptides and estrogen replacement for severe postmenopausal vertebral osteoporosis:prediction of long-term responses in spine and femur. J Bone Miner Metab 2001;19:102–114.

107. Body J, Gaich G, Scheele W, et al. A randomized double-blind trial to compare the efficacy of teri-paratide [recombinant human parathyroid hormone (1–34)] with alendronate in psotmenopausal women with osteoporosis. J Clin Endocrinol Metab 2002;87:4528–4535.

108. Rittmaster R, Bolognese M, Ettinger M, et al. Enhancement of bone mass in osteoporotic women with parathyroid hormone followed by alendronate. J Clin Endocrinol Metab 2000;85:2129–2134.

109. Vahle JL, Sato M, Long GG, et al. Skeletal changes in rats given daily subcutaneous injections of recombinant human parathyroid hormone (1–34) for 2 years and relevance to human safety. Toxicol Pathol 2002;30:312–321.

110. Ettinger B, San Martin J, Crans G, Pavo I. Differential effects of teriparatide on BMD after treatment with raloxifene or alendronate. J Bone Miner Res 2004;19:745–751.

111. Lindsay R, Cosman F, Lobo R, et al. Addition of alendronate to ongoing hormone replacement ther-apy in the treatment of osteoporosis: a randomized, controlled clinical trial. J Clin Endocrinol Metab 1999;84:3076–3081.

112. Bone H, Greenspan S, McKeever C, et al. Alendronate and estrogen effects in postmenopausal women with low bone mineral density. J Clin Endocrinol Metab 2000;85:720–726.

113. Palomba S, Orio F, Colao A, et al. Effect of estrogen replacement plus low-dose alendronate treat-ment on bone density in surgically postmenopausal women with osteoporosis. J Clin Endocrinol Metab 2002; 87:1502–1508.

114. Harris S, Eriksen EF, Davidson M, et al. Effect of combined risedronate and hormone replacement therapies on bone mineral density in postmenopausal women. J Clin Endocrinol Metab 2001;86: 1890–1897.

115. Greenspan S, Emkey R, Bone H, et al. Significant differential effects of alendronate, estrogen, or combination therapy on the rate of bone loss after discontinuation of treatment with postmenopausal osteoporosis. Ann Intern Med 2002;137:875–883.

116. Johnell O, Scheele W, Lu Y, Reginster J, Need A, Seeman, E. Additive effects of raloxifene and alendronate on bone density and biochemical markers of bone remodeling in postmenopausal women with osteoporosis. J Clin Endocrinol Metab 2002;87:985–992.

117. Sambrook PN, Geusens P, Ribot C, et al. Alendronate produced greater effects than raloxifene on bone density and bone turnover in postmenopausal women with low bone density: results of EFFECT (Efficacy of Fosamax versus Evista Comparison Trial) International. J Intern Med 2004;255:503–511.

118. Downs RW Jr, Bell N, Ettinger M, et al. Comparison of alendronate and intranasal calcitonin for treatment of osteoporosis in postmenopausal women. J Clin Endocrinol Metab 2000;85:1783–1788.

119. Finkelstein JS, Hayes A, Hunzelman JL, et al. The effects of parathyroid hormone, alendronate, or both in men with osteoporosis. N Engl J Med 2003;349: 1216–1226.

120. Black D, Greenspan SL, Ensrud KE, et al. The effects of parathyroid hormone and alendronate alone or in combination in postmenopausal osteoporosis. N Engl J Med 2003;349:1207–1215.

121. Kanis JA, Johnell O, DeLaet C, et al. A meta-analysis of previous fracture and subsequent fracture risk. Bone 2004;35:375-382.

122. Siminoski K, Jiang G, Adachi JD, et al. Accuracy of height loss during prospective monitoring for detection of incident vertebral fractures. Osteoporos Int 2005;16:403–410.

123. Watts N, Harris S, Genant HK. Treatment of painful osteoporotic vertebral fractures with percuta-neous vertebroplasty or kyphoplasty. Osteoporos Int 2001;12:429–437.

124. Lopes NM, Lopes VK. Paraplegia complicating percutaneous vertebroplasty for osteoporotic verte-bral fracture: case report. Arq Neuropsiquiatr 2004;62:879–881.

125. Legroux-Gerot I, Lormeau C, Boutry N, Cotten A, Duquesnoy B, Corter B. Long-term follow-up of vertebral osteoporotic fractures treated by percutaneous vertebroplasty. Clin Rheumatol 2004;23: 310–317.

126. Kim SH, Kang HS, Choi JA, Ahn JM. Risk factors of new compression fractures in adjacent verte-brae after percutaneous vertebroplasty. Acta Radiol 2004;45:440–445.

127. Mussolino ME, Looker AC, Madans JH, Langlois JA, Orwoll ES. Risk factors for hip fracture in white men: the NHANES I epidemiologic follow-up study. J Bone Miner Res 1998;13:918–924.

128. Seeman E, Bianchi G, Adami S, Kanis J, Khosla S, Orwoll E. Osteoporosis in men-consensus is premature. Calcif Tissue Int 2004;75:120–122.

129. Baillie SP, Davison CE, Johnson FJ, Francis RM. Pathogenesis of vertebral crush fractures in men. Age Ageing1992; 21:139–141.

130. Ebeling PR, Wark JD, Yeung SS, et al. Effects of calcitriol or calcium on bone mineral density, bone turnover, and fractures in men with primary osteoporosis: a two-year randomized, double-blind, double placebo study. J Clin Endocrinol Metab 2001;86:4098–4103.

131. Amory JK, Watts NB, Easley KA, et al. Exogenous testosterone or testosterone with finasteride increases bone mineral density in older men with low serum testosterone. J Clin Endocrinol Metab 2004;89:503–510.

132. Gonelli S, Cepollaro C, Montagnani A, et al. Alendronate treatment in men with primary osteoporosis: a three-year longitudinal study. Calcif Tissue Int 2003;73:133–139.

133. Orwoll E, Ettinger M, Weiss S, et al. Alendronate for the treatment of osteoporosis in men. N Engl J Med 2000;343:604–610.

134. Trovas GP, Lyritis GP, Galanos A, Raptou P, Constantelou, E. A randomized trial of nasal spray salmon calcitonin in men with idiopathic osteoporosis: effects on bone mineral density and bone markers. J Bone Miner Res 2002;17:521–527.

135. Orwoll E, Scheele W, Adami PS, et al. The effect of teriparatide [human parathyroid hormone (1–34)] therapy on bone mineral density in men with osteoporosis. J Bone Miner Res 2003;18:9–17.

136. Kurland ES, Cosman F, McMahon DJ, Rosen CJ, Lindsay R, Bilezikian JP. Therapy of idiopathic osteoporosis in men with parathyroid hormone: effects on bone mineral density and bone markers. J Clin Endocrinol Metab 2000;85:3069–3076.

137. Kaufman JM, Orwoll E, Goemaere S, et al. Teriparatide effects on vertebral fractures and bone mineral density in men with osteoporosis: treatment and discontinuation of therapy. Osteoporos Int 2005;16:510–516.

138. Smith MR, Fallon MA, Lee H, Finkelstein JS. Raloxifene to prevent gonadotropin-releasing hormone agonist-induced bone loss in men with prostate cancer: a randomized controlled trial. J Clin Endocrinol Metab 2004;89:3841–3846.

139. Diamond TH, Winters J, Smith A, et al. The antiosteoporotic efficacy of intravenous pamidronate in men with prostate carcinoma receiving combined androgen blockade: a double blind, randomized, placebo-controlled crossover study. Cancer 2001;92:1444–1450.

140. Smith MR, Eastham J, Gleason DM, Shasha D, Tchekmedyian S, Zinner N. Randomized controlled trial of zoledronic acid to prevent bone loss in men receiving androgen deprivation therapy for non-metastatic prostate cancer. J Urol 2003;169:2008–2012.

141. Canalis E, Bilezikian JP, Angeli A, Giustina A. Perspectives on glucocorticoid-induced osteoporosis. Bone 2004;34:595–598.

142. Homik JE, Cranney A, Shea B, et al. A metaanalysis on the use of bisphosphonates in corticosteroid induced osteoporosis. J Rheumatol 1999;26:1148–1157.

143. Adachi JD, Bensen WG, Brown J, et al. Intermittent etidronate therapy to prevent corticosteroid-induced osteoporosis. N Engl J Med 1997;337:382–387.

144. Homik J, Cranney A, Shea B, et al. Bisphosphonates for steroid-induced osteoporosis (Cochrane Review). In: The Cochrane Library, Issue 4. Oxford: Update Software, 2002.

145. Saag KG, Emkey R, Schnitzer T, et al. Alendronate for the prevention and treatment of glucocorticoid-induced osteoporosis. Glucocorticoid-Induced Osteoporosis Intervention Study Group. N Engl J Med 1998;339:292–299.

146. Adachi JD, Saag KG, Delmas PD, et al. Two-year effects of alendronate on bone mineral density and vertebral fracture in patients receiving glucocorticoids: a randomized, double-blind, placebo-controlled extension trial. Arthritis Rheum 2001;44:202–211.

147. Reid DM, Adami S, Devogelaer JP, Chines, A. Risedronate increases bone density and reduced vertebral fracture risk within one year in men on corticosteroid therapy. Calcif Tissue Int 2001;69:242–247.

148. Cohen D, Adachi JD. The treatment of glucocorticoid-induced osteoporosis. J Steroid Biochem Mol Biol 2004;88:337–349.

23

The Neuroendocrinology of Medically Unexplained Syndromes

The Example of Chronic Fatigue Syndrome

Jason W. Busse, DC, MSc

CONTENTS

INTRODUCTION

Physical symptoms account for more than half of all outpatient visits in the United States each year, and yet one-third to half of all such presentations lack a clear physical explanation *(1,2)*. Such conditions are labeled on the basis of excluding known disease and as a group they have been designated as functional somatic syndromes or medically unexplained syndromes *(3,4)*. One such medically unexplained syndrome is chronic fatigue syndrome (CFS) *(5,6)*, a relatively common condition of unclear origin that is estimated to affect as many as 400 per 100,000 adults with increased prevalence among minorities, women, and persons in lower-income brackets *(7)*. CFS is associated with disability and poor health-related quality of life and is characterized by disabling fatigue of at least 6 mo in duration *(5–8)*.

Of all the medically unexplained syndromes CFS has arguably been the focus of most neuroendocrine investigation, and as such we have elected to focus on this syndrome for this chapter; however, some authors have postulated that labels assigned to medically unexplained syndromes are an artifact of medical specialization *(see* Fig. 1) *(3,4,9)*. Diagnostic criteria for these syndromes frequently overlap, patients often meet the criteria for multiple syndromes, and similarities in patient characteristics, prognosis, and response to treatment are common *(3,4,10,11)*. We would, thus, pro-

From: *Contemporary Endocrinology: Evidence-Based Endocrinology*
Edited by: V. M. Montori © Mayo Foundation for Medical Education and Research

Allergy	Multiple Chemical Sensitivity/Idiopathic Environmental Intolerance, Post-Combat Syndromes, Sick Building Syndrome
Cardiology	Atypical or Non-Cardiac Chest Pain
Dentistry	Atypical Facial Pain, Temporomandibular Joint Syndrome
Ear, Nose, and Throat	Globus Syndrome
Gastroenterology	Irritable Bowel Syndrome, Non-Ulcer Dyspepsia
Gynaecology	Chronic Pelvic Pain, Premenstrual Syndrome
Infectious Diseases	Candidiasis Hypersensitivity, Chronic Fatigue Syndrome, Chronic Lyme Disease
Neurology	Chronic Tension Headache
Physical Medicine	Chronic Whiplash, Chronic Repetition Strain Injury
Respiratory Medicine	Hyperventilation Syndrome
Rheumatology	Fibromyalgia, Myofascial Pain Syndrome
Urology	Interstitial Cystitis

Fig. 1. Medically unexplained syndromes by medical specialty. (Modified from refs. *3* and *4*.)

pose that clinicians should not view CFS and similar disorders in isolation, but consider that syndrome-specific research findings may be relevant to other unexplained multisymptom illnesses.

Stress and Chronic Fatigue Syndrome

The impact of stress on the neuroendocrine system is firmly established, and report of stressful events prior to the onset of CFS is common. Theorell et al. *(12)* interviewed 46 individuals with CFS and 46 matched controls and reported excess prevalence of both infections and negative life events during the quarter year preceding the onset of CFS. Hatcher and House have recently reported the results of a case control study that found patients with CFS were more likely to experience severe events and difficulties in the 3 mo (odds ratio [OR] = 9; 95% confidence interval [CI] 3.2–25.1) and year (OR = 4.3; 95% CI 1.8–10.2) prior to onset of their illness than population controls. In the 3 mo prior to onset 19 of the 64 patients (30%) experienced a dilemma compared to none of the controls *(13)*.

There is evidence that certain personality types generate higher levels of stress than others. Individuals with CFS have been found to rate themselves higher than controls on the "hard-driving" and "many outside interests" of the Bortner type A personality scale *(14)*. Individuals with CFS have also been found to adopt confrontational coping styles and to rate themselves highly on an "action proneness" scale *(14,15)*. CFS has been found to be associated with a defensive high anxious coping style *(16)*, which may directly affect physical well being through the hypothalamic-pituitary-adrenal (HPA)-axis *(17)*.

With respect to animal models, studies of rats have shown that neuroendocrine changes in response to stress can persist long after the stressful event has resolved *(18)*.

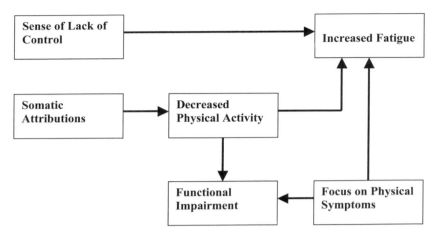

Fig. 2. A validated model of chronic fatigue syndrome. (Modified with permission from ref. *21.*)

Biologists studying the effects of stress in fish populations have identified strong correlations between social stress and reactions along the HPA-axis. Studies have shown that social subordination leads to chronic stress, related to a reduction in aggressive interactions and to lack of control *(19,20).*

Such findings compliment the model validated by Vercoulen et al. to explain the perpetuation of CFS (*see* Fig. 2) *(21).* Their model was able to account for the experience of fatigue amongst CFS sufferers through three factors: (1) focusing on bodily symptoms, (2) low physical activity, and (3) low sense of control. Patients with CFS are more likely than depressed patients and normal controls to interpret symptoms (characteristic of CFS) in terms of physical illness, and least likely to interpret symptoms in terms of negative emotional states *(22).* Attributing symptoms to underlying physical pathology results in low levels of physical activity, which in turn amplifies fatigue severity *(21).* Given the role of the neuroendocrine system in mediating stress, and the association between stress and CFS, research on this area has been very active.

THE NEUROENDOCRINE SYSTEM
AND CHRONIC FATIGUE SYNDROME

CFS is associated with pathophysiologic abnormalities across multiple domains, suggesting that the etiology is complex and multifactorial. A number of central nervous system (CNS) pathways have been implicated in the etiology of CFS and the role of the neuroendocrine system has been the focus of much debate in this regard (*see* Fig. 3) *(23).*

There has been particular interest in the neuroendocrinology of CFS for a number of reasons. There are many similarities between the clinical presentation of CFS and depression, and the latter has established neuroendocrine abnormalities characterized by excess production cortisol and abnormal dexamethasone suppression *(24).* CFS also shares many features of clinical conditions characterized by lack of cortisol, such as Addison's disease *(25),* and fatigue is the most common complaint following bilateral adrenalectomy *(26).*

The neuroendocrine system is made up of a combination of the central nervous and hormonal systems, and is under particular onslaught in our modern life. The HPA-axis

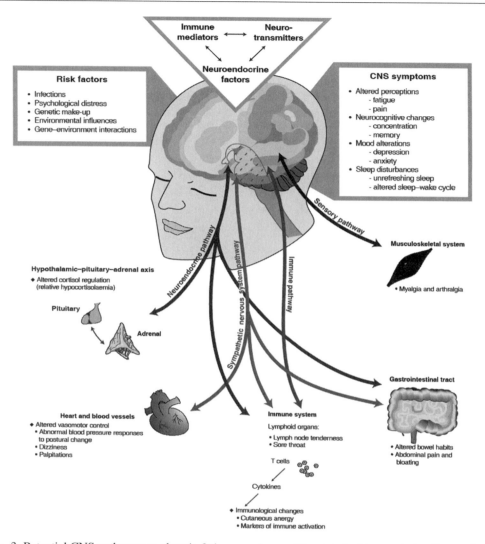

Fig. 3. Potential CNS pathways to chronic fatigue syndrome. (Reprinted with permission from ref. *23*.)

is the classical neuroendocrine system that responds to both physical and mental stress by, ultimately, producing corticosteroids. The HPA-axis includes parts of the hypothalamus, the anterior lobe of the pituitary gland, the adrenal cortices, hormones, systems that transport hormones and feedback mechanisms that transport cortisol from adrenal glands back to the hypothalamus and to other parts of the brain (*see* Fig. 4) *(27)*.

When subject to stress, the hypothalamus releases corticotropin-releasing hormone (CRH) that is transported to the anterior lobe of the pituitary. In the anterior pituitary gland, CRH stimulates release of stored adrenocorticotropic hormone (ACTH), which is transported to the adrenal gland where it rapidly stimulates biosynthesis of corticosteroids. CRH also acts to increase sympathetic nervous function. The HPA-axis is down-regulated by glucocorticoid receptors that are activated in response to plasma cortisol levels, forming a negative feedback loop.

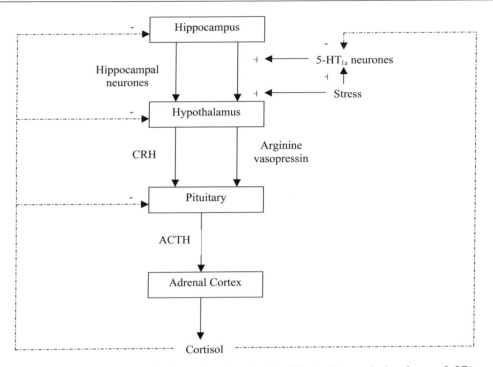

Fig. 4. The Hypothalamo-pituitary-adrenal axis. (Modified with permission from ref. *27*.)

Increased production of cortisol mediates alarm reactions to stress, facilitating a general adaptation in which alarm reactions are suppressed, and allowing the body to attempt countermeasures. Glococorticoids, such as cortisol, serve important functions including modulation of stress reactions but they can be damaging. Atrophy of the hippocampus in humans and animals exposed to severe stress is believed to be caused by the presence of excessive stress-induced glococorticoids. Deficiencies of the hippocampus are believed to reduce the memory resources available to help a body formulate appropriate reactions to stress. As can be seen from Fig. 4 there are a number of sites where abnormalities could arise in the HPA-axis, leading to increased or decreased levels of plasma cortisol.

STUDIES OF CHRONIC FATIGUE SYNDROME AND THE NEUROENDOCRINE SYSTEM

The Hypothalamic-Pituitary-Adrenal Axis

Most studies, but not all, *(28–31)* have found that approximately one-third of adult CFS patients exhibit mild hypocortisolism *(32–40)*. Low-plasma cortisol, linked with CRH deficiency, may provide some explanation for CFS patient's struggle to respond to stressors and to the demands of everyday life *(41)*. However, central CRH deficiency is impossible to demonstrate directly in humans, and evidence to support this model can only be acquired indirectly. Demitrack et al. *(42)* investigated differences in HPA-axis function between CFS patients and normal controls. They reported that basal levels of ACTH were elevated and found that in response to ovine CRH challenge the maximal response of the adrenal glands to ACTH appeared to be blunted. However, many subjects had co-morbid psychiatric disorders that may have influenced results.

Scott and colleagues reported on ovine CRH challenge in CFS patients without psychiatric co-morbidity and found normal basal levels of ACTH, but attenuated ACTH and cortisol responses, suggesting possible downregulation of CHR receptors on the pituitary (43). Cleare et al. (39) conducted a similar study that also excluded CFS patients with psychiatric co-morbidity, but using human CRH, and found normal ACTH responses but blunted cortisol responses.

Arginine vasopressin and CRH act synergistically at the pituitary to activate ACTH secretion and Altemus and colleagues have found that in response to a vasopressin infusion CFS patients demonstrate a blunted ACTH response and a more rapid cortisol response vs controls (44). These authors suggested that low levels of hypothalamic CRH may be the cause, but there also exists preliminary evidence to consider either upregulation of pituitary arginine vasopressin receptors or a deficit in endogenous arginine vasopressin (43,45,46).

There is some evidence to suggest that the adrenal cortex of some CFS patients may be hypersensitive to ACTH but that endogenous pituitary output of ACTH may be impaired (42,47); other studies have failed to support this hypothesis (48). Studies investigating the insulin stress test have generally failed to support primary adrenal insufficiency as a cause of CFS (32,39,49,50). Hypocortisolism may also result from enhanced negative feedback of corticosteroid receptors on either the hypothalamus or pituitary, and results to date generally support this hypothesis (31,51).

Other Neuroendocrine Factors

The possible role of growth hormone (32,52), plasma leptin (53), and melatonin (54) in the genesis of CFS have been explored; however, no compelling evidence has yet been forthcoming. Further, the only randomized controlled trial (RCT) to date that investigated the role of growth hormone replacement in managing symptoms associated with CFS found no improvements in quality of life scores over placebo (55).

Dehydroepiandrostenedione (DHEA) is an adrenal steroid that is conjugated to sulfate to form dehydroepiandrostenedione-sulfate (DHEAS) before its release into the circulation. Reported measures of DHEA or DHEAS within CFS populations have been inconsistent, with studies reporting low-basal levels, normal levels, or even elevated levels of these steroids (56–62). Based on the findings of certain studies some investigators have suggested that DHEA may have a role in either the genesis or propagation of CFS (59). Himmel and Seligman explored the effect of DHEA administration on 23 women with CFS that exhibited low levels of DHEA at baseline and reported modest improvements in mood, pain, and fatigue (63). These results have not been replicated in a controlled trial.

Neurotransmitters

The central serotonin neurotransmitter hydroxytryptamine 5-(HT) is able to activate the HPA-axis, and there is some evidence to suggest that individuals with CFS exhibit increased sensitivity to 5-HT mediated hypothalamic activation via up-regulation of 5-HT_{1A} receptors in the hypothalamus. This finding, however, come from a trial that exposed CFS patients to buspirone and measured prolactin secretion (64). Buspirone is largely a 5-HT_{1A} receptor partial agonist but also acts at dopamine D2 receptors, which poses a potential problem in that D2 receptors may also mediate prolactic secretion. To clarify this issue Sharpe and colleagues performed an experiment measuring both prolactin and growth hormone secretion, as growth hormone secretion is more likely to be influenced by 5-HT$_{1A}$ receptor alone. This study found normal growth hormone levels and an elevated prolactin response, suggesting that abnormalities in dopamine, not serotonin, neurotransmission may explain the enhanced prolactin response associated with CFS (65).

Another trial made use of a more specific 5-HT$_{1A}$ partial agonist, ipsapirone, and found evidence to suggest that serotonergic activation of the HPA-axis is defective in CFS (66). Other studies have explored the impact of D-fenfluramine (a selective 5-HT releasing agent) on individuals with CFS, and found evidence of enhanced serotonergic responses (67,68). However, these results have not been replicated in all studies (69,70), possibly a result of methodological issues (71).

Other neurotransmitters have not been as well studied in CFS populations. Demitrack et al. (72) have found that levels of the noradrenaline metabolite MHPG are normal in the cerebrospinal fluid of CFS patients, but lower than usual in the plasma. There is limited evidence to suggest that CFS patients may express up-regulated cholinergic receptors (73).

Chronic Fatigue Syndrome and Depression

Twenty-five to fifty percent of CFS patients present with co-morbid clinical depression, 50–75% have a history of depression, and depression is an established risk factor for development of CFS (74–77). However, in spite of the similarities in clinical presentation, neuroendocrine abnormalities associated with CFS provide evidence that the syndrome is distinct from depression. Many CFS patients exhibit mild hypocortisolism (78) as opposed to hypercortisolism with depression, and dexamethasone suppression, that is commonplace in clinical depression, is very rare in CFS (79). Further, individuals with CFS tend to demonstrate findings consistent with up-regulation of the serotonergic system, which may lead to lowered plasma cortisol levels (33,66–68). These results suggest that although CFS is often complicated by co-morbid depression (80) that CFS is distinct from depression, which is characterized by hypercortisolism and downregulation of the serotonergic system (67).

There is a reasonable hypothesis to explain the association between the established risk of prior episodes of depression and the development of CFS. Animal studies have shown that chronic stress may lead to long standing abnormalities in HPA-axis function (81), and humans subjected to chronic stressors have demonstrated HPA-axis perturbations long after the stress has resolved (82). Heim et al. (83) have proposed that a persistent lack of cortisol availability in traumatized or chronically stressed individuals may promote an increased vulnerability for the development of stress-related bodily disorders, such as CFS. Thus, it can be reasonably hypothesized that previous episodes of depression or chronic stress may leave so-called "endocrine scars" that increase the risk for the development of CFS (84).

Neuroendocrine Abnormalities and Chronic Fatigue Syndrome: Cause or Effect?

An important limitation of most studies on the neuroendocrinology of CFS is that they explore populations with long-standing illness, which does not allow for an understanding of whether neuroendocrine abnormalities associated with CFS are a cause or a consequence of the illness *(85)*. Both disturbance in sleep and physical deconditioning, which are common in CFS, have been found to affect the HPA-axis *(85)*. Further, the identified neuroendocrine abnormalities are nonspecific to CFS and have also been associated with burnout syndrome *(86)* and chronic pelvic pain *(87)*, and found in individuals with histories of childhood sexual abuse *(88)*.

Vedhara et al. *(89)* observed a reduction in basal HPA activity in students undergoing an exam in comparisons to the same population during a nonexam period. Leese et al. *(90)* have replicated neuroendocrine abnormalities associated with CFS in normal subjects after 5 d of night shift work. As a result of these findings, they concluded that abnormal neuroendocrine findings in CFS may be the consequence of disrupted sleep and social routine. Recent prospective studies of cohorts at high risk for developing CFS have found that there are no neuroendocrine abnormalities present during the early stages of the developing illness *(91,92)*. These studies also found no evidence that an initial abnormal stress response was implicated in the development of chronic fatigue *(91,92)*. These results suggest that neuroendocrine abnormalities associated with CFS are a result of the illness rather than a cause.

TREATMENT IMPLICATIONS FOR CHRONIC FATIGUE SYNDROME

If, as some studies have suggested, hypocortisolaemia is of causal importance with regards to symptoms associated with CFS, then treatment with hydrocortisone replacement should be of benefit. McKenzie and colleagues pursued a placebo-controlled RCT in which they prescribed hydrocortisone in a pattern approximating the normal diurnal variation in cortisol *(93)*. The authors found that treatment produced modest benefits on a global health scale but not on other outcomes and concluded that, "the degree of adrenal suppression precludes [hydrocortisone's] practical use for CFS" *(93)*. Cleare et al. *(39,53,94)* provided low-dose hydrocortisone or placebo to 32 CFS patients, in a cross-over RCT, and noted improvement in self-reported fatigue among a subgroup of responders ($n = 9$) with no adrenal suppression. However, the study explored short-term results only, and the authors cautioned that long-term results were needed before determining the clinical utility of hydrocortisone therapy *(94)*. Further, there is often no association between cortisol parameters and symptom severity described by CFS patients *(50)*. Neither fludrocortisone *(95,96)* nor combination therapy of hydrocortisone and fludrocortisone *(97)* or growth hormone *(55)* have been found ineffective in the treatment of CFS.

No compelling evidence exists for the efficacy of drug therapy, including antidepressants *(98)*; however, management of CFS with antidepressants is supported by virtue of three considerations: (1) up to 50% of cases of CFS present with co-morbid depression, (2) limited evidence to suggest deregulation of 5-HT and other monoamine receptors, and (3) the restorative effect of antidepressants on HPA-axis function *(27)*. Clinicians should be aware however that practical use of antidepressants in CFS patients may be complicated by the nocebo response *(99)*.

A recent systematic review has concluded that current evidence best supports treatment of CFS with cognitive behavioral therapy and graduated exercise *(100)*. There is evidence from a study of 60 patients with CFS that treatment with cognitive behavioral therapy does lead to increases in salivary cortisol levels and improved response of the HPA-axis to CRH *(85)*. Muscle strength and fatiguability are normal in patients with CFS *(101)*, and a case report by Sharma and colleagues found that successful treatment of CFS with graduated exercise led to objective improvements in neuroendocrine function *(102)*. These findings reinforce data suggesting that CFS is not a primary neuroendocrine disorder, and that abnormalities of the neuroendocrine system in this population are reversible through therapy targeting illness attributions, negative cognitions, and maladaptive coping strategies.

Prevention of Chronic Fatigue Syndrome

The evolving model for CFS suggests that there may be a role for preventing high-risk populations from developing this syndrome. And, as with CFS, there is evidence that the development of other medically unexplained syndromes is strongly influenced by personality style and underlying coping mechanisms. In a large, population-based prospective study, McBeth and colleagues *(103)* found that individuals who were free of chronic widespread pain were at increased future risk of its development if they displayed features of somatization. Castro et al. *(104)* exposed 51 healthy volunteers to a placebo motor vehicle accident, and found that 20% reported development of a whiplash injury. Ten percent continued to report symptoms of whiplash at 4 wk, and reporting of symptoms at any time point was highly correlated with certain psychological profiles. Cognitive-behavioral stress management training has been shown to reduce the neuroendocrine stress response to an acute stressor in healthy subjects *(105)* and the identification of populations at high risk for developing CFS may suggest a role for preventative cognitive-behavioral therapy.

Patients with unexplained symptoms need a name for their illness and clinicians need discrete diagnoses *(106)*; however, it has also been suggested that the manner in which individuals presenting to clinicians with medically unexplained syndromes are managed may strongly influence the course of their illness *(107)*. Clinicians whom promote a symptom-focused approach to medically unexplained syndromes (e.g., sleep for fatigue and avoidance of activity for exercise intolerance) may inadvertently promote illness and disability *(108)*—the so called "medicalization of misery *(109)*"—vs clinicians who rule out objective medical disease and promote an approach to treatment that focuses on functional gains vs symptom-relief.

Further, the role of social factors in the development and perpetuation of medically unexplained syndromes has been demonstrated. Using as an example chronic or "late" whiplash syndrome, investigators have found that in countries lacking medicolegal industries to service such syndromes that they are essentially unheard of *(110–112)*. Other investigators have found that the elimination of compensation for pain and suffering is associated with a markedly decreased incidence and improved prognosis of whiplash injury *(113)*. Such findings suggest that modifying social factors may be essential in preventing the development and progression of medically unexplained syndromes.

SUMMARY

Given current evidence it is unlikely that a single biological explanation will emerge to explain the symptoms and behavioral abnormalities that characterize CFS. Rather, it seems more reasonable to consider CFS as the final common pathway of chronic exhaustion that is arrived at following a complex series of biopsychosocial events *(84,114)*.

There are neuroendocrine abnormalities associated with some CFS patients, at least in the populations represented in the trials we have described; most consistently involving hypocortisolism, enhanced negative feedback of the HPA-axis, and impaired response of the HPA-axis to activation *(71)*. The etiology of these abnormalities remains unclear, but in the vast majority of cases they are not the result of a primary neuroendocrine disorder. The neuroendocrine abnormalities typically described are nonspecific and appear to occur later in the illness, probably as a response to certain features of the illness such as sleep disturbance, inactivity, and physical deconditioning. Psychiatric co-morbidity may also offer an explanation for the neuroendocrine abnormalities described in some studies. To better inform the role of the neuroendocrine system in CFS large prospective cohort studies are required of populations at high risk for development of CFS, as well as testing of CFS patients for neuroendocrine abnormalities following recovery.

With regard to management, current evidence supports treatment of CFS with cognitive behavioral therapy and graduated exercise; there is some data to suggest that these therapies may reverse neuroendocrine abnormalities associated with CFS. Furthermore, there may be a role for preventing high-risk populations from developing CFS via education for clinicians attending to patients with medically unexplained symptoms, provision of cognitive-behavioral therapy to high-risk populations, and through revising social policy to reduce the impact of environmental factors.

REFERENCES

1. Kroenke K. Studying symptoms: sampling and measurement issues. Ann Intern Med 2001;134:844–853.
2. Nimnuan C, Hotopf M, Wessely S. Medically unexplained symptoms: an epidemiological study in seven specialities. J Psychosom Res 2001;51:361–367.
3. Barsky AJ, Borus JF. Functional somatic syndromes. Ann Intern Med 1999;130:10–21.
4. Wessely S, Nimnuan C, Sharpe M. Functional somatic syndromes: one or many? Lancet 1999;354: 936–939.
5. Hardt J, Buchwald D, Wilks D, Sharpe M, Nix WA, Egle UT. Health-related quality of life in patients with chronic fatigue syndrome: an international study. J Psychosom Res 2001;51:431–434.
6. Fukuda K, Straus SE, Hickie I, Sharpe MC, Dobbins JG, Komaroff A, for the International Chronic Fatigue Syndrome Study Group. The chronic fatigue syndrome: a comprehensive approach to its definition and study. Ann Intern Med 1994;121:953–959.
7. Jason LA, Richman JA, Rademaker AW, et al. A community-based study of chronic fatigue syndrome. Arch Intern Med 1999;159:2129–2137.
8. Wessely S. Chronic fatigue: symptom and syndrome. Ann Intern Med 2001;134:838–843.
9. Nimnuan C, Rabe-Hesketh S, Wessely S, Hotopf M. How many functional somatic syndromes? J Psychosom Res 2001;51:549–557.
10. Buchwald D, Garrity D. Comparison of patients with chronic fatigue syndrome, fibromyalgia, and multiple chemical sensitivities. Arch Intern Med 1994;154:2049–2053.
11. Aaron LA, Buchwald D. A review of the evidence for overlap among medically unexplained clinical conditions. Ann Intern Med 2001;134:868–881.
12. Theorell T, Blomkvist V, Lindh G, Evengard B. Critical life events, infections, and symptoms during the year preceding chronic fatigue syndrome (CFS): an examination of CFS patients and subjects with a nonspecific life crisis. Psychosom Med 1999;61:304–310.
13. Hatcher S, House A. Life events, difficulties and dilemmas in the onset of chronic fatigue syndrome: a case-control study. Psychol Med 2003;33:1185–1192.
14. Lewis S, Cooper CL, Bennett D. Psychosocial factors and chronic fatigue syndrome. Psychol Med 1994;24:661–671.
15. Van Houdenhove B, Onghena P, Neerinckx E, Hellin J. Does high 'action-proneness' make people more vulnerable to chronic fatigue syndrome? A controlled psychometric study. J Psychosom Res 1995;39:633–640.

16. Creswell C, Chalder T. Defensive coping styles in chronic fatigue syndrome. J Psychosom Res 2001; 51:607–610.
17. Jamner LD, Schwartz GE, Leigh H. The relationship between repressive and defensive coping styles and monocyte, eosinophile, and serum glucose levels: support for the opioid peptide hypothesis of repression. Psychosom Med 1988;50:567–575.
18. Brennan FX, Ottenweller JE, Seifu Y, Zhu G, Servatius RJ. Persistent stress-induced elevations of urinary corticosterone in rats. Physiol Behav 2000;71:441–446.
19. Sloman KA, Metcalfe NB, Taylor AC, Gilmour KM. Plasma cortisol concentrations before and after social stress in rainbow trout and brown trout. Physiol Biochem Zool 2001;74:383–389.
20. Winberg S, Lepage O. Elevation of brain 5-HT activity, POMC expression, and plasma cortisol in socially subordinate rainbow trout. Am J Physiol 1998;274:R645–R654.
21. Vercoulen JH, Swanink CM, Galama JM, et al. The persistence of fatigue in chronic fatigue syndrome and multiple sclerosis: development of a model. J Psychosom Res 1998;45:507–517.
22. Dendy C, Cooper M, Sharpe M. Interpretation of symptoms in chronic fatigue syndrome. Behav Res Ther 2001;39:1369–1380.
23. Working Group of the Royal Australasian College of Physicians. Chronic fatigue syndrome. Clinical practice guidelines—2002. Med J Aust 2002;176:S23–S56.
24. Barden N. Implication of the hypothalamic-pituitary-adrenal axis in the physiopathology of depression. J Psychiatry Neurosci 2004;29:185–193.
25. Brosnan CM, Gowing NF. Addison's disease. BMJ 1996;312:1085–1087.
26. O'Riordain DS, Farley DR, Young WF Jr, Grant CS, van Heerden JA. Long-term outcome of bilateral adrenalectomy in patients with Cushing's syndrome. Surgery 1994;116:1093–1094.
27. Cleare AJ, Wessely SC. Chronic fatigue syndrome: a stress disorder? Br J Hosp Med 1996;55: 571–574.
28. MacHale SM, Cavanagh JT, Bennie J, Carroll S, Goodwin GM, Lawrie SM. Diurnal variation of adrenocortical activity in chronic fatigue syndrome. Neuropsychobiology 1998;38:213–217.
29. Hamilos DL, Nutter D, Gershtenson J, et al. Core body temperature is normal in chronic fatigue syndrome. Biol Psychiatry 1998;43:293–302.
30. Young AH, Sharpe M, Clements A, Dowling B, Hawton KE, Cowen PJ. Basal activity of the hypothalamic-pituitary-adrenal axis in patients with the chronic fatigue syndrome (neurasthenia). Biol Psychiatry 1998;43:236–237.
31. Gaab J, Huster D, Peisen R, et al. Low-dose dexamethasone suppression test in chronic fatigue syndrome and health. Psychosom Med 2002;64:311–318.
32. Moorkens G, Berwaerts J, Wynants H, Abs R. Characterization of pituitary function with emphasis on GH secretion in the chronic fatigue syndrome. Clin Endocrinol 2000;53:99–106.
33. Parker AJ, Wessely S, Cleare AJ. The neuroendocrinology of chronic fatigue syndrome and fibromyalgia. Psychol Med 2001;31:1331–1345.
34. Cleare AJ, Blair D, Chambers S, Wessely S. Urinary free cortisol in chronic fatigue syndrome. Am J Psychiatry 2001;158:641–643.
35. Roberts AD, Wessely S, Chalder T, Papadopoulos A, Cleare AJ. Salivary cortisol response to awakening in chronic fatigue syndrome. Br J Psychiatry 2004;184:136–141.
36. Demitrack MA, Dale JK, Straus SE, et al. Evidence for impaired activation of the hypothalamic-pituitary-adrenal axis in patients with chronic fatigue syndrome. J Clin Endocrinol Metab 1991;73: 1224–1234.
37. Poteliakhoff A. Adrenocortical activity and some clinical findings in acute and chronic fatigue. J Psychosom Res 1981;25:91–95.
38. Scott LV, Dinan TG. Urinary free cortisol excretion in chronic fatigue syndrome, major depression and in healthy volunteers. J Affect Disord 1998;47:49–54.
39. Cleare AJ, Miell J, Heap E, et al. Hypothalamo-pituitary-adrenal axis dysfunction in chronic fatigue syndrome, and the effects of low-dose hydrocortisone therapy. J Clin Endocrinol Metab 2001; 86: 3545–3554.
40. Strickland P, Morriss R, Wearden A, Deakin B. A comparison of salivary cortisol in chronic fatigue syndrome, community depression and healthy controls. J Affect Disord. 1998;47:191–194.
41. Van Houdenhove B, Neerinckx E, Onghena P, Vingerhoets A, Lysens R, Vertommen H. Daily hassles reported by chronic fatigue syndrome and fibromyalgia patients in tertiary care: a controlled quantitative and qualitative study. Psychother Psychosom 2002;71:207–213.

42. Demitrack MA, Dale JK, Straus SE, et al. Evidence for impaired activation of the hypothalamic-pituitary-adrenal axis in patients with chronic fatigue syndrome. J Clin Endocrinol Metab 1991;73: 1224–1234.

43. Scott LV, Medbak S, Dinan TG. Blunted adrenocorticotropin and cortisol responses to corticotropin-releasing hormone stimulation in chronic fatigue syndrome. Acta Psychiatr Scand 1998;97:450–457.

44. Altemus M, Dale JK, Michelson D, Demitrack MA, Gold PW, Straus SE. Abnormalities in response to vasopressin infusion in chronic fatigue syndrome. Psychoneuroendocrinology 2001;26:175–188.

45. Scott LV, Medbak S, Dinan TG. Desmopressin augments pituitary-adrenal responsivity to corticotropin-releasing hormone in subjects with chronic fatigue syndrome and in healthy volunteers. Biol Psychiatry 1999;45:1447–1454.

46. Bakheit AM, Behan PO, Watson WS, Morton JJ. Abnormal arginine-vasopressin secretion and water metabolism in patients with postviral fatigue syndrome. Acta Neurol Scand 1993;87:234–238.

47. Scott LV, Medbak S, Dinan TG. The low dose ACTH test in chronic fatigue syndrome and in health. Clin Endocrinol (Oxf) 1998;48:733–737.

48. Hudson M, Cleare AJ. The 1microg short Synacthen test in chronic fatigue syndrome. Clin Endocrinol (Oxf). 1999;51:625–630.

49. Gaab J, Huster D, Peisen R, et al. Hypothalamic-pituitary-adrenal axis reactivity in chronic fatigue syndrome and health under psychological, physiological, and pharmacological stimulation. Psychosom Med 2002;64:951–962.

50. Gaab J, Engert V, Heitz V, Schad T, Schurmeyer TH, Ehlert U. Associations between neuroendocrine responses to the Insulin Tolerance Test and patient characteristics in chronic fatigue syndrome. J Psychosom Res 2004;56:419–424.

51. Lavelle E, Dinan TG. Hypothalamic-pituitary-adrenal axis function in chronic fatigue syndrome: a study of feedback mechanisms. Royal College of Surgeons of Ireland Research Meeting, Dublin, Ireland, 1996.

52. Cleare AJ, Sookdeo SS, Jones J, O'Keane V, Miell JP. Integrity of the growth hormone/insulin-like growth factor system is maintained in patients with chronic fatigue syndrome. J Clin Endocrinol Metab 2000;85:1433–1439.

53. Cleare AJ, O'Keane V, Miell J. Plasma leptin in chronic fatigue syndrome and a placebo-controlled study of the effects of low-dose hydrocortisone on leptin secretion. Clin Endocrinol 2001;55: 113–119.

54. Korszun A, Sackett-Lundeen L, Papadopoulos E, et al. Melatonin levels in women with fibromyalgia and chronic fatigue syndrome. J Rheumatol 1999;26:2675–2680.

55. Moorkens G, Wynants H, Abs R. Effect of growth hormone treatment in patients with chronic fatigue syndrome: a preliminary study. Growth Horm IGF Res 1998;8:131–133.

56. Kuratsune H, Yamaguti K, Sawada M, et al. Dehydroepiandrosterone sulfate deficiency in chronic fatigue syndrome. Int J Mol Med 1998;1:143–146.

57. De Becker P, De Meirleir K, Joos E, et al. Dehydroepiandrosterone (DHEA) response to i.v. ACTH in patients with chronic fatigue syndrome. Horm Metab Res 1999;31:18–21.

58. Scott LV, Salahuddin F, Cooney J, Svec F, Dinan TG. Differences in adrenal steroid profile in chronic fatigue syndrome, in depression and in health. J Affect Disord 1999;54:129–137.

59. Scott LV, Svec F, Dinan T. A preliminary study of dehydroepiandrosterone response to low-dose ACTH in chronic fatigue syndrome and in healthy subjects. Psychiatry Res 2000;97:21–28.

60. Ottenweller JE, Sisto SA, McCarty RC, Natelson BH. Hormonal responses to exercise in chronic fatigue syndrome. Neuropsychobiology 2001;43:34–41.

61. van Rensburg SJ, Potocnik FC, Kiss T, et al. Serum concentrations of some metals and steroids in patients with chronic fatigue syndrome with reference to neurological and cognitive abnormalities. Brain Res Bull 2001;55:319–325.

62. Cleare AJ, O'Keane V, Miell JP. Levels of DHEA and DHEAS and responses to CRH stimulation and hydrocortisone treatment in chronic fatigue syndrome. Psychoneuroendocrinology 2004;29:724–732.

63. Himmel P, Seligman TM. A pilot study employing dehydroepiandrosterone (DHEA) in the treatment of chronic fatigue syndrome. J Clin Rheumatol 1999;5:56–59.

64. Bakheit AM, Behan PO, Dinan TG, Gray CE, O'Keane V. Possible upregulation of hypothalamic 5-hydroxytryptamine receptors in patients with postviral fatigue syndrome. BMJ 1992;304:1010–1012.

65. Sharpe M, Clements A, Hawton K, Young AH, Sargent P, Cowen PJ. Increased prolactin response to buspirone in chronic fatigue syndrome. J Affect Disord 1996;41:71–76.

66. Dinan TG, Majeed T, Lavelle E, Scott LV, Berti C, Behan P. Blunted serotonin-mediated activation of the hypothalamic-pituitary-adrenal axis in chronic fatigue syndrome. Psychoneuroendocrinology 1997; 22:261–267.

67. Cleare AJ, Bearn J, Allain T, et al. Contrasting neuroendocrine responses in depression and chronic fatigue syndrome. J Affect Disord 1995;34:283–239.

68. Sharpe M, Hawton K, Clements A, Cowen PJ. Increased brain serotonin function in men with chronic fatigue syndrome. BMJ 1997;315:164–165.

69. Bearn J, Allain T, Coskeran P, et al. Neuroendocrine responses to d-fenfluramine and insulin-induced hypoglycemia in chronic fatigue syndrome. Biol Psychiatry 1995;37:245–252.

70. Yatham LN, Morehouse RL, Chisholm BT, Haase DA, MacDonald DD, Marrie TJ. Neuroendocrine assessment of serotonin (5-HT) function in chronic fatigue syndrome. Can J Psychiatry 1995;40: 93–96.

71. Cleare AJ. The neuroendocrinology of chronic fatigue syndrome. Endocr Rev 2003;24:236–252.

72. Demitrack MA, Gold PW, Dale JK, Krahn DD, Kling MA, Straus SE. Plasma and cerebrospinal fluid monoamine metabolism in patients with chronic fatigue syndrome: preliminary findings. Biol Psychiatry 1992;32:1065–1077.

73. Chaudhuri A, Majeed T, Dinan T, Behan PO. Chronic fatigue syndrome: a disorder of central cholinergic neurotransmission. J Chronic Fatigue Syndr 1997;3:3–16.

74. Wessely S, Chalder T, Hirsch S, Wallace P, Wright D. Psychological symptoms, somatic symptoms, and psychiatric disorder in chronic fatigue and chronic fatigue syndrome: a prospective study in the primary care setting. Am J Psychiatry 1996;153:1050–1059.

75. Manu P, Matthews DA, Lane TJ, et al. Depression among patients with a chief complaint of chronic fatigue. J Affect Disord 1989;17:165–172.

76. Wessely S, Chalder T, Hirsch S, Pawlikowska T, Wallace P, Wright DJ. Postinfectious fatigue: prospective cohort study in primary care. Lancet 1995;345:1333–1338.

77. David AS. Postviral fatigue syndrome and psychiatry. Br Med Bull 1991;47:966–988.

78. Harvey A, Purdie G, Bushnell J, Ellis P. Are cortisol levels low in chronic fatigue syndrome? Third International Clinical and Scientific Meeting on CFS/ME. Sydney, Australia, 2001.

79. Taerk GS, Toner BB, Salit IE, Garfinkel PE, Ozersky S. Depression in patients with neuromyasthenia (benign myalgic encephalomyelitis). Int J Psychiatry Med 1987;17:49–56.

80. Wessely S, Chalder T, Hirsch S, Wallace P, Wright D. Psychological symptoms, somatic symptoms, and psychiatric disorder in chronic fatigue and chronic fatigue syndrome: a prospective study in the primary care setting. Am J Psychiatry 1996;153:1050–1059.

81. McEwen BS. Neuroendocrine interactions. In: Bloom FE, Kupfer DJ, eds. Psychopharmacology: the Fourth Generation of Progress. Raven Press, New York, pp. 705–718.

82. De Bellis MD, Chrousos GP, Dorn LD, et al. Hypothalamic-pituitary-adrenal axis dysregulation in sexually abused girls. J Clin Endocrinol Metab 1994;78:249–255.

83. Heim C, Ehlert U, Hellhammer DH. The potential role of hypocortisolism in the pathophysiology of stress-related bodily disorders. Psychoneuroendocrinology 2000;25:1–35.

84. Wessely S, Hotopf M, Sharpe M. The neurobiology of CFS. In: Wessely HM, Sharpe M, eds. Chronic Fatigue and its Syndromes. Oxford University Press, Oxford, 1998, pp. 250–276.

85. Cleare AJ. The neuroendocrinology of chronic fatigue syndrome. Endocr Rev 2003;24:236–252.

86. Pruessner JC, Hellhammer DH, Kirschbaum C. Burnout, perceived stress, and cortisol responses to awakening. Psychosom Med 1999;61:197–204.

87. Heim C, Ehlert U, Hanker JP, Hellhammer DH. Abuse-related posttraumatic stress disorder and alterations of the hypothalamic-pituitary-adrenal axis in women with chronic pelvic pain. Psychosom Med 1998;60:309–318.

88. Stein MB, Yehuda R, Koverola C, Hanna C. Enhanced dexamethasone suppression of plasma cortisol in adult women traumatized by childhood sexual abuse. Biol Psychiatry 1997;42:680–686.

89. Vedhara K, Hyde J, Gilchrist ID, Tytherleigh M, Plummer S. Acute stress, memory, attention and cortisol. Psychoneuroendocrinology 2000;25:535–549.

90. Leese G, Chattington P, Fraser W, Vora J, Edwards R, Williams G. Short-term night-shift working mimics the pituitary-adrenocortical dysfunction in chronic fatigue syndrome. J Clin Endocrinol Metab 1996;81:1867–1870.

91. Candy B, Chalder T, Cleare AJ, et al. Predictors of fatigue following the onset of infectious mononucleosis. Psychol Med 2003;33:847–855.

92. Cleare AJ. The HPA axis and the genesis of chronic fatigue syndrome. Trends Endocrinol Metab 200; 15:55–59.
93. McKenzie R, O'Fallon A, Dale J, et al. Low-dose hydrocortisone for treatment of chronic fatigue syndrome: a randomized controlled trial. JAMA 1998;280:1061–1606.
94. Cleare AJ, Heap E, Malhi GS, Wessely S, O'Keane V, Miell J. Low-dose hydrocortisone in chronic fatigue syndrome: a randomised crossover trial. Lancet 1999;353:455–458.
95. Peterson PK, Pheley A, Schroeppel J, et al. A preliminary placebo-controlled crossover trial of fludrocortisone for chronic fatigue syndrome. Arch Intern Med 1998;158:908–914.
96. Rowe PC, Calkins H, DeBusk K, et al. Fludrocortisone acetate to treat neurally mediated hypotension in chronic fatigue syndrome: a randomized controlled trial. JAMA 2001;285:52–59.
97. Blockmans D, Persoons P, Van Houdenhove B, Lejeune M, Bobbaers H. Combination therapy with hydrocortisone and fludrocortisone does not improve symptoms in chronic fatigue syndrome: a randomized, placebo-controlled, double-blind, crossover study. Am J Med 2003;114:736–741.
98. Reid S, Chalder T, Cleare A, Hotopf M, Wessely S. Chronic fatigue syndrome. BMJ 2000;320:292–296.
99. Barsky AJ, Saintfort R, Rogers MP, Borus JF. Nonspecific medication side effects and the nocebo phenomenon. JAMA 2002;287:622–627.
100. Whiting P, Bagnall AM, Sowden AJ, Cornell JE, Mulrow CD, Ramirez G. Interventions for the treatment and management of chronic fatigue syndrome: a systematic review. JAMA 2001;286:1360–1368.
101. Stokes MJ, Cooper RG, Edwards RH. Normal muscle strength and fatigability in patients with effort syndromes. BMJ 1988;297:1014–1017.
102. Sharma A, Oyebode F, Kendall MJ, Jones DA. Recovery from chronic fatigue syndrome associated with changes in neuroendocrine function. J R Soc Med 2001;94:26–27.
103. McBeth J, Macfarlane GJ, Benjamin S, Silman AJ. Features of somatization predict the onset of chronic widespread pain: results of a large population-based study. Arthritis Rheum 2001;44:940–946.
104. Castro WH, Meyer SJ, Becke ME, et al. No stress—no whiplash? Prevalence of "whiplash" symptoms following exposure to a placebo rear-end collision. Int J Legal Med 2001;114:316–322.
105. Gaab J, Blattler N, Menzi T, Pabst B, Stoyer S, Ehlert U. Randomized controlled evaluation of the effects of cognitive-behavioral stress management on cortisol responses to acute stress in healthy subjects. Psychoneuroendocrinology 2003;28:767–779.
106. Wessely S. Chronic fatigue: symptom and syndrome. Ann Intern Med 2001;134:838–843.
107. Staudenmayer H. Clinical consequences of the EI/MCS "diagnosis": two paths. Regul Toxicol Pharmacol 1996;24:S96–S110.
108. Sharpe M, Wessely S. Putting the rest cure to rest—again. BMJ 1998;316:796.
109. Hadler NM. "Fibromyalgia" and the medicalization of misery. J Rheumatol 2003;30:1668–1670.
110. Schrader H, Obelieniene D, Bovim G, et al. Natural evolution of late whiplash syndrome outside the medicolegal context. Lancet 1996;347:1207–1211.
111. Obelieniene D, Schrader H, Bovim G, Miseviciene I, Sand T. Pain after whiplash: a prospective controlled inception cohort study. J Neurol Neurosurg Psychiatry 1999;66:279–283.
112. Partheni M, Constantoyannis C, Ferrari R, Nikiforidis G, Voulgaris S, Papadakis N. A prospective cohort study of the outcome of acute whiplash injury in Greece. Clin Exp Rheumatol 2000;18:67–70.
113. Cassidy JD, Carroll LJ, Cote P, Lemstra M, Berglund A, Nygren A. Effect of eliminating compensation for pain and suffering on the outcome of insurance claims for whiplash injury. N Engl J Med 2000;342:1179–1186.
114. Demitrack MA. The psychobiology of chronic fatigue: the central nervous system as a final common pathway. In: Demitrack MA, Abbey SE, eds. Chronic Fatigue Syndrome: An Integrative Approach to Evaluation and Treatment. Guilford Press, New York, 1996, pp. 72–112.

Index